Coronary Artery Disease

Proceedings of the A. N. Richards Symposium sponsored by the Physiological Society of Philadelphia—May 7–8, 1981.

Coronary Artery Disease

Edited by

WILLIAM P. SANTAMORE, PH.D.

Bockus Institute
Graduate Hospital
Philadelphia, Pennsylvania

ALFRED A. BOVE, M.D., PH.D.

Mayo Clinic
Rochester, Minnesota

With 73 illustrations and 24 tables

Urban & Schwarzenberg
Baltimore-Munich 1982

Urban & Schwarzenberg, Inc.
7 E. Redwood Street
Baltimore, Maryland 21202
USA

Urban & Schwarzenberg
Pettenkoferstrasse 18
D–8000 München 2
West Germany

© Urban & Schwarzenberg 1982

All rights including that of translation, reserved. No part of this publication may be reproduced, stored in a retrieval system, or transmitted in any other form or by any means, electronic, mechanical, recording, or otherwise without the prior written permission of the publisher.

Printed in the United States of America

Notices

The Editors (or Author(s)) and the Publisher of this work have made every effort to ensure that the drug dosage schedules herein are accurate and in accord with the standards accepted at the time of publication. The reader is strongly advised, however, to check the product information sheet included in the package of each drug he or she plans to administer to be certain that changes have not been made in the recommended dose or in the contraindications for administration.

The publishers have made an extensive effort to trace original copyright holders for permission to use borrowed material. If any have been overlooked, it will be corrected at the first reprint.

Library of Congress Cataloging in Publication Data

Coronary artery disease.

Proceedings of the A.N. Richards Symposium held May 7–8, 1981 in Philadelphia, sponsored by the Physiological Society of Philadelphia.
Includes index.
1. Coronary heart disease—Congresses. I. Bove, Alfred A. II. Santamore, William P. III. A.N. Richards Symposium (1981: Philadelphia, Pa.) IV. Physiological Society of Philadelphia. [DNLM: 1. Coronary diseases—Congresses. W3 R114 1981c / WG 300 A531c 1981]
RC685.C6C628   616.1'23   81-19731
ISBN 0-8067-1761-0   AACR2

Cover design : Thea Glidden
Compositor : Brushwood Graphics
Printer : Universal Lithographers
Copy preparation : Sally MacLeod
Kimberly Apple
Production and design : John Cronin
Detlev Moos

ISBN 0-8067-1761-0 Baltimore

ISBN 3-541-71761-0 Munich

Dedications

To my wife, Kathy, and David, Joana, and Mia for your love and support.

Bill

To my wife, Sandy, and Jacqueline, Christopher, and Andrew for your patience.

Fred

Acknowledgments

This symposium was supported by the Physiological Society of Philadelphia and by the generous contributions of the following companies:

American Critical Care
American Cyanamid Co.
Boehringer Ingelheim Ltd.
Bristol Laboratories
E. I. DuPont de Nemours & Co.
E. R. Squibb
Hoechst-Roussel Pharmaceuticals Inc.
ICI Americas Inc.
Ives Laboratories, Inc.
Mead Johnson and Company
Merck, Sharp & Dohme Research Labs.
McNeil Laboratories, Inc.
Norwich-Eaton Pharmaceuticals
Pennwalt Corporation
Sandoz, Inc.
Schering Corporation
The Upjohn Company
USV Pharmaceutical Corporation
Wallace Laboratories
Warner-Lambert
Wyeth Laboratories

Contents

Contributors and Participants xii
Introduction xvii

SECTION I Basic Coronary Physiology
              Robert M. Berne, Chairperson

Physiology of Smooth Muscle 3
   Thomas M. Butler and Marion J. Siegman
Mechanical Aspects of Large Coronary Arteries 19
   Robert H. Cox
The Regulation of Coronary Blood Flow 39
   Robert M. Berne and Rafael Rubio
Discussion 53

SECTION II Drug Effects on Coronary Vessels
              Martin M. Winbury, Chairperson

Proximal and Distal Coronary Arteries 63
   Martin M. Winbury
Blood-Blood Vessel Wall Interaction 79
   James W. Aiken
Calcium Entry Blocking Agents: Actions and Utility
in Ischemic Heart Disease 93
   James L. Perhach, Jr., William Diamantis, Joseph P. Buckley,
   R. Duane Sofia and Bhagavan S. Jandhyala
Effects of Pharmacologic Agents on Isolated Human Arteries 103
   Robert Ginsburg, Michael R. Bristow, John S. Schroeder,
   Edward B. Stinson and Donald C. Harrison
Discussion 117

Section III Etiology of Coronary Artery Disease
K. Lance Gould, Chairperson

The Hemodynamic Basis of Coronary Artherosclerosis 129
  Meyer Texon
The Pathogenesis of Atherosclerosis 139
  Russell Ross
Discussion 149

Section IV Hemodynamic Consequences of Coronary Artery Disease
K. Lance Gould, Chairperson

Alterations in the Severity of Coronary Stenosis:
Effects of Intraluminal Pressure and Proximal Coronary
Vasoconstriction 157
  William P. Santamore and Alfred A. Bove
Hemodynamics of Coronary Stenoses 173
  K. Lance Gould and Katherine O. Kelley
Dynamics of Human Coronary Stenosis:
Interactions Among Stenosis Flow, Distending Pressure
and Vasomotor Tone 199
  B. Greg Brown, Robert B. Petersen, Cynthia D. Pierce,
  Edward L. Bolson and Harold T. Dodge
Discussion 215

Section V Current Clinical Aspects of Coronary Artery Disease
James F. Spann, Chairperson

Coronary Artery Spasm and Atherosclerosis 223
  Attilio Maseri
Diagnosis and Treatment of Coronary Artery Spasm 233
  Carl J. Pepine, Robert L. Feldman and C. Richard Conti
Thromboxane A_2 in Coronary Artery Disease 247
  Paul Walinsky, Mark Lebenthal, J. Bryan Smith and Alan M. Lefer
Intracoronary Thrombolysis: A New Treatment for
Myocardial Infarction 255
  James F. Spann

Lifestyle Patterns as a Defense Against Coronary
Heart Disease 263
   Ralph S. Paffenbarger, Jr.
Discussion 275

SECTION VI **Symposium Summary**

Current Concepts About Coronary Artery Disease 283
   Alfred A. Bove and William P. Santamore

Index 291

Contributors and Participants

James W. Aiken, Ph.D.
Experimental Biology Research
The Upjohn Company
Kalamazoo, Michigan

Robert M. Berne, M.D.
Department of Physiology
University of Virginia
School of Medicine
Charlottesville, Virginia

Edward L. Bolson, M.D.
Cardiology Section
University of Washington
School of Medicine
Seattle, Washington

Alfred A. Bove, M.D., Ph.D.
Cardiology Section
Temple University
Philadelphia, Pennsylvania

Michael R. Bristow, M.D.
Division of Cardiology and Department of Cardiovascular Surgery
Stanford University Medical Center
Stanford, California

B. Greg Brown, M.D., Ph.D.
Cardiology Section
Wadsworth V.A. Hospital
Los Angeles, California

Joseph P. Buckley, Ph.D.
University of Houston
Houston, Texas

Thomas M. Butler, Ph.D.
Department of Physiology
Jefferson Medical College
Thomas Jefferson University
Philadelphia, Pennsylvania

C. Richard Conti, M.D.
Department of Medicine
University of Florida, and
  the V.A. Medical Center
Gainesville, Florida

Robert H. Cox, Ph.D.
Bockus Research Institute
The Graduate Hospital and
  Department of Physiology
University of Pennsylvania
Philadelphia, Pennsylvania

William Diamantis, Ph.D.
Wallace Laboratories
Cranbury, New Jersey

Harold T. Dodge, M.D.
Cardiology Section
University of Washington
School of Medicine
Seattle, Washington

Robert L. Feldman, M.D.
Department of Medicine
Division of Cardiology
University of Florida, and
 the V.A. Medical Center
Gainesville, Florida

Robert Ginsburg, M.D.
Division of Cardiology and Department of Cardiovascular Surgery
Stanford University Medical Center
Stanford, California

K. Lance Gould, M.D.
Division of Cardiology
Department of Medicine
University of Texas Medical School at Houston
Houston, Texas

Donald C. Harrison, M.D.
Division of Cardiology and Department of Cardiovascular Surgery
Stanford University Medical Center
Stanford, California

Bhagavan S. Jandhyala, Ph.D.
College of Pharmacy
University of Houston
Houston, Texas

Katharine O. Kelley, B.S.
Division of Cardiology
Department of Medicine
University of Texas Medical School at Houston
Houston, Texas

Mark Lebenthal, M.D.
Jefferson Medical College
Philadelphia, Pennsylvania

Alan M. Lefer, Ph.D.
Department of Physiology
Jefferson Medical College
Philadelphia, Pennsylvania

Attilio Maseri, M.D.
University of London
Royal Postgraduate Medical School
London, United Kingdom

Ralph S. Paffenbarger, Jr., M.D.
Stanford University School of Medicine
Stanford, California

Carl J. Pepine, M.D.
Department of Medicine
Division of Cardiology
University of Florida, and
 the V.A. Medical Center
Gainesville, Florida

James L. Perhach, Jr., Ph.D.
Wallace Laboratories
Cranbury, New Jersey

Robert B. Petersen, Ph.D.
Cardiology Section
University of Washington School of Medicine
Seattle, Washington

Cynthia D. Pierce, B.S.
Cardiology Section
University of Washington
  School of Medicine
Seattle, Washington

Russell Ross, M.D.
Departments of Pathology and
  Biochemistry
University of Washington
  School of Medicine
Seattle, Washington

Rafael Rubio, Ph.D.
Department of Physiology
University of Virginia
  School of Medicine
Charlottesville, Virginia

William P. Santamore, Ph.D.
Cardiology Section
Temple University
Philadelphia, Pennsylvania

John S. Schroeder, M.D.
Division of Cardiology and Department of Cardiovascular Surgery
Stanford University Medical Center
Stanford, California

Marion J. Siegman, Ph.D.
Department of Physiology
Jefferson Medical College
Thomas Jefferson University
Philadelphia, Pennsylvania

J. Bryan Smith, Ph.D.
Jefferson Medical College
Thomas Jefferson University
Philadelphia, Pennsylvania

R. Duane Sofia, Ph.D.
Wallace Laboratories
Cranbury, New Jersey

James F. Spann, M.D.
Department of Medicine
Temple University School of
  Medicine
Philadelphia, Pennsylvania

Edward B. Stinson, M.D.
Division of Cardiology and
  Department of Cardiovascular
  Surgery
Stanford University Medical
  Center
Stanford, California

Meyer Texon, M.D.
Department of Forensic Medicine
New York University Medical
  Center
New York, New York

Paul Walinsky, M.D.
Jefferson Medical College
Thomas Jefferson University
Philadelphia, Pennsylvania

Martin M. Winbury, Ph.D.
Warner-Lambert Company
Ann Arbor, Michigan

Introduction

The chapters of this book are from the presentations given at the A.N. Richards Symposium of the Philadelphia Physiological Society.

In developing this symposium we hoped to provide a review of recent developments in coronary artery physiology. Many recent studies are moving us away from the concept of fixed concentric stenoses that develop over many decades, toward the concept that stenoses are dynamic and can affect myocardial perfusion by vasoactivity even when no change in myocardial oxygen demand occurs.

To develop an understanding of the contribution of large vessel vasoactivity to coronary disease, angina and myocardial infarction, the symposium began with a general overview of basic coronary physiology. Chapter 3 deals with control of the coronary circulation and with the factors that regulate coronary vascular resistance. Regulation at this level involves arteriolar tone and much of the control is locally mediated. There are two resistances to deal with in the coronary circulation. The relationship between arteriolar (distal resistance) responses and large artery (proximal resistance) responses to vasoactive compounds and to relaxing agents such as nitroglycerin and calcium-blocking drugs requires attention. Properties of the large coronary vessels are provided in Chapters 1 and 2. We are interested chiefly in the large artery responses in this symposium, but the microvascular responses must be understood to gain a proper perspective. Smooth muscle physiology is an important component of the knowledge needed to understand coronary artery function. Chapter 1 examines the properties of coronary smooth muscle. To examine such properties, one may study the intact artery in vitro and in vivo or measure responses in vascular segments mounted in a muscle bath. The isolated vascular ring studies provide information on drug effects. A significant species dependence often causes confusion about drug responsiveness. Rabbit aorta may act differently to vasoactive agents and to vascular relaxing drugs than the rat aorta, the dog coronary artery or the human coronary artery. Studies in animal models are needed to develop an understanding of drug and hormonal responses and useful information on drug action has come from these studies. Chapters 1 and 2 review the effects of drugs on coronary smooth muscle, and in

Chapter 7 the responses in human coronary arteries are provided from studies on the hearts of transplant patients.

At present, smooth muscle-constricting agents such as norepinephrine, histamine, angiotensin, certain of the prostaglandins and possibly acetylcholine are considered to be constrictors of large coronary vessels in man. These compounds are released endogenously by one or another stimulus and raise a number of questions concerning the etiology of clinical coronary spasm. In some cases, specific inhibitors of these mediators are available and are in need of further study. On the other hand, nonspecific relaxing drugs such as nitrates and Ca^{2+}-channel blocks appear to be effective even when receptor-specific constriction occurs. Chapter 6 reveals the pharmacology of the calcium-channel blockers.

The data available to date on large vessel coronary vasomotion suggest that significant caliber changes are a frequent event in the normal function of the coronary arteries.

An important goal of the symposium was to address the question of whether coronary vasoactivity contributes to the atherosclerotic process. Those experienced in clinical coronary arteriography have seen fluctuations in the caliber of the large coronary arteries under a number of conditions including emotional stress. One wonders whether this constant vasomotion and the hydraulic changes thus induced contributed to the development of local vessel wall injury, accumulation of lipid and, ultimately, focal narrowing of the artery. Clincial coronary arteriography has demonstrated patients in the catheterization laboratory who had minor wall irregularities that progressed to high grade obstructive lesions in a few years. These lesions develop more rapidly than one would expect, even if the atherosclerotic process began early in life and progressed relentlessly. The current concepts on the etiology of atherosclerosis are presented in Chapters 8 and 9. It is evident that atherosclerosis is not a single-factor disease, and that atherosclerosis and its effects on the myocardium must be considered separately. From the data of these chapters, it is evident that a combination of mechanical and biochemical events ultimately produces an occlusive coronary lesion, and a combination of vasoconstriction and thrombosis completes the process and causes myocardial infarction. Among the data available in the book are some, but not all, of the pieces of this complex puzzle.

Chapters 10, 11, and 12 examine the relationship of coronary vasomotion to events such as myocardial infarction, angina, and sudden death. These chapters present convincing data on the vasoactive aspects of coronary disease and provide some insight into the hemodynamics of stenoses that are compliant enough to undergo local vasomotion. Chapter 10 provides data on both passive and active stenoses in vitro and the hemodynamics of coronary stenoses in intact dogs, while Chapters 11 and 12 extend the concepts from animal studies to man. From these data it is clear that both vasomotion and passive diameter changes resulting from altered local pressures drastically affect the flow in the coronary artery.

From these in vivo and in vitro studies, it is possible to hypothesize a number of conditions based on stenotic hemodynamics that appear to fit the clinical pattern of angina, infarct and sudden death at least as well as, and sometimes better than, the fixed lesion demand/supply concept. Clearly the lumen of a stenosis in man and animals can become wider or narrower under a variety of stimuli. These fluctuations might be the true nature of coronary disease, or at least, may be an important component of the process.

The symposium also considered hormonal effects that might contribute to coronary vasomotion or spasm. Chapter 5, on the contribution of prostaglandins to the vasoactivity, provides useful information in this area. From this chapter we find that a constant communication goes on between the blood and the vessel wall. The process of platelet activation from whatever cause produces vasoconstrictor prostaglandins. Blood-borne elements probably contribute to instability in stenoses and the circumstances that cause interaction between a stenosis and a blood-borne mediators of constriction need to be examined.

The final chapters provide the clinical correlation needed to link the basic studies with clinical observations and approaches to therapy. Chapter 16 provides a clinical overview of the pathophysiology, prognosis and therapy in patients with coronary disease and infarction, and clinical experience with coronary spasm is provided in Chapters 13 and 14. The current interest in the platelet and in the role of thromboxanes in coronary spasm is reviewed in Chapter 15.

The symposium and this book close with a preview of the epidemiology of coronary disease. If coronary disease involves a dynamic vasoactive process in the large coronary arteries, and angina and infarction are in part related to coronary vasomotion, then new relationships must be developed between coronary incidence and physical activity, smoking, hypertension and other risk factors. It would be of interest, for example, to know if long term physical activity alters the coronary smooth muscle response to vasoconstrictor stimuli or how smoking affects the caliber of atherosclerotic lesions in the coronary arteries.

This symposium provides some new data on coronary disease that have changed our concepts and should change the approach to patients with coronary disease as well as research in this area. A field of medicine that was thought to be well understood has recently become a new area for research. New data has already provided improved care of patients with coronary disease. Both basic and clinical studies in this area are providing input to the care of patients, but there is much more to be understood in this disease. In the subsequent chapters, the new ideas are presented and verified, and a view is provided of the direction our knowledge is moving toward in the future.

Finally, we would like to thank the many people who helped make this symposium and this volume possible: Dr. Gerald Kelliher and the Board of the Philadelphia Physiological Society; Drs. R. Berne, M. Winbury, K. L. Gould and J. Spann, who served as Session Chairpersons; Mrs. Gloria Spector for her help and assistance in arranging this symposium; Mr. John Michele, Paul Thomas, Robert Kent, Thomas Vinciquerra, Mrs. Grace Wilson and Sandy Gordon for their assistance during the symposium, Ms. Grace M. Stuart for her help in preparing this volume; and Ms. Katherine P. Santamore for her editorial assistance.

July, 1981

WILLIAM P. SANTAMORE
ALFRED A. BOVE

Temple University
Philadelphia, Pennsylvania

Section I

Basic Coronary Physiology

Robert M. Berne, *Chairperson*

Physiology of Smooth Muscle

Thomas M. Butler and Marion J. Siegman

Introduction

This chapter deals with some basic structural, biochemical and physiological aspects of smooth muscle. Although little of the material is derived directly from work on coronary smooth muscle, its relevance to coronary artery disease comes from the thesis that many of these processes are quite similar in diverse smooth muscles. Only after additional research will it be possible to address the problem of subtle, or perhaps not so subtle, differences in the basic properties of smooth muscles from different tissues.

In this chapter we give a short description of the ultrastructure of smooth muscle followed by a discussion of current ideas as to how the interaction of contractile proteins is regulated by calcium concentrations in the cell. Finally, some experiments are presented that partially characterize the mechanism by which energy derived from splitting of ATP is transduced into a mechanical output by smooth muscle.

Smooth Muscle Ultrastructure

The ultrastructure of vascular smooth muscle has recently been reviewed in detail by Somlyo (1980). Figures 1 and 2 show different magnifications of transverse sections of smooth muscle cells from rabbit portal anterior mesenteric vein. The cells are dominated by a regular array of thick filaments. These filaments are 15–18 nm in diameter and contain myosin. From longitudinal sections it has been determined that the thick filaments are approximately 2.2 μm in length and are tapered at both ends (Ashton et al., 1975). The thin, actin-containing filaments are 6–8 nm in diameter and are made up of G-actin monomers polymerized into a two-stranded helical filament. The thin filament also contains tropomyosin, but there is no troponin present in smooth muscle. The proposed mechanisms for calcium regulation of the contractile proteins in the absence of an equivalent of the striated muscle troponin-regulation system are discussed later.

There is a much higher actin content relative to myosin content in smooth than in striated muscle. Murphy et al. (1974) showed that the molar ratio of actin to myosin in the hog carotid artery was 36 compared to only 4 in skeletal muscle. There is also evidence that arterial smooth muscle has a higher actin to myosin ratio than does nonarterial smooth muscle (Cohen and Murphy, 1979).

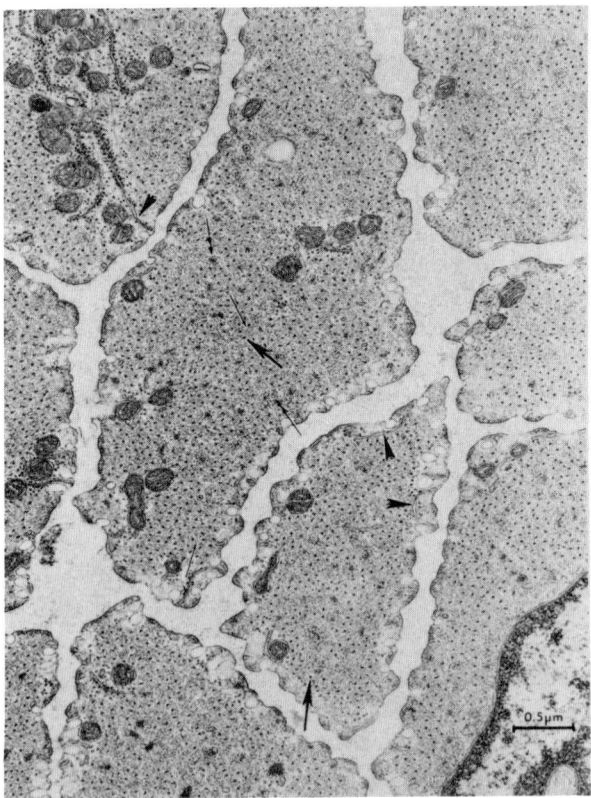

Fig. 1. Transverse section of smooth muscle cells from the rabbit portal anterior mesenteric vein. Thick (large arrows) and thin (small arrows) filaments are seen. Double arrows show groups of intermediate filaments while the arrow heads show elements of sarcoplasmic reticulum. From Somlyo et. al., 1973. Reprinted with permission from *Philosophical Transactions*, Royal Society of London.

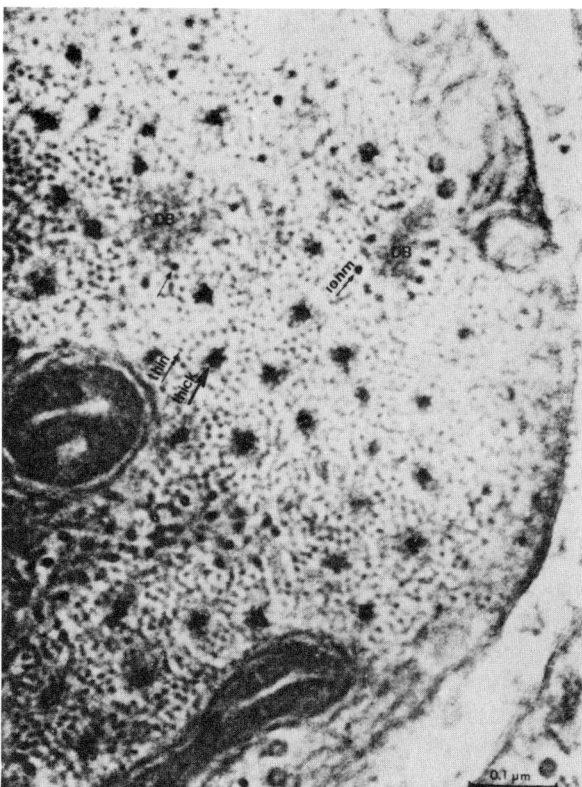

Figure 2. Thick transverse section of a smooth muscle cell from the rabbit portal anterior mesenteric vein. Thick, thin and intermediate filaments are identified. Also shown are cytoplasmic dense bodies (DB). From Somlyo et al., 1976. Reprinted with permission by Cold Spring Harbor Laboratory.

The third major filament system in smooth muscle is the 10 nm or intermediate filament. These filaments are composed of the protein desmin, which has a molecular mass of approximately 55,000 daltons. The intermediate filaments are not continuous with thick or thin filaments; their function, other than presumably being of a structured nature, is not known. It has been shown, however, that there is a disproportionate increase in the number of intermediate filaments in hypertrophied smooth muscle cells (Gabella, 1979; Berner et al., 1981).

Another characteristic of the ultrastructure of smooth muscle is the presence of amorphous structures known as dense bodies. There are both cytoplasmic and membrane-bound dense bodies. Thin filaments insert into dense bodies (see Fig. 3). The dense body thus seems to be analogous to the Z line in striated muscle. It has recently been found with myosin S_1 decoration of thin filaments

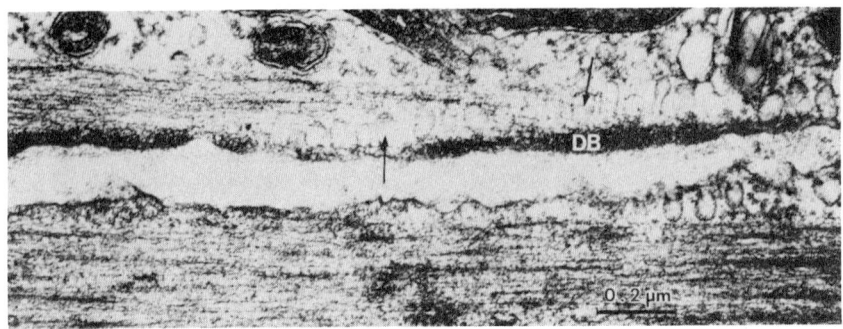

Figure 3. Thick longitudinal section of smooth muscle cells showing thin filaments (arrows) inserting into a membrane-bound dense body (DB). From Ashton et al., 1975. Reprinted with permission from *Journal of Molecular Biology*. Copyright: Academic Press Inc. (London) Ltd.

that the polarity of the actin-containing filament is different on one side of the cytoplasmic dense body than on the other (Bond et al., 1981). This is similar to that which occurs at the Z line in striated muscle.

Figure 4 shows a diagram of the smooth muscle myosin molecule. The molecule has two major subunits (heavy chains), which form a coiled coil. The association of the tail portions of the molecules form the backbone of the thick filament. Although other association patterns have been suggested (Craig and Megerman, 1977), it is generally thought that myosin-filament organization in smooth muscle is similar structurally to that in skeletal muscle. This involves initial tail-to-tail aggregation of myosin molecules followed by head-to-tail aggregation, which gives rise to a bipolar filament.

Part of the myosin molecule extends out from the filament, and is referred to as the crossbridge portion. It contains two S_1 subunits of myosin, each of which has an ATP hydrolysis site and actin-binding site. There are two light chains of 17,000 and 20,000 daltons associated with each head. The 20,000-dalton light chain can be phosphorylated by a calcium-dependent protein kinase, and this phosphorylation has been implicated in the calcium regulation of the muscle.

Suzuki et al. (1978) have shown that phosphorylation of the light chain also assists in myosin assembly into filaments in vitro. These authors suggested that in the resting muscle myosin exists as individual molecules, which aggregate into filaments after phosphorylation. In collaboration with Drs. A. P. and A. V. Somlyo we have shown this not to be the case (Somlyo et al., 1981), because, at rest, quick-frozen rabbit portal anterior mesenteric vein showed less than 5% of the myosin light chain phosphorylated while normal arrays of thick filaments could be observed in paired muscles frozen identically and processed for electron microscopy by freeze substitution.

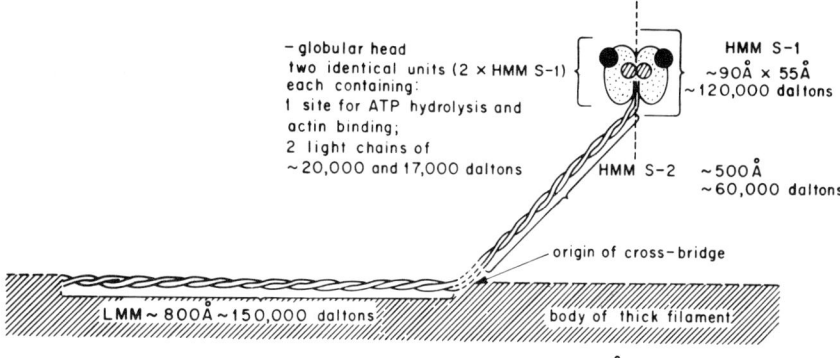

Figure 4. Diagram of a smooth muscle myosin molecule. From Hartshorne and Gorecka, 1980. Reprinted with permission of the American Physiological Society.

Figure 5 shows a diagramatic sketch of the crossbridge cycle representing some of the steps in the mechanochemical transduction process in muscle. This particular diagram represents striated muscle because Z bands are shown, but substitution of dense bodies and removal of troponin makes this figure applicable to smooth muscle. The basic idea is that each crossbridge cycle involves the attachment of the crossbridge to actin, a power stroke during which filaments slide past each other, and a subsequent detachment of the

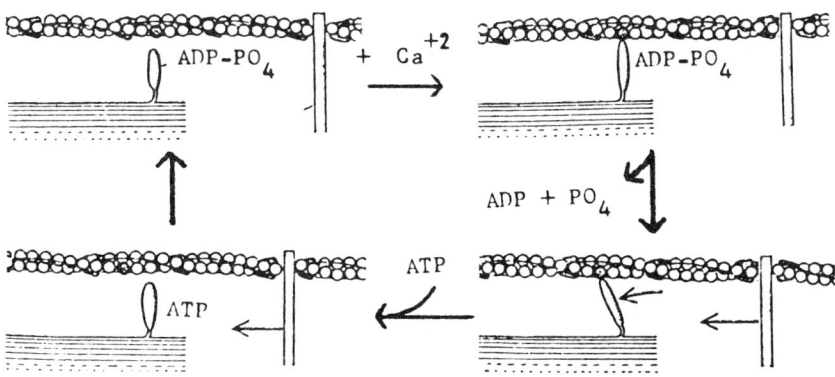

Figure 5. Diagram of a possible sequence of steps in the crossbridge cycle. The upper left panel represents the muscle at rest when crossbridges are detached. When the calcium concentration rises, the crossbridge binds to actin. It then releases the products of ATP hydrolysis and goes through a power stroke, which results in the relative sliding of filaments. The crossbridge detaches with ATP binding to myosin. The ATP is hydrolysed and the cycle starts again if there is sufficient Ca^{2+} present.

crossbridge. Although the figure shows that each cycle involves the splitting of one molecule of ATP, possibly there is multiple hydrolysis for each cycle.

Very little work has been done on the kinetics of the actin-myosin interaction in isolated smooth muscle proteins. It is known that the intrinsic rate of actin-activated myosin ATPase activity is lower in smooth than in skeletal muscle (see Hartshorne and Gorecka, 1980, for review). Indirect evidence suggests that there are some novel crossbridge states in smooth muscle. Siegman et al., (1976) described a calcium-dependent state in resting smooth muscle, which was interpreted to mean that the crossbridge could stop in the attached state before the power stroke. Dillon et al., (1981) have suggested that the crossbridge can stop in the attached state, but after the power stroke.

Calcium Regulation of Actin-activated Myosin ATPase Activity

There are two current theories concerning the calcium regulation of the actin-myosin interaction in smooth muscle. The first involves a calcium-dependent phosphorylation of the myosin molecule, and the second, which was put forward by Professor Ebashi, is a thin-filament-associated calcium-binding protein called leiotonin.

Figure 6 shows the proposed mechanism based on myosin light chain phosphorylation. At rest, the calcium concentration is low and myosin is in the unphosphorylated state. The catalytic subunit of the myosin light chain kinase is inactive. When calcium increases, it binds to calmodulin and the calcium-calmodulin complex binds to and activates the catalytic subunit of the light chain kinase. Myosin is phosphorylated and can then interact with actin and split ATP. Relaxation is achieved through the action of a myosin light chain phosphatase, which dephosphorylates the myosin. An interesting side light of this mechanism is that the kinase itself can be phosphorylated by a cyclic AMP-dependent protein kinase (Adelstein et al., 1978). In the phosphorylated state the affinity of the light chain kinase for the calcium-calmodulin complex is lower, so at a particular calcium concentration the presence of cyclic AMP would tend to reduce the quantity of active myosin light chain kinase and thus reduce actin-myosin interaction.

The mechanism of calcium regulation proposed by Ebashi is based on a thin filament-associated regulatory protein called leiotonin (for review, see Nonomura and Ebashi, 1980). Leiotonin binds calcium directly and activates the actin-myosin system directly. There is only one leiotonin molecule for every 60 actin monomers in smooth muscle. The mode of action of leiotonin has not been established.

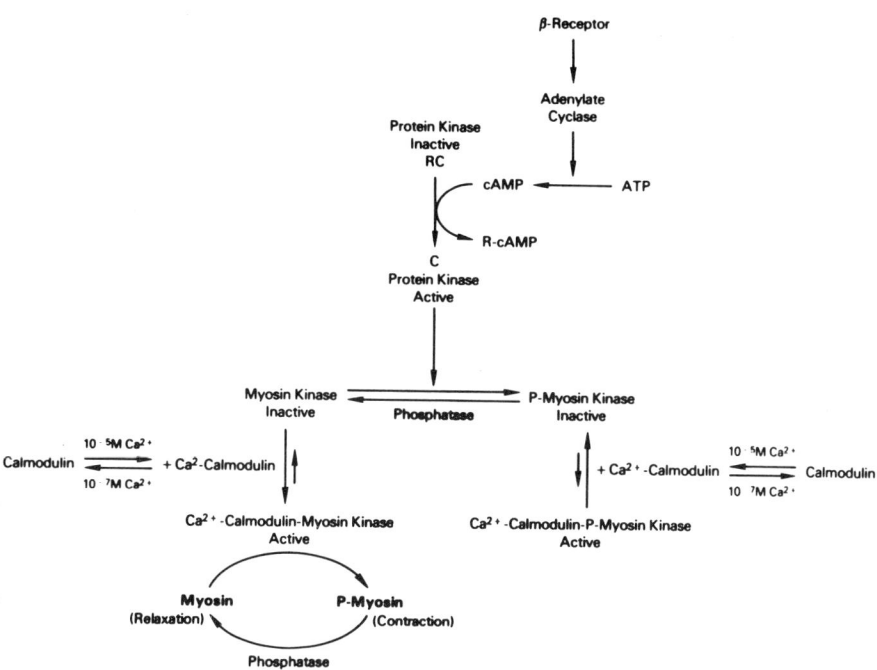

Figure 6. Postulated scheme of regulation of smooth muscle actomysin ATPase activity by a calcium-dependent phosphorylation of the 20,000-dalton myosin light chain. From Conti and Adelstein (1980). Reprinted by permission.

Actin-Myosin Interaction not Involving ATP Splitting

Siegman et al., (1976) and Butler et al., (1976) reported a calcium-dependent resistance to stretch in smooth muscle. This is illustrated in Figure 7. A quick stretch of about 10% ℓ_0 in a resting muscle caused force to increase and then decrease over time. This resistance to stretch and subsequent stress relaxation decreased in the absence of extracellular calcium, and it could be restored when calcium was added back. The resistance to stretch had the same length dependence as active tension under isometric conditions. Furthermore, the presence or absence of calcium did not have any effect on steadystate force generated by the muscle. The small change in steadystate force shown in Figure 7 is a hysteresis that occurs whether or not calcium is removed. Panel C shows that when calcium is added back and resistance to stretch increases, steadystate force does not. This observation was consistent with the presence of attached bridges in the resting muscle that would resist stretch, but that

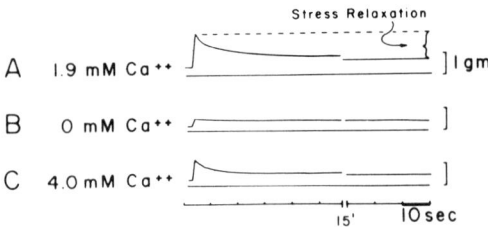

Fig. 7. Force response to a length change of 10% ℓ_o in the resting rabbit tenia coli. Muscle was bathed in 1.9 mM Ca^{2+} -Krebs solution (a), then 0 mM Ca^{2+} -Krebs (2 mM EGTA) solution for 0.5 hour (b) and finally 4mM Ca^{2+} -Krebs solution for 1 hour (c) muscle length at which maximum isometric force development occurs. From Siegman et al., 1976. Reprinted with permission of the American Physiological Society.

would not generate a net steadystate force. Stretching of the muscle at rest would thus result in the straining of attached bridges and stress relaxation would reflect the temporary detachment of the strained crossbridges and reformation under unstrained conditions. This crossbridge phenomenon does not depend on phosphorylation of the myosin light chain because changes in extracellular calcium did not change the degree of light chain phosphorylation in the resting muscle. We have also shown that maintenance of such attached crossbridges requires little, if any, energy input (Mooers, Siegman and Butler, unpublished observation).

Dillon et al., (1981) have reported experiments that led them to conclude that there is a "latch" state of crossbridges in smooth muscle. Their observation was that the velocity of contraction decreased during a continued contracture even though force maintenance did not. The characteristics of the latch state are that the crossbridge remains attached and maintains force, but cycles very slowly. They also showed that the maximum velocity of contraction showed the same time course as did phosphorylation of the 20,000 dalton myosin light chain. This suggested that phosphorylation determines the velocity of contraction and crossbridge cycling but does not determine force maintenance.

Thus, it seems that in contrast to skeletal muscle the smooth muscle crossbridge cycle can stop in states that involve a variety of actin-myosin interactions. The functional significance of such multiple states has not been fully realized.

High Energy Phosphate Usage in Contracting Smooth Muscle

The mechanochemical transduction process can be probed by determination of the different relationships among energy utilizations and mechanical outputs in smooth muscle under a variety of mechancial conditions. In this section, energetics experiments are described that utilize a tenia coli preparation. The muscle was treated so that high energy phosphate usage could be determined directly from net changes in phosphocreatine and adenine nucleotide contents (Butler et al., 1978). The muscles were stimulated electrically at 18°C and the chemical contents were normalized to the total creatine (Ct) content of the muscle, which is approximately 2.7 μmol/g, wet weight.

Energetics of Isometric Contractions

Figure 8 shows total high energy phosphate usage during single isometric tetani of different durations compared to paired unstimulated controls. Upon stimulation, the rate of chemical energy usage increased, and it did not change

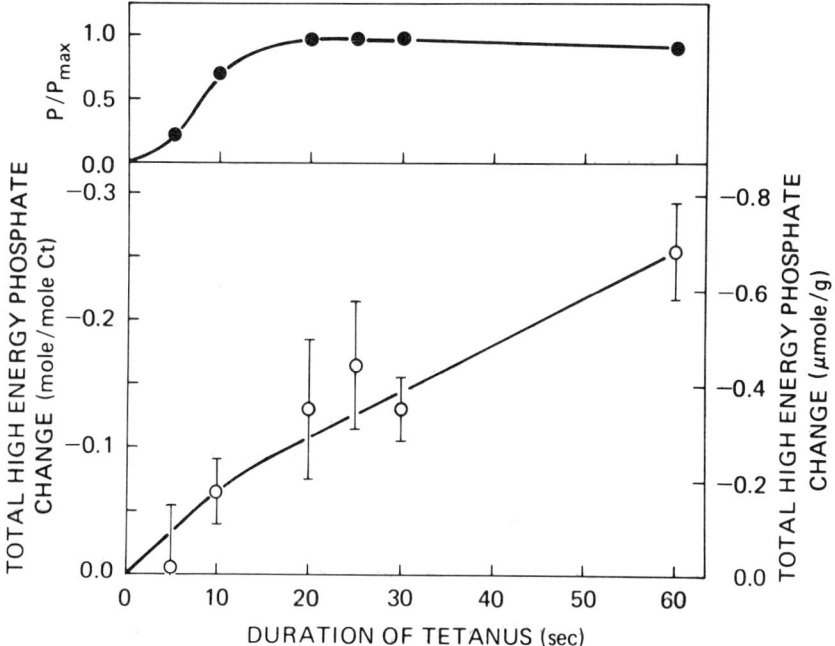

Fig. 8. Total high energy phosphate usage (O) during single isometric tetani of different durations in the rabbit tuenia coli at 84% l_0 and 18°C. The top panel shows the force response during the stimulation. From Butler et al., 1978. Reprinted with permission of the American Physiological Society.

significantly in tetani of different durations. There was a possibility, however, that the average rate was higher during the early stages of the tetanus when force was increasing. A different experimental design was used to investigate this.

Each smooth muscle was divided into three segments. One was stimulated for 25 sec and frozen; one was stimulated for 60 sec; and the third was an unstimulated control frozen 25 sec after the equilibration period. In this way energy usage for force development and force maintenance was obtained in paired muscle. Figure 9 shows that the average rate of energy usage during the period of force development is significantly greater than that during force maintenance. Because of the experimental design, the rate of energy usage for force maintenance includes the resting metabolism of the muscle while the value for force development does not. The resting metabolism is about 30% of the total energy cost during the period of isometric force maintenance. Correction for resting metabolism reveals that the energy usage during force development is more than fourfold higher than that during subsequent force maintenance. Siegman et al., (1980) have shown that this high rate of energy usage during the early part of the tetanus is not due only to the internal work done against the series elasticity. Rather there seems to be an energetically expensive process associated with the initial activation of the muscle.

The degree of phosphorylation of the 20,000-dalton light chain during isometric tetani is shown in Figure 10. At rest, the phosphorylation was 11%. Upon stimulation, degree of phosphorylation increased to 32% at 5 sec and then decreased slightly with continued stimulation. Phosphorylation peaked before force development. The relative degrees of phosphorylation during force development and subsequent force maintenance are not proportional to the relative rates of ATP utilization during these times. The average phosphorylation during the first 25 sec of contraction is 27% and it averages 24% during the subsequent 35 sec while the average rate of energy usage varies by fourfold. Some questions raised by this phosphorylation data are: 1) What are the other 70% of myosins doing if they do not cycle without being

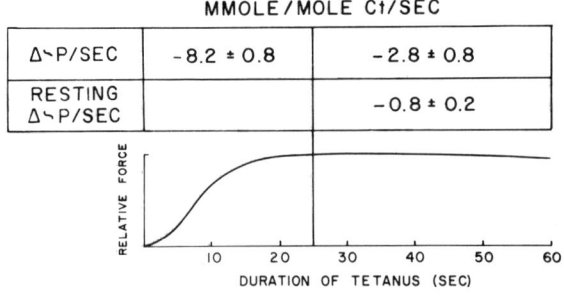

Fig. 9. Average rate of energy usage ($\triangle \sim P$) during different phases of an isometric tetanus in the rabbit tenia coli at 18°C. The rate shown for 35-60 sec of stimulation includes the resting energy usage of the muscle.

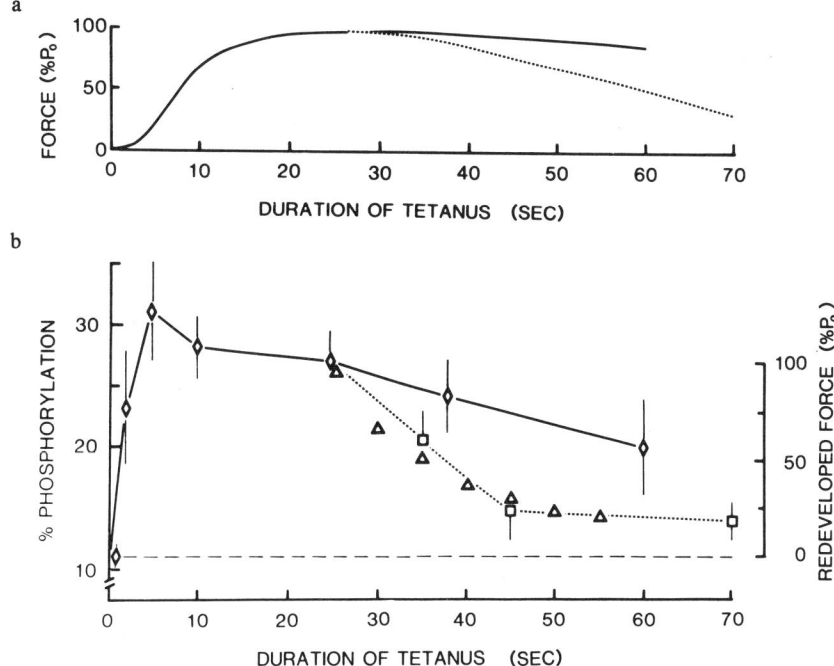

Fig. 10. Degree of phosphorylation of the 20,000-dalton myosin light chain during contraction of the rabbit tenia coli. a) The solid line shows the force response to a supramaximal stimulation under isometric conditions at ℓ_0, while the broken line shows the force response during relaxation from a 25-sec tetanus. b) Degree of phosphorylation at different times during an isometric tetanus at ℓ_0 ($\diamond$), and during relaxation following a 25-sec tetanus, ($\square$). also shown is the relative active force redeveloped following a 1% ℓ_0 quick-release during relaxation from a 25-sec tetanus ($\triangle$). Data for degree of phosphorylation are shown ± standard error. The standard errors for the redeveloped force data are smaller than the data points.

phosphorylated? and 2) Do the same 30% of the myosin S_1 subunits remain phosphorylated or does that population change?

Siegman et al., (1980) also determined the relative myosin contents in the frog sartorius and rabbit tenia coli. The reason that the frog sartorius was chosen is that it is the classical muscle in the field of skeletal muscle energetics. There is a 3.3 times higher myosin content per gram, wet weight, in the skeletal muscle and about a 500 times different in average rate of energy utilization during isometric force maintenance at 18–20°C (Siegman et al., 1980). If it is assumed that each myosin molecule is a crossbridge and that one crossbridge cycle involves the splitting of one molecule of ATP, it is possible to calculate an average crossbridge cycle duration by dividing the molar myosin content by the rate of ATP utilization. This gives an average crossbridge cycle time of

50 msec for the sartorius and 7.5 sec for the smooth muscle. This 150-fold difference is reasonably consistent with the observed difference in isolated actin-activated myosin ATPase activities in smooth and fast twitch skeletal muscles.

The term "economy" or the force per cross-sectional area divided by the rate of energy utilization is used to compare the energy requirements for force maintenance in different muscles (See Rüegg, 1971). Measured economies for the frog sartorius and rabbit tenia coli are 10 and 700 $(N/cm^2)/(\mu mol/g/sec)$, respectively. This high economy of force maintenance in smooth muscle is undoubtedly due in part to its very much slower crossbridge cycle. Ashton et al., (1975) have also reported a 40% longer myosin filament in smooth muscle. This could give rise to a greater number of crossbridges arranged mechanically in parallel and could contribute to the high economy.

Energetics of Relaxation

Siegman et al., (1980) showed that the high energy phosphate usage during relaxation was very low in smooth muscle. It was of interest, however, to determine the relative energy usage associated with force maintenance during stimulation and relaxation. Figure 11 shows the design that was used. Isometrically held muscles were either stimulated for 60 sec or stimulated for

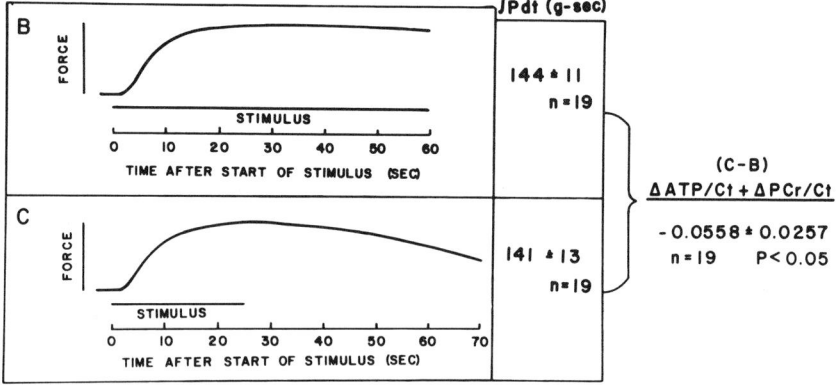

Fig. 11. Energy cost of force maintenance during stimulation and relaxation. The muscle represented in Panel B maintained the same $\int P \cdot dt$ as those in Panel C. The muscles in Panel B used significantly more energy to maintain this force than those in Panel C.

25 sec and allowed to relax for 45 sec. The $\int P \cdot dt$ was the same in these two designs; the muscle shown in Panel B was maintaining force while being stimulated, while the muscle shown in Panel C maintained a large fraction of its force during relaxation. In paired comparisons, the energy usage was greater in muscles maintaining force during the stimulation. Thus force can be exerted with a lower expenditure of energy during relaxation than when it is maintained during stimulation. We have suggested that this very high economy during relaxation is a result of decreasing calcium levels with crossbridges reverting to the attached but noncycling state, which was described earlier.

Figure 10 also shows the degree of phosphorylation of the light chain during relaxation. The muscles were stimulated for 25 sec and then allowed to relax for 10, 20 or 45 sec. The degree of phosphorylation declines more rapidly than does force. This is consistent with the finding that the rate of energy usage also decreased more quickly than force. The ability of the muscle to redevelop force after a quick release was also determined (see fig. 10). This measure of active state shows approximately the same rate of decline as does phosphorylation during relaxation. These data are consistent with the concept that degree of phosphorylation determines rate of energy utilization and active state, but not force output during relaxation.

Therefore, although the degree of light chain phosphorylation alone does not seem to determine the relative rate of energy usage during the development and maintenance of isometric force, it is possible that crossbridge cycling during relaxation is determined solely by degree of light chain phosphorylation.

Energetics of Shortening in Smooth Muscles

All of the energetics data that have been discussed so far have dealt with isometric conditions. We have also determined the energy usage in smooth muscles shortening and doing external work.

The first question that was addressed was: Do muscles that shorten and do work have a greater total energy output than muscles stimulated under isometric conditions? Fenn has observed this in skeletal muscle more than 50 years ago (Fenn, 1923). The design for the shortening experiment was similar to that used for determining the energy usage for 35 sec of isometric force maintenance. The experimental muscle was stimulated isometrically for 20 sec and then subjected to an isovelocity shortening of $5 \times 10^{-3} \ell_0$/sec. Total duration of the shortening was 35 sec. The control muscle was stimulated isometrically for 20 sec. The average rate of energy usage during the isovelocity shortening was 5.6 ± 0.8 mmol/mol of Ct·sec) compared to 2.0 ± 0.8 mmol/(mol of Ct·sec) for maintenance of isometric force during the shortening is a direct demonstration of the Fenn effect in smooth muscle. So, under certain conditions when smooth muscle shortens and does external work, crossbridges cycle faster than under isometric conditions. There is no change in degree of light chain phosphorylation during the shortening.

Interestingly, if the same experiment is done except that the shortening is started from the beginning of the tetanus, there is no increase in energy usage above the isometric case. It was initially thought that this might have been due to the fact that the energy usage was so high during the initial phase of the isometric tetanus. If the same energy-requiring process were occurring during the shortening then it might override the effect of the shortening. A way of testing this was to look at the work output per mole of high energy phosphate used. If this extra energy-utilizing process during the first part of the tetanus also occurred during the shortening, then the work per high energy phosphate used would be lower when the shortening started from the beginning of the tetanus. In other words, there would be an energy usage that had nothing to do with work production. This is not the case because the work per ATP used is actually higher during shortening from the beginning of the tetanus than shortening from the plateau (4.2 versus 2.8 kJ/mol). This suggests that the high rate of energy usage during the development of isometric force is actually due to crossbridge cycling, and that if the muscle is shortening this energy can be transduced into work. This means that the process responsible for the high rate of crossbridge cycling must shut down later during the maintenance of isometric force. Regulation of crossbridge cycling by degree of light chain phosphorylation cannot alone account for such an observation.

A final note is that the values for work per mole of ATP utilized are quite low in both of these cases. Similar experiments on frog skeletal muscle give values of 15–20 kJ/mol (Kushmerick and Davies, 1969; Curtin et al., 1974). We are currently determining efficiencies for mammalian skeletal muscle. It is clear, however, that the high economy of force maintenance in smooth muscle occurs in spite of a low efficiency of active external work production.

Summary

Smooth muscle contraction occurs through the sliding of actin and myosin-containing filaments by means of the energy derived from ATP splitting by the crossbridge. In contrast to the striated muscle case, there is evidence that the crossbridge cycle can stop in a variety of attached or detached states in smooth muscle. The crossbridge cycle is very slow and there is an associated high economy of isometric force maintenance. This occurs in spite of a low efficiency of active external work production. Finally, there is a large volume of evidence that the calcium-dependent phosphorylation of the 20,000-dalton myosin light chain is involved in the regulation of actin-myosin interaction in smooth muscle, but recent data from energetics and mechanics experiments suggest that a mechanism in addition to phosphorylaction must also operate.

Acknowledgments

This work was supported in part by National Institutes of Health Grant HL 15835 to the Pennsylvania Muscle Institute and National Science Foundation Grant PCM 7912618.

References

Aldelstein, R.S., Conti, M.A., Hathaway, D.R. and Klee, C.B. 1978. Phosphorylation of smooth muscle myosin light chain kinase by the catalytic subunit of adenosine 3':5'-monophosphate-dependent protein kinase. J Biol Chem 253:8347–8350

Ashton, F.T., Somlyo, A.V. and Somlyo, A.P. 1975. The contractile apparatus of vascular smooth muscle: intermediate high voltage stereo electron microscopy. J Mol Biol 98:17–29

Berner, P.F., Somlyo, A.V. and Somlyo, A.P. 1981. Hypertrophy-induced increase of intermediate filaments in vascular smooth muscle. J Cell Biol 88:96–101

Bond, M., Somlyo, A.V., Butler, T.M. and Somlyo, A.P. 1981. Dense bodies, actin polarity and the state of myosin in vertebrate brate smooth muscle. Abstract, VII International Biophysics Congress, Mexico City, Mexico

Butler, T.M. and Siegman, M.J. 1982. Chemical energetics of contraction in mammalian smooth muscle. Fed. Proc. in Press

Butler, T.M., and Siegman, M.J. and Davies, R.E. 1976. Rigor and resistance to stretch in vertebrae smooth muscle. Am J Physiol 231: 1509–1504

Butler, T.M., Siegman, M.J., Mooers, S.U. and Davies, R.E. 1978. Chemical energetics of single isometric tetani in mammalian smooth muscle. Am J Physiol 235: C1–C7

Cohen, D.M. and Murphy, R.A. 1979. Cellular thin filament protein contents and force generation in porcine arteries and veins. Circ Res 45:661–665

Conti, M.A. and Adelstein, R.S. 1980. Phosphorylation by cyclic adenosine 3':5'-monophosphate-dependent protein kinase regulates myosin light chain kinase. Fed Proc 39:1569–1573

Craig, R. and Megerman, J. 1977. Assembly of smooth muscle myosin into side-polar filaments. J Cell Biol 75:990–996.

Curtin, N.A., Gilbert, C., Kretzschmar, K.M. and Wilkie, D.R. 1974. The effect of the performance of work on total energy output and metabolism during muscular contraction. J Physiol 238:455–472

Dillon, P.F., Aksoy, M.O., Driska, S.P. and Murphy, R.A. 1981. Myosin phosphorylation and the crossbridge cycle in arterial smooth muscle. Science 211:495–497

Fenn, W.D. 1923. A quantitative comparison between energy liberated and the work performed by the isolated sartorius muscle of the frog. J Physiol 58:175–203

Gabella, G. 1979. Hypertrophic smooth muscle. IV. Myofilaments, intermediate filaments and some mechanical properties. Cell Tissue Res 201:277–288

Hartshorne, D.J. and Gorecka, A. 1980. Biochemistry of the contratile proteins of smooth muscle. In: *Handbook of Physiology,* Sec. 2. *The Cardiovascular System* Vol. II. *Vascular Smooth Muscle.* eds. D.F. Bohr, A.P. Somlyo and H.V. Sparks, pp. 93–120. Bethesda: American Physiology Society

Kushmerick, M.J. and Davies, R.E. 1969. The chemical energetics of muscle contraction. II. The chemistry, efficiency and power of maximally working sartorius muscles. Proc Soc Lond (Biol) 190: 315–321.

Murphy, R.A., Herlihy, J.T. and Megerman, J. 1974. Force generating capacity and contractile protein content of arterial smooth muscle. J Gen Physiol 64:691–705

Nonomura, Y. and Ebashi, S. 1980. Calcium regulatory mechanism in vertebrate smooth muscle. Biomed Res 1:1–14

Rüegg, J.C. 1971. Smooth muscle tone. Physiol Rev 51:201–248

Siegman, M.J., Butler, T.M., Mooers, S.U. and Davies, R.E. 1976. Calcium-dependent resistance to stretch and stress relaxation in resting smooth muscle. Am J Physiol 231:1501–1508.

Siegman, M.J., Butler, T.M., Mooers, S.U. and Davies, R.E. 1980. Chemical energetics of force development, force maintenance and relaxation in mammalian smooth muscle. J Gen Physiol 76: 609–629.

Somlyo, A.V. 1980. Ultrastructure of vascular smooth muscle. In: *Handbook of Physiology,* Sec 2. *The Cardiovascular System.* Vol. II. *Vascular Smooth Muscle.* eds., D.F. Bohr, A.P. Somlyo and H.V. Sparks, pp. 33–67. Bethesda: American Physiological Society.

Somlyo, A.V., Butler, T.M., Bond, M., Berner, P.F. and Somlyo, A.P. 1981. The state of myosin in isoproterenol-relaxed vascular smooth muscle. Abstract, Eighth International Congress of Pharmacology, Tokyo, Japan

Somlyo, A.P., Devine, C.E., Somlyo, A.V. and Rice, R.V. 1973. Filament organization in vertebrate smooth muscle. Philos Trans R Soc Lond Ser. B 265:223–229

Somlyo, A.P., Somlyo, A.V., Ashton, F.T. and Valieres, J. 1976. Vertebrate smooth muscle ultrastructure and function. In: *Cell Motility.* eds. R. Goldman, T. Pollard and J. Rosenbaum. Cold Spring Harbor, N.Y.: Cold Spring Harbor Labs. Vol. 3 Book A, pp. 165–183

Suzuki, H., Onishi, H., Takabashi, K., and Watanabe, S. 1978. Structure and function of chicken gizzard myosin. J. Biochem (Tokyo) 84:1529–1542

Mechanical Aspects of Large Coronary Arteries

Robert H. Cox

Introduction

The large coronary arteries are primarily involved in the distribution of coronary blood flow throughout the heart. That is, they act primarily as conduits for blood flow distribution. The importance of the coronary vasculature extends beyond this purely conduit function, however. Coronary arteries are the site of disease processes (Buccino and McIntosh, 1979; Brest et al., 1972), acute pathophysiological reactions (Luchi et al., 1979) and regulatory mechanics (Olsson, 1981). The functions of the coronary arteries in this regard are primarily determined by their mechanical properties. The mechanical properties of arteries in general are determined by the principle constituents of the blood vessel wall including connective tissue, vascular smooth muscle cells, endothelial cells and autonomic innervation.

In considering the mechanical properties of coronary arteries, it is convenient to divide them into two categories: passive mechanics and active mechanics. Passive mechanics refer to the properties of arteries in the absence of extrinsic smooth muscle activation, while active mechanics refer to the properties of arteries with some level of smooth muscle activation. The level of activation depends on a number of factors including the agent used for activation, its concentration as well as the intrinsic properties of the contractile system in the muscle and the properties of passive tissue elements with which they are connected.

Passive Mechanics

The passive mechanics of coronary arteries are important for several reasons. First of all, they contribute to vascular elasticity and arterial compliance as do all the vessels in the arterial tree. The passive mechanical properties of arteries are also an important determinant of the structural component of vascular resistance (Folkow, 1978; Snyder et al., 1975). The structural component of vascular resistance has an important influence on the maximum vasodilation capacity of a vascular bed as well as an indirect effect on a subsequent response of a vascular bed to vasomotor influences. Passive mechanical properties of mural coronary arteries have an important impact on the response of these vessels to the compressive effect of the myocardium during systolic contraction. And lastly, the passive mechanical properties of arteries are important determinants of the initial conditions for smooth muscle contractions. This factor arises because of the sliding filament nature of the organization of the myofilaments in smooth muscle (Murphy, 1976) and the influence of filament overlap on subsequent mechanical responses of the contractile machinery to activation.

Nonlinear Properties

One of the fundamental properties of arteries in general is the nonlinear nature of arterial wall elasticity. As the arterial wall is stretched, the resistance to stretch progressively increases as stretch is continued (Roy, 1881). This characteristic is manifest as a nonlinear relationship between measures of load and wall deformation. An example of a representation of these properties is given in Figure 1, which shows the relationship between passive values of tangential wall stress and strain, which represents the direction of wall circumference. Shown in this figure is a comparison of passive mechanical properties for arteries from a variety of arterial sites that represent secondary branches of the aorta and are vessels of similar size. Substantial differences exist in values of passive mechanics for these various arterial sites. They all demonstrate a qualitatively similar variation. Values of the elastic modulus, which are determined from the slope of the stress-strain curve, are low at small values of stress or strain. Increases in strain are associated with progressive increases in the slope of the stress-strain curve. The magnitude of the slope increases dramatically beyond values of stress and strain associated with physiological values of arterial pressure.

The relative position of the various stress-strain curves can be taken as a measure of stiffness. For example, the data from the mesenteric artery at the extreme left of this group would be considered to be the stiffest of the five

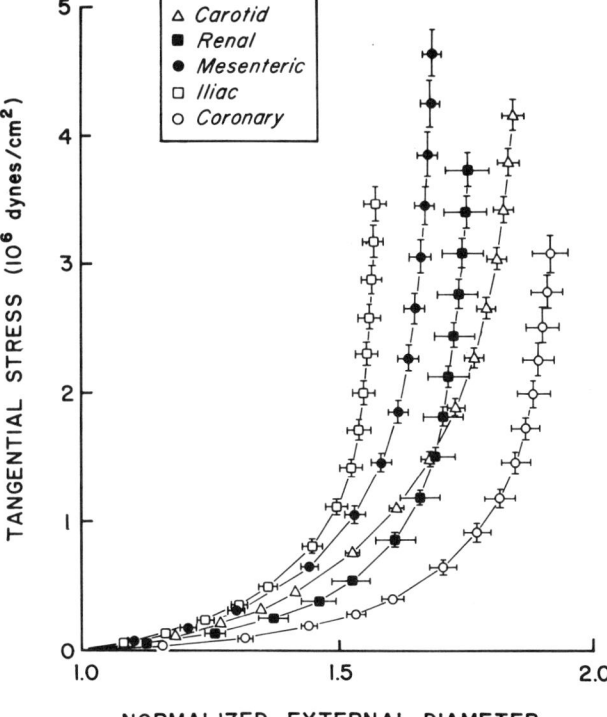

Fig. 1. Summary of passive tangential stress/normalized external diameter relations for five arterial sites identified in the insert. Diameter was normalized by dividing each diameter value by the value at zero pressure. Symbols are means while horizontal and vertical bars represent ± SEM (from Cox, 1978a).

arterial sites. The coronary artery data at the extreme right side of this graph would be considered as the most compliant of the five arterial sites.

It is generally considered that the passive mechanical properties of the arterial wall are primarily determined by their connective tissue content (Fischer and Llaurado, 1966). A summary of connective tissue content of the arteries shown in Figure 1 is given in Table 1. A cursory examination of the data in Table 1 does not provide much insight into the relationship between connective tissue composition and the passive mechanical properties of these five arterial sites. The mesenteric artery, which from a mechanical point of view in Figure 1 is the stiffest of the five sites, has the lowest ration of collagen-to-elastin content. The coronary artery, which on the basis of Figure 1 is the most compliant of the arterial sites, has the highest ratio of collagen-to-elastin content.

Collagen is considered to be a highly cross-linked protein with a high intrinsic elastic modulus of the order of 10^9 dyn/cm^2. Elastin, on the other hand, is an amorphous protein with high extensibility and a relatively low

Table 1. Connective Tissue Content and Water Distribution in Canine Arteries.

	% Dry Weight		
	Collagen	Elastin	C+E
Coronary	55.8 ± 1.6	20.4 ± 0.6	76.2 ± 2.7
Carotid	51.9 ± 1.0	26.2 ± 0.8	76.4 ± 2.2
Renal	47.1 ± 0.9	29.2 ± 1.0	75.9 ± 1.5
Iliac	46.3 ± 0.9	35.5 ± 0.8	81.8 ± 1.2
Mesenteric	43.9 ± 0.9	33.1 ± 0.8	76.9 ± 1.4

Legend: C, collagen; E, elastin; H_2O, total water content; ^{60}Co-space, extracellular water volume using ^{60}Co-EDTA as a marker; cell, cell water volume = $H_2O - {}^{60}$Co-space.

elastic modulus of the order of 10^6 dyn/cm^2. It has been suggested that the relative amount of collagen and elastin are measures of the relative stiffness of different arteries (Fischer and Llaurado, 1966). This concept of connective tissue content does not fit well with the data presented in Figure 1.

This concept arises out of the classic explanation for the nonlinear nature of vascular elasticity (Burton, 1954). Roach and Burton (1957) tried to describe the nonlinear nature of arterial elasticity in terms of contributions of collagen and elastin elements in the arterial wall. This explanation was based upon experimental results in which they attempted to selectively remove either collagen or elastin by chemical treatment of arterial wall segments (Roach and Burton, 1957). These concepts were subsequently supported by histological studies conducted by Wolinsky and Glagov (1964). The classical view based upon the above work holds that the low stress mechanical properties of arteries are primarily determined by the elastin network. At low values of stress or strain collagen does not contribute to supporting loads within the arterial wall, and collagen fibers are slack. As the wall is stretched collagen fibers are progressively recruited to support wall load. As a consequence, the stiffness of the arterial wall increases in proportion to the number of collagen fibers supporting wall load. At high degrees of extension all the collagen fibers in the wall are contributing to the support of wall load. Elastin fibers under this condition simply act to distribute wall load uniformly throughout the wall by virtue of their highly extensible nature.

This concept would suggest, therefore, that the low stress passive mechanical properties of arteries are primarily determined by the elastin component, while high wall stress values of mechanical properties are primarily determined by the collagen components. An attempt has been made to quantitatively test this concept (Cox, 1978a). Figure 2 shows a summary of the

	% Wet Weight		
C/E	H_2O	^{60}Co-space	Cell
2.75 ± 0.11	82.0 ± 0.6	65.9 ± 1.3	16.2 ± 0.7
1.98 ± 0.08	75.3 ± 0.4	53.7 ± 1.8	21.6 ± 1.8
1.65 ± 0.06	75.8 ± 0.3	52.1 ± 1.5	23.2 ± 1.5
1.32 ± 0.04	73.8 ± 0.4	49.8 ± 2.1	24.0 ± 2.1
1.33 ± 0.04	73.8 ± 0.4	44.9 ± 1.8	28.9 ± 2.1

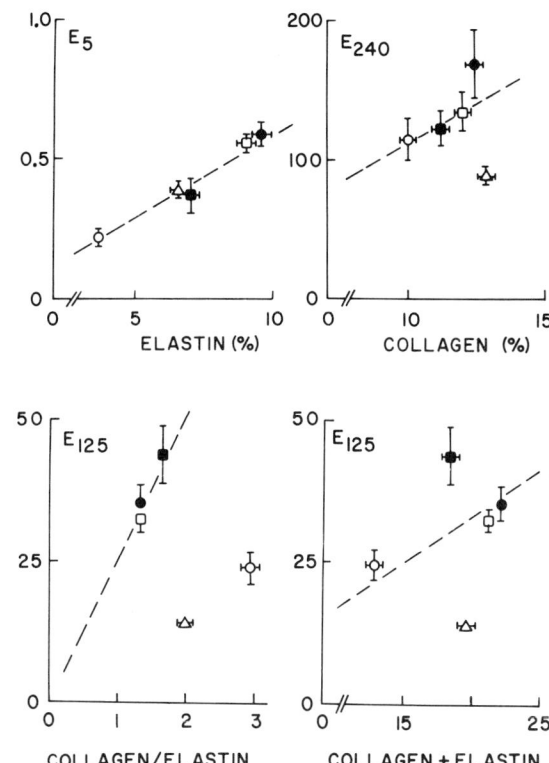

Fig. 2. Correlation of values of incremental elastic modulus with connective tissue factors. Upper left: correlation of low wall stress elastic modulus (E_5) with elastic content. Upper right: correlation of high wall stress modulus (E_{240}) with collagen content. Lower left: correlation of a physiological value of elastic modulus (E_{125}) with collagen/elastin ratio. Lower right: correlation of a physiological value of elastic modulus (E_{125}) with collagen plus elastin. All connective tissue values are given on a wet-weight basis. Subscripts of E represent values of transmural pressure in millimeters of mercury. Symbols represent means while horizontal and vertical bars represent ±1 SEM. Symbols represent: □, iliac artery; ●, mesenteric artery; △, carotid artery; ■, renal artery; and ○, coronary artery (from Cox, 1978a).

correlation between values of the arterial wall elastic modulus and different measures of the connective tissue composition of these arteries. As indicated in the upper left panel, there is an excellent agreement between the low wall stress elastic modulus of these arteries and their elastic content. This is clear support of the concept of Roach and Burton (1957) and Wolinsky and Glagov (1964). High wall stress values of elastic modulus are compared with the collagen content in the upper right panel. Although there is a reasonable relationship between some values in the figure, data from several vessels including the carotid and iliac do not fit as well. A relatively poor correlation was found to exist between physiological values of incremental elastic modulus and the ratio of collagen-to-elastin content as shown in the lower left panel. In particular, data for the carotid and coronary artery were well out of line with the data from other arterial sites. This result suggests that the functional ratio of collagen-to-elastin content for these sites is much too high compared to the chemical ratio of collagen-to-elastin based upon the

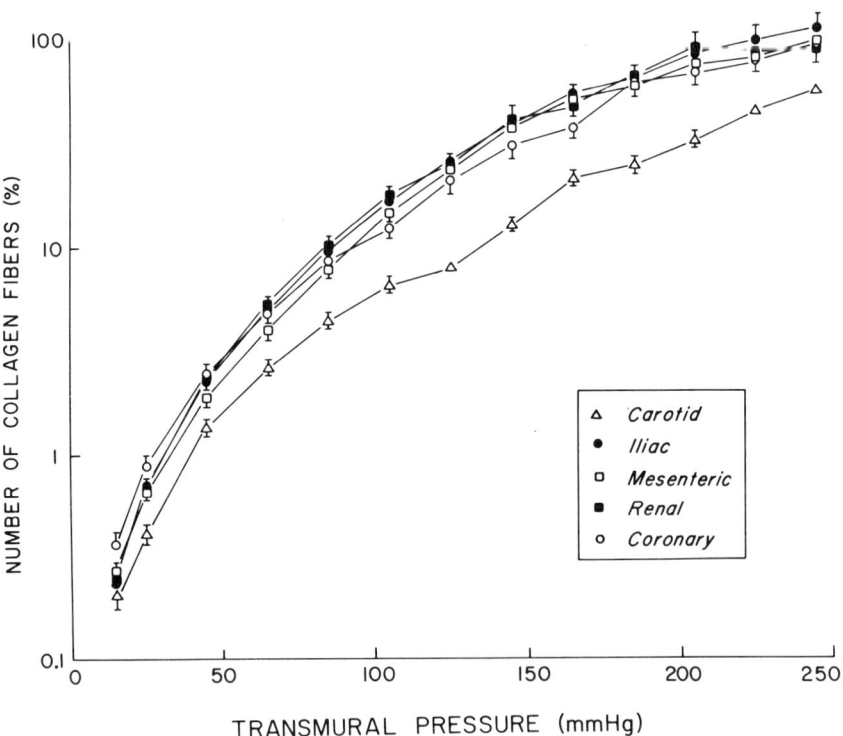

Fig. 3. Variation of f_c, number of fibers supporting wall stress, with transmural pressure for several arterial sites. Symbol representation is defined in the figure (from Cox, 1978a).

correlation for other arterial sites. The data in the lower right panel shows the relationship between physiological values of incremental elastic modulus and total connective tissue content, that is, collagen plus elastin. This relationship is better than that shown in the lower left panel but again data for the renal artery and the carotid artery fall somewhat outside the limits of those obtained for other arterial sites.

The concept of the contribution of collagen-to-elastin to arterial wall mechanics can be formalized in an analytical relationship as follows (Cox, 1978a). The effective elastic modulus of the arterial wall can be related to the connective tissue content of the wall and the mechanical properties of the collagen and elastin matrices as:

$$E_{inc} = E_e W_e + f_c E_c W_c$$

In this relationship, E_e and E_c represent the elastic modulus of the elastin and collagen matrices, respectively. W_e and W_c represent the chemically determined elastin and collagen content, respectively. The term f_c represents the fraction of collagen fibers that support wall load at any given level of stretch. As a result of this relationship, the incremental elastic modulus E_{inc} becomes a function of wall stretch. According to the concepts of Roach and Burton (1957), values for f_c would vary from 0 at low values of stretch to a value of 1 at high values of wall stretch.

Experimental data derived from measurements of mechanical properties of arteries shown in Figure 1 were used to compute the variation of f_c with transmural pressure. This is summarized in Figure 3. In this figure the relative number of collagen fibers supporting wall load is given as a function of transmural pressure. Data for all the arterial sites except the carotid are very close together. The fact that the carotid deviated most from the correlations shown in Figure 2 would have produced an anticipation of this result. These results suggest that at equivalent values of transmural pressure a smaller fraction of collagen contributes to the support of wall loads in the carotid artery.

When the data at high and low values of wall stretch are used with chemical content, data values of elastic modulus for elastin and collagen can be calculated. The computed value for the elastic modulus of elastin was approximately 3×10^2 dyn/cm^2 and a value of $1.2 \times$ dyn/cm^2 was attained for collagen. These values agree well with data published in the literature from more direct measurements of collagen and elastin containing structures such as tendon and ligament (Burton, 1954).

More recent studies have applied this simplistic model to a variety of different situations. Measurements of passive mechanical properties of arteries from puppies during growth and development have suggested differences in values of elastic modulus for the elastin and collagen matrix during maturation (Cox, 1979). Values of elastic modulus for both elastin and collagen matrices were considerably smaller in younger animals than for those obtained from adults. This concept is consistent with the concept of a maturation-associated increase in cross-linking of proteins in the connective tissue matrix contributing to an apparent increase in the stiffness of these structures.

A comparison of values of passive mechanics with collagen and elastin content for carotid arteries from different animal species has also been performed (Cox, 1979). From this analysis species differences in the mechanical properties of collagen and elastin matrices have been suggested. Values for the elastic modulus of elastin for the rat and dog carotid artery were approximately twice that determined for the rabbit carotid. In addition, values of elastic modulus for the collagen matrix were approximately twice as high in a rabbit as compared to the rat and the dog.

One limitation to the usefulness of this equation is its relatively simplistic nature. For example, this equation assumes that adventitial and medial collagen contribute in a qualitatively similar way to the mechanical properties of the arterial wall. Some evidence does exist that suggests that this may in fact not be true (Burton, 1954; Cox, 1980). The possibility exists that adventitial connective tissue by virtue of a very loose-knit organization may be of less importance to the determination of arterial wall mechanical properties than medial connective tissue. In addition, recent studies of the biochemistry of collagen and elastin point to the potential for substantial differences in connective tissue of different arteries, especially related to pathological situations. Such factors as collagen polymorphism, variability of amino acid composition of various polypeptide chains and the nature of intramolecular cross-links may significantly influence the mechanical properties of connective tissue matrices in different arteries of the same subject (Prockop et. al., 1979a, b; Eyre, 1980; Sandberg et al., 1981). Additional alterations at the same arterial site in a subject may be affected by different pathological situations (Fuller et al., 1972; Brecher et al., 1978).

Active Mechanics

Activation of vascular smooth muscle produces substantial effects on measures of arterial wall mechanics. Figure 4 shows a summary of pressure-diameter relations obtained from six arterial sites under active (norepinephrine) and passive conditions. The relative area between these two curves delineates the overall range of control of arterial smooth muscle on the properties of these various blood vessels. It is apparent that substantial differences exist in the effectiveness of smooth muscle in different arteries. The

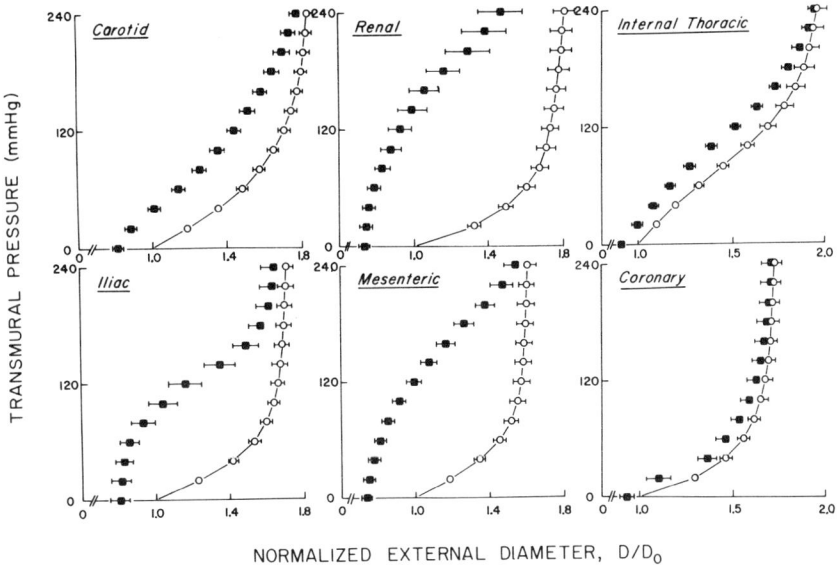

Fig. 4. Summary of pressure-diameter data for various arterial sites under active (■) and passive conditions (○). Symbols are means and horizontal bars ±1 SEM. Active curves were obtained with 145 mM K$^+$ and passive curves with 0 mM Ca^{2+} and 2 mM EGTA (from Cox, 1978b).

largest potential range of control is found in the renal artery while the smallest is found in the coronary artery.

The effects of activation of smooth muscle on arterial wall mechanics can be considered from two points of view. In the first (the elastomeric point of view), the contribution of smooth muscle to arterial wall properties can be measured in terms of its effect on arterial wall stress-strain relations (i.e., nonlinear elasticity). In the second (the muscle point of view), the contribution of arterial smooth muscle can be measured in terms of two basic mechanical properties of muscle systems, that is, force development and shortening.

Elastometric Approach

A representation of the effect of activation of smooth muscle on the mechanical properties of arteries by the elastomeric representation in shown in Figure 5. This figure shows the effect of activation of vascular smooth muscle on the relationship between incremental elastic modulus and transmural pressure for canine coronary arteries. At specific values of transmural

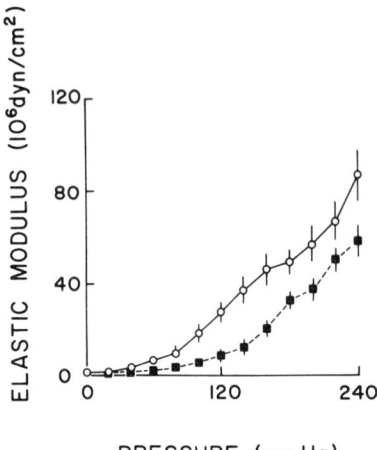

Fig. 5. Effects of smooth muscle activation on the variation of incremental elastic modulus with transmural pressure for canine left circumflex coronary arteries. Data are given for conditions of active (■) and passive (○) smooth muscle as given in Figure 4. Symbols are mean values while vertical lines are ±1 SEM.

pressure, vascular smooth muscle activation consistently produces a reduction in values of incremental elastic modulus (Laszt, 1968). The magnitude of this reduction is strongly dependent upon the value of transmural pressure. For values of pressure in the physiological range, the maximum effect of activation reduces elastic modulus to about 40% of its passive value. Although this effect of smooth muscle activation may appear to be paradoxical, it has a very simple explanation. Activation of vascular smooth muscle at constant pressure decrease the diameter of the arterial wall. The contribution of passive wall components, collagen and elastin, to the total elastic modulus of the arterial wall in this situation is reduced by virtue of nonlinear elasticity. Under activated conditions, the elastic modulus represents the increased contribution from activated muscle and a decreased contribution from passive wall elements. The contribution of the former factor usually predominates so that the effective modulus is decreased. When measurements are made under conditions of constant wall diameter values of incremental elastic modulus are consistently increased by activation (Cox, 1976). This increase represents the contribution of smooth muscle to arterial wall stiffness.

Muscle Approach

The effects of activation of vascular smooth muscle can also be represented in terms of classical concepts of muscular mechanics. The mechanical effect of interaction between myofilaments in muscle can be given in terms of force development at constant muscle length or shortening responses under constant muscle load. These are so-called isometric force development and isotonic shortening characteristics of muscle.

Isometric Force Development

Figure 6 shows a summary of values of isometric force development by smooth muscle at a variety of arterial sites. A consistent behavior exists for all these sites that is qualitatively similar. An optimum value of diameter (muscle length) exists at which the isometric response to activation is maximum. At values of diameter above and below the optimum, active force development decreases. This muscle-length dependence of active force development is cited as primary evidence for the existance of a sliding filament form of contraction in arterial smooth muscle (Murphy, 1976). A significant quantitative dif-

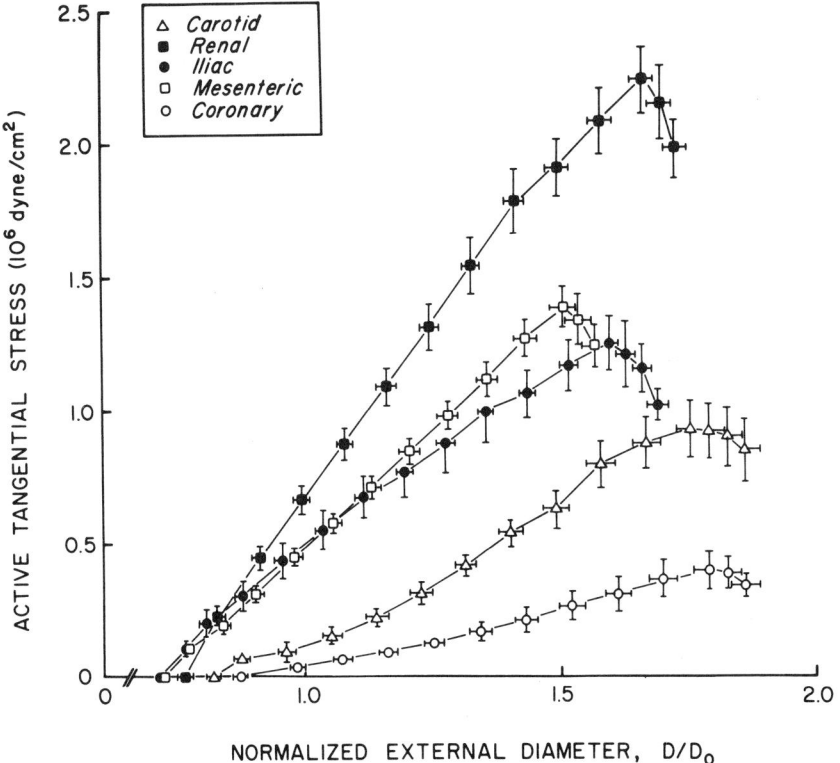

Fig. 6. Variation of active values of tangential wall stress with external diameter for several canine arteries. Diameter was normalized by dividing by the diameter value at zero pressure for passive conditions. Symbols are identified in the insert and represent means, with bars representing ± 1 SEM. Active responses were obtained with 145 mM K$^+$.

Table 2. Active Force Development and Relative Cell Content of Canine Arteries.

Site	$\triangle$F/wall (10^3 dyn/cm^2)	Cell (%)	$\triangle$F/cell (10^3 dyn/cm^2)
Coronary	395 ± 72	20.5 ± 1.8	1935 ± 365
Carotid	920 ± 107	26.8 ± 2.1	3443 ± 375
Renal	2230 ± 125	29.3 ± 2.1	7605 ± 445
Iliac	1243 ± 102	29.1 ± 2.3	4285 ± 360
Mesenteric	1380 ± 77	35.3 ± 2.3	3915 ± 235

Legend: $\triangle$F, maximum active force development normalized by wall cross-sectional area and cell cross-sectional area.

ference exists between the maximum force development capacity of arterial smooth muscle from different sites. As shown in Figure 6, force development for the renal artery was largest while that for the coronary artery was smallest of the sites studied. Although numerous factors could potentially contribute to these differences, the most obvious one relates to the relative cell content or more appropriately to the contractile protein content of these arteries.

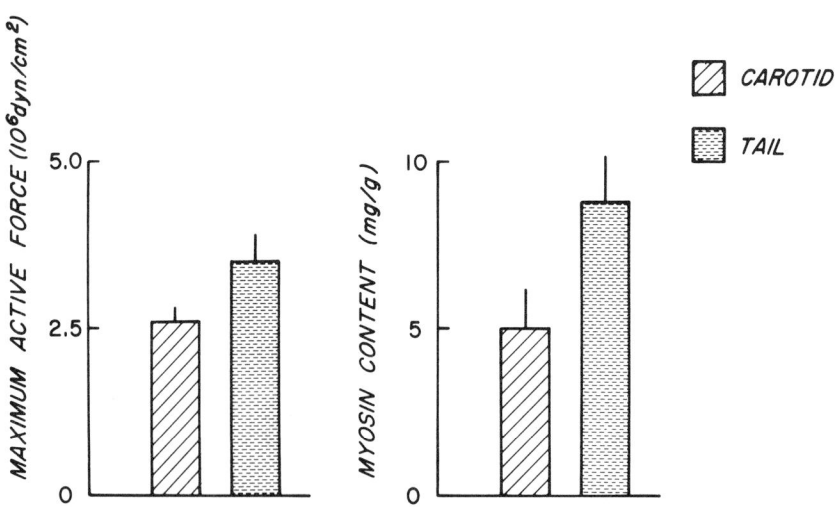

Fig. 7. Comparison of values of maximum active force normalized by wall cross-sectional area and myosin content of carotid and tail arteries from Wistar rats. Bars are means and vertical bars are 1 SEM. Active responses were obtained with 145 mM K$^+$. Myosin contents are expressed on the basis of amount per gram of tissue, wet weight.

Table 2 contains the summary of values of relative cell volume of a number of arterial sites. When maximum values of force development are corrected for differences in relative cell content, the relative ordering of active force development among the various sites remains approximately the same. It is clear, therefore, that differences in cell content alone cannot explain the differences in active force development.

A summary of values of contractile protein content obtained from a variety of sites in the arterial tree of the pig (Cohen and Murphy, 1979) is given in Table 3. Similar data of this sort are not yet available for arterial sites in the dog. Assuming the general principles apply to various animal species, the results in Table 3 suggest that no substantial difference exists in values of contractile protein content from different arterial sites in the dog.

In contrast, recent studies of contractile protein content of rat arteries shows a significant difference for the carotid and tail arteries of this animal (Cox and Chacko, 1981). The myosin content of the tail artery is substantially larger than that of the carotid artery. In addition, maximal force development in response to 145 mM K$^+$ activation was likewise larger in the tail artery as compared to the carotid. These data are summarized in Figure 7. The relative contribution of differences in contractile protein content and properties in different arterial smooth muscles is not clear. Whether the data from the rat described above are an exception and the data from the pig the rule is yet to be determined.

Isotonic Shortening

The ability of activated smooth muscle to shorten is another primary property of contractile systems. Smooth muscle cells are circumferentially distributed through the wall of arteries. Connections exist between various cells including cell-to-cell connections as well as cell-to-extracellular matrix ones. These

Table 3. Contractile Protein Content of Pig Arteries.

Vessel	Myosin (mg/g)	Actin (mg/g)	Tropomyosin (mg/g)	A/M	T/A
Coronary	20.6 ± 3.4	60.6 ± 11.9	16.0 ± 2.6	2.94	0.78
Carotid	19.8 ± 3.3	48.5 ± 6.1	13.5 ± 1.8	2.45	0.68
Renal	15.1 ± 1.0	43.2 ± 4.6	10.8 ± 1.4	2.86	0.72
Femoral	19.4 ± 1.6	58.7 ± 6.2	14.0 ± 1.4	3.03	0.72
Aorta	18.3 ± 1.2	40.9 ± 3.6	12.5 ± 1.9	2.23	0.68
Pulmonary	19.0 ± 3.9	46.3 ± 6.2	11.6 ± 2.0	2.53	0.63

Legend: A/M, ratio of actin to myosin content; T/A, ratio of tropomyosin to actin content.

connections serve to couple individual cellular responses with activation to produce total wall responses. The analog of smooth muscle cell shortening is constriction of the arterial wall and reduction in lumen size. The ability of smooth muscle cells to modulate wall dimensions varies substantially with initial muscle length and with different arterial sites. A summary of values of constriction response from various arterial sites is given in Figure 8. Again, large variations in constriction capacity can be seen as well as the strong

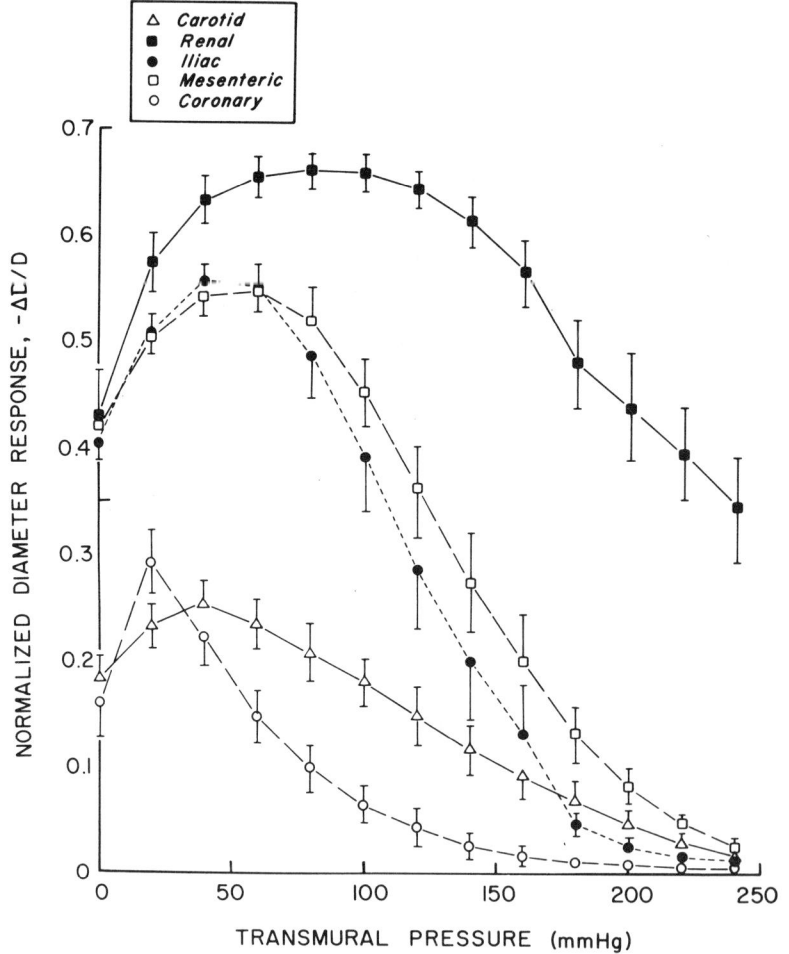

Fig. 8. Variation of active midwall diamter response to 145 mM K$^+$ with transmural pressure at several different sites identified in the insert. The active diameter response represents the difference in values of midwall diameter under active and passive conditions divided by the passive value. Symbols are means and bars are ±1 SEM.

dependence on transmural pressure. An optimum range of transmural pressure exists at which values of constriction capacity are maximum. At higher and lower values of transmural pressure constriction capacity decreases. Consistent with the data given in Figure 4, the total constriction capacity of smooth muscle in the coronary artery is much smaller than that of other arterial sites such as the renal and mesenteric artery.

From the physiological point of view this measure of muscle function is probably more appropriate to the role of the arterial wall in the regulation of arterial blood pressure and the distribution of cardiac output than are the measures of isometric force development shown in Figure 6. It is the effect of smooth muscle through variations in the degree of activation to control lumen dimensions that the regulatory influences of arteries are manifest in the intact circulation. It is of interest in this regard that most studies of the pharmacology and physiology of arterial smooth muscle are conducted using isometric force development.

Series Elasticity

Activated muscle (including vascular muscle) behaves mechanically as if a nonlinear elastic element were functionally coupled in series with the contractile system (Hill, 1950). This property has come to be known as series elasticity and the functional structures as series elastic elements. Recent studies in skeletal muscle have documented that series elasticity is a characteristic of the crossbridges between contractile filaments (Huxley, 1974). The situation in smooth muscle, however, is more complicated perhaps as a result of a different organization of the contractile system and the extensive intra- and intercellular connections that exist (Murphy, 1976; Cox, 1980). Series elastic elements of smooth muscle are more compliant than those of skeletal muscle by nearly an order of magnitude (Cox, 1978b).

A summary of the properties of series elastic elements of arteries from several sites are summarized in Figure 9. This figure shows the relation between incremental modulus and tangential wall stress during isometric contractions at a muscle length near L_{max}, the optimum length for maximum force development. The slope of these curves is a relative measure of the compliance of the series elastic elements, i.e., the steeper the slope, the greater the stiffness. Substantial differences exist in series elasticity at these various arterial sites (Cox, 1978b). No obvious relationship, however, could be found between values of the maximum series elastic element extension associated with smooth muscle activation and the connective tissue content or maximum active responses of these sites (Table 4).

The properties of series elastic elements in arterial smooth muscle were found to be strongly dependent upon muscle length (Cox, 1978c). Incremental active stiffness was not uniquely related to active wall stress. This suggests that

Table 4. Summary of Regional Variation of Arterial Smooth Muscle Properties.

Site	$\triangle \sigma_{max}$ (10^3 dyn/cm^2)	$-\triangle D/D_0$ (%)	$\triangle L_{se}$ (%L_{max})	Collagen/ Elastin
Coronary	387 ± 57	20.6 ± 2.9	3.5 ± 0.6	3.0 ± 0.3
Internal Thoracic	612 ± 74	15.4 ± 1.3	20.4 ± 2.4	1.2 ± 0.1
Carotid	1085 ± 135	36.9 ± 4.0	17.7 ± 2.7	2.1 ± 0.1
Iliac	1720 ± 209	50.8 ± 2.2	6.0 ± 1.0	1.6 ± 0.2
Mesenteric	1722 ± 143	57.0 ± 2.3	3.7 ± 0.5	1.4 ± 0.1
Renal	2142 ± 270	63.1 ± 3.3	5.3 ± 0.9	2.0 ± 0.2

Legend: $\triangle \sigma_{max}$, maximum active stress response; $-\triangle D/D_0$, maximum constriction response; $\triangle L_{se}$, maximum series elastic element extension with active stress development; L_{max}, length for maximum force development.

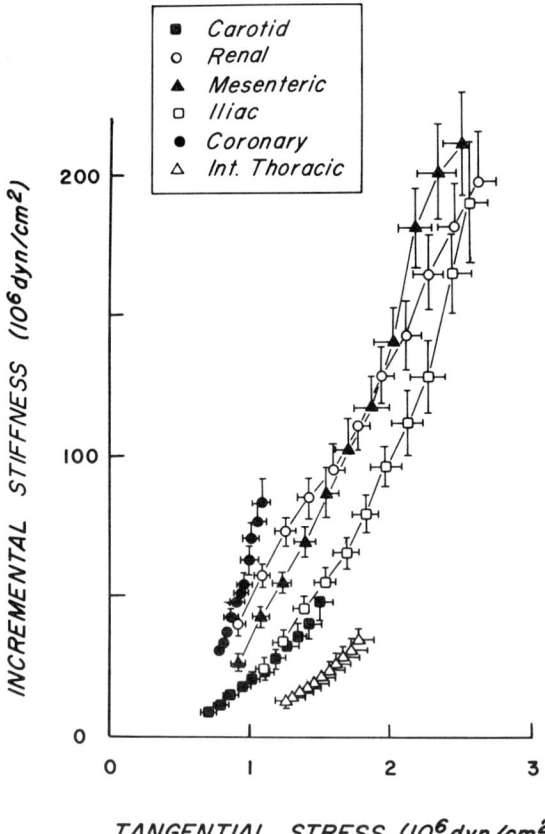

Fig. 9. Comparison of values of series elasticity for different arterial sites. Shown is the variation of incremental stiffness with tangential wall stress during isometric contractions from L_{max}, the optimum muscle length for force development. Symbols are means and bars are ±1 SEM (from Cox, 1978b).

the site of series elasticity in smooth muscle is not completely in the filament crossbridges or incremental active stiffness would be a unique function of active stress, independent of muscle length. A portion of series elasticity in smooth muscle series elasticity must reside outside the contractile filaments (Cox, 1978c; Mulvaney, 1979).

Series elastic elements act to distort the intrinsic properties of the contractile system by virtue of their interconnections. Force generation from any initial muscle length is decreased as is total shortening capacity by the series elastic elements (Cox, 1978d). This distortion is governed by the relative stiffness of the series elastic elements: the stiffer the series elastic elements, the smaller the distortion.

In Vivo Studies

Although these measures of in vitro mechanics are important for an understanding of the basic physiology of the arterial wall, in vivo studies may be more relevant to a determination of the role of the arterial wall in the regulation of circulatory regional vascular function. In recent years a number of studies have been conducted to evaluate the role of coronary artery smooth muscle in the control of coronary circulation. These experiments documented that stimulating sympathetic nerve supply to the coronary vasculature produces an effect on the mechanical properties of those structures (Gerova et al., 1979). This supports the concept that coronary arteries have a contractile system that may be reflexly regulated (Feigl, 1968). More recently, studies have been conducted using unanesthetized animals that have been chronically instrumented for the measurement of pressure and diameter in large extramural epicardial coronary arteries (Vatner et al., 1980; Tomoike et al., 1981). These experiments have used intraarterial methoxamine to activate coronary artery smooth muscle and intraarterial nitroglycerine to relax coronary artery smooth muscle (Vatner et al., 1980). These studies have documented a large potential range of control of coronary artery smooth muscle over arterial properties. Methoxamine given to conscious resting animals produced a 9% reduction in diameter of the left circumflex coronary artery. Nitroglycerin produced a 3% increase in wall diameter. These results show not only a large range of control but also the presence of a significant amount of resting tone of coronary artery smooth muscle. The relative significance of this smooth muscle in the production of coronary spasm and in contributing to acute angina has not been studied.

In addition to their role as a conduit system, the coronary arteries play an important role in the matching of the metabolic supply and demand in the heart. They perform this function by regulating the total coronary blood flow and its distribution within the heart. A variety of neural humoral factors are known to influence the functional properties of coronary arteries. These various signals are integrated at the level of the smooth muscle cell membrane in the coronary vasculature to mediate this regulation.

Several lines of evidence suggest an important role of the adrenergic innervation to the coronary arteries in mediating regulatory responses. Coronary artery smooth muscle cells have thick and thin filaments that are qualitatively organized in a manner similar to that of other smooth muscle cells. Nonspecific activation of coronary artery smooth muscle by high potassium, for example, elicits contractile responses as either force development or shortening (Cox, 1978b). Coronary artery smooth muscle cell membranes possess adrenergic receptors as they respond to a variety of alpha- and beta-adrenergic agonists (Feigl, 1967; Mekata and Niu, 1969; Van Breeman and Siegel, 1980; Hamilton and Feigl, 1976). Coronary arteries also possess postganglionic innervation from the sympathetic nervous system. Adrenergic nerve endings had been identified in the wall of coronary arteries (Denn and Stone, 1976) and catecholamine fluorescence has been shown to exist near the medial adventitial border in coronary arteries as well (Dolezel et al., 1978). Mechanical response of coronary arteries can be elicited by stimulating sympathetic nerves to the heart (Kalsner, 1979; Uchida and Murao, 1975; Gerova et al., 1979). Other studies have indicated that these neural pathways can be reflexly activated to produce vasomotor responses in the coronary vasculature (Feigl, 1968).

In spite of this overwhelming evidence documenting a functional adrenergic innervation to the coronary vasculature its role in the control and regulation of the coronary vascular system is obscure and controversial. The coronary vasculature is also highly sensitive to locally produced metabolically related vasodilator factors (Olsson, 1981). These local factors appear to be more directly involved in the metabolic matching of supply and demand in the coronary vasculature. Because of the importance of the local metabolically related factors in this regard the contribution of adrenergic mediated regulatory influences may be overshadowed (Mohrman and Feigl, 1978).

Acknowledgment

The author's research summarized in this manuscript has been supported by Research Grants HL 17840, HL 23348 and HL 23779 from the National Heart, Lung and Blood Institute of the United States Public Health Service.

References

Brecher, P., Chan, C. T., Franzblau, C., Faris, B. and Chobian, A. V. 1978. Effects of hypertension and its reversal on aortic metabolism in the rat. Circ Res 43:561–569

Brest, A. N., Harrer, W. V. and Schatz, J. 1972. The small coronary arteries. In *Atherosclerosis and Coronary Heart Disease*, eds. W. Likoff, B. L. Segal, W. Insull, Jr., and J. H. Moyer, pp. 122–128. New York: Grune & Stratton, Inc:

Buccino, R. A. and McIntosh, H. D. 1979. The role of aortocoronary bypass surgery in the management of coronary artery disease. In *Atherosclerosis Reviews*, Vol. 6, eds. A. M. Gotto and R. Paoletti, pp. 29–104. New York: Raven Press

Burton, A. C. 1954. Relation of structure to function of the tissues of the wall of blood vessels. Physiol Rev 34:619–642

Cohen, D. M. and Murphy, R. A. 1979. Relation of structure to function of the tissues of the wall of blood vessels. Physiol Rev 34: 316–642

Cohen, D. M. and Murphy, R. A. 1979. Cellular thin filament protein contents and force generation in porcine arteries and veins. Circ Res 45: 661–665

Cox, R. H. 1976. Effects of norepinephrine on mechanics of arteries in vitro. Am J Physiol 231:420–425

Cox, R. H. 1978a. Passive mechanics and connective tissue composition of canine arteries. Am J Physiol 234:H533–H541

Cox, R. H. 1978b. Regional variation of series elasticity in canine arterial smooth muscles. Am J Physiol 234:H542–H551

Cox, R. H. 1978c. Influence of muscle length on series elasticity in arterial smooth muscle. Am J Physiol 234:C146–C154

Cox, R. H. 1978d. Arterial smooth muscle mechanics. In *The Arterial System*, eds. R. D. Bauer and R. Busse, pp. 63–79. New York: Springer-Verlag

Cox, R. H. 1979. Regional, species, and age related variations in the mechanical properties of arteries. Biorheology 16: 85–94.

Cox, R. H. 1980. The mechanism of force transduction between vascular smooth muscle cells. In *Vascular Neuroeffector Mechanisms*, eds. J. A. Bevan, T. Godfraind, R. A. Maxwell, and P. M. Vanhoutte, pp. 192–99. New York: Raven Press.

Cox, R. H. and Chacko, S. 1981. Comparison of force development and contractile protein content of rat carotid and tail arteries. IRCS Med Sci, Biochem, 9:733–734

Denn, M. J. and Stone, H. L. 1976. Autonomic innervation of dog coronary arteries. J Appl Physiol 41:30–35

Dolezel, S., Gerova, M., Gero, J., Sladek, T. and Vasku, J. 1978. Adrenergic innervation of the coronary arteries and the myocardium. Acta Anat 100:306–316

Eyre, D. 1980. Collagen: Molecular diversity in the body's protein scaffold. Science 207:1315–1322

Feigel, E. O. 1967. Sympathetic control of coronary circulation. Circ Res 20: 262–270

Feigel, E. O. 1968. Carotid sinus reflex control of coronary blood flow. Circ Res 23:223–237

Fischer, G. M. and Llaurado, J. G. 1966. Collagen and elastin content in canine arteries selected from functionally different vascular beds. Circ Res 19: 394–399

Folkow, B. 1978. Cardiovascular structural adaptation: Its role in the initiation and maintenance of primary hypertension. Clin Sci Mol Med 55:3s–22s

Fuller, G. C., Miller, E., Farber, T. and Vanloon, E. 1972. Aortic connective tissue changes in miniature pigs fed a lipid-rich diet. Connect Tissue Res 1:217–220

Gerova, M., Barta, E. and Gero, J. 1979. Sympathetic control of major coronary artery diameter in the dog. Circ Res 44:459–467

Hamilton, F. N. and Feigl, E. O. 1976. Coronary vascular sympathetic beta-receptor innervation. Am J Physiol 230:1569–1576

Hill, A. V. 1950. The series elastic component of muscle. Proc Soc Biol 137: 273–280

Huxley, A. F. 1974. Muscular contraction. J Physiol 243:1–43

Kalsner, S. 1979. The effects of periarterial nerve activation on coronary vessel tone in an isolated and perfused slab of beef ventricle. Can J Physiol Pharmacol 57:291–297

Laszt, L. 1968. Untersuchungen über die elastischen Eigenschaften der Blutgefasse im Ruhe- und im Kontraktionszustand. Angiologia 5:14–27

Luchi, R. J., Chahine, R. A. and Raizner, A. E. 1979. Coronary artery spasm. Ann Int Med 91:441–449

Mekata, H. and Niu, H. 1969. Electrical and mechanical responses of coronary artery smooth muscle to catecholamines. Jpn J Physiol 19:599–608

Mohrman, D. E. and Feigl, E. O. 1978. Competition between sympathetic vasoconstriction and metabolic vasodilation in the canine coronary circulation. Circ Res 42:79–86

Mulvaney, M. J. 1979. The undamped and damped series elastic components of a vascular smooth muscle. Biophys J 26:401–413

Murphy, R. A. 1976. Contractile system function in mammalian smooth muscle. Blood Vessels 13:1–23

Olsson, R. A. 1981. Local factors regulating cardiac and skeletal muscle blood flow. Ann Rev Physiol 43:385–395

Prockop, D. J., Kivirikko, K. I., Tuderman, L. and Guzman, N. A. 1979a. The biosynthesis of collagen and its disorders. I. Engl J Med 301:13–23

Prockop, D. J., Kivirikko, K. I., Tuderman, L. and Guzman, N.A. 1979b. The biosynthesis of collagen and its disorders. II. Engl J Med 301:77–85

Roach, M. R. and Burton, A. C. 1957. The reason for the shape of the distensibility curves of arteries. Can J Biochem Physiol 35:681–690

Roy, C. S. 1881. The elastic properties of the arterial wall. J. Physiol 3:125–159

Sandberg, L. B., Soskel, N. T. and Leslie, J. G. 1981. Elastin structure, biosynthesis, and relation to disease states. Engl J Med 304:566–579

Snyder, R., Downey, J. M. and Kirk, E. S. 1975. The active and passive components of extravascular coronary resistance. Cardiovasc Res 9:161–166

Tomoike, H., Ootsubo, H., Sakai, K., Kikuchi, Y. and Nakamura, M. 1981. Continuous measurement of coronary artery diameter in situ. Am J Physiol 240:H73–H79

Uchida, Y. and Murao, S. 1975. Sustained decrease in coronary blood flow and excitation of cardiac sensory fibers following sympathetic stimulation. Jpn Heart J 16:265–279

Van Breeman, C. and Siegel, B. 1980. The mechanism of α-adrenergic activation of the dog coronary artery. Circ Res 46:426–429

Vatner, S. R., Pagani, M., Manders, W. T. and Pasipoularides, A. D. 1980. Alpha adrenergic vasoconstriction and nitroglycerine vasodilation of large coronary arteries in the conscious dog. J Clin Invest 65:5–14

Wolinsky, H. and Glagov, S. 1964. Structural basis for the static mechanical properties of the aortic media. Circ Res 14:400–413

The Regulation of Coronary Blood Flow

Robert M. Berne and Rafael Rubio

Introduction

Research on the coronary circulation has been active and has recently accelerated with the advent of new flow-metering devices and chemical techniques for studies on animals and the development of sophisticated noninvasive or minimally invasive investigative procedures for studies on humans. It is not within the scope of this brief review to discuss methodology, morphology (macroscopic to ultramicroscopic) of the coronary vasculature, pathophysiology or vasoactive drugs. These subjects, as well as many detailed aspects of proposed mechanisms of coronary blood flow (CBF) regulation, have been amply dealt with in previous reviews (Berne, 1964; Berne, 1974; Rubio and Berne, 1975; Berne, 1975; Rubio and Berne, 1978; Belloni, 1979; Berne and Rubio, 1979) and are in part covered by other participants in this symposium. Hence, this review briefly summarizes the more accepted views of factors involved in the regulation of CBF and focuses on some of the newer and more controversial aspects of the subject.

For convenience one can divide the factors that influence CBF into three major categories—mechanical, neural and metabolic. It is also conceivable that a fourth mechanism, the myogenic response, operates in adjustments of coronary vascular resistance when coronary perfusion is abruptly changed. A myogenic mechanism is characterized by a prompt relaxation of the coronary vascular smooth muscle in response to a rapid incease in coronary transmural pressure and a prompt constriction in response to a rapid reduction in coronary transmural pressure. This could account for the phenomenon of autoregulation of CBF; that is a constant CBF in the face of changes in perfusion pressure. Changes in coronary vascular resistance suggesting a myogenic mechanism have been observed after brief (1 or 2 cardiac cycle) coronary occlusions (Eikens and Wilcken, 1974). However, it has not been established that a myogenic response occurs in the coronary vascular bed because metabolic changes that affect CBF can occur within a single cardiac cycle (Thompson et al., 1980; Schwartz et al., 1981). Furthermore, a myogenic mechanism would probably not be involved in the physiological regulation of CBF because blood pressure (coronary perfusion pressure) rarely undergoes abrupt changes in the normal state because of the buffering capacity of the baroreceptor reflex.

Mechanical Factors

Of the mechanical factors, such as perfusion pressure (which is of course essential for CBF), blood viscosity and mechanical properties of the microvessels, the one that has been most thoroughly studied is *extravascular compression* produced by the contraction of the heart. Since the early work of Anrep et al., (1931) it has been recognized that left CBF is greater in diastole than in systole and this difference in left CBF during the cardiac cycle is inversely related to the extravascular pressure developed by the contracting left ventricle (Gregg, 1963). In contrast to the thick walled left ventricle, the thin walled right ventricle develops relatively little extravascular resistance and consequently blood flow is greater during systole when perfusion pressure is greatest. An estimate of the magnitude of left ventricular extravascular resistance to CBF can be obtained by inducing abrupt cessation of the heart beat (peripheral vagus nerve stimulation or ventricular fibrillation with maintenance of a constant perfusion pressure) and measuring the increment in CBF (Sabiston and Gregg, 1957). Any procedure that increases the duration of systole at the expense of diastole (tachycardia) or enhances the developed tension of the left ventricle (e.g., stellate ganglion stimulation) increases the extravascular resistance to CBF, whereas the opposite effect on CBF is obtained with interventions that reduce heart rate or contractile force. In a single cardiac cycle left coronary arterial inflow often ceases or is reversed during early systole, whereas coronary sinus outflow is increased during this phase of the cycle because of compression of the veins. Studies of the microcirculation corroborate the gross flow changes; red cell velocity decreases in arterioles and increases in capillaries and venules during systole and exhibits opposite flow patterns during diastole (Tillmanns et al., 1974).

In a steady state condition it is conceivable that, with periods of increased or decreased ventricular pressure, the altered myocardial pressure (tissue pressure) could compress or decompress, respectively, the thin walled microvessels either directly or via movement of fluid into and out of the interstitial space and hence be responsible for autoregulation of blood flow (Rodbard, 1971). However, experiments in which perfusion pressure was increased when the coronary resistance vessels were maximally dilated with dipyridamole failed to show autoregulation of CBF despite increments in intramyocardial pressure (Driscol et al., 1964).

Because the endocardium is in direct contact with the ventricular cavity it is affected by ventricular pressure to a greater extent than are the more distal segments of the left ventricular wall. Hence, there is a pressure gradient across the left ventricular wall; pressure is highest at the endocardial surface and lowest at the epicardial surface of the free wall of the left ventricle. Such a ventricular transmural pressure gradient could result in a lesser blood flow, per unit weight, to the endocardium than to the epicardium. However, studies with diffusable traces such as ^{86}Rb or ^{133}Xe, or with labeled microspheres indicated that blood flow to the endocardial and epicardial regions of the heart was essentially equal (Cutarelli and Levy, 1963; Baggar, 1977; Domenech et al., 1969). Only when diastolic CBF is greatly reduced by increments in left ventricular diastolic pressure, enhanced extravascular compression or marked decreases in the duration of diastole is the ratio of endocardial to epicardial blood flow decreased (Buckberg and Kattus, 1973). It appears that the endocardial resistance vessels exhibit less tone than do the epicardial vessels, thereby compensating for the difference in extravascular pressure. Therefore, they have less vasodilator reserve and under certain types of cardiac stress the endocardium is more vulnerable to ischemic damage than is the epicardium.

Recently, considerable attention has been focused on the observation that when diastole is greatly prolonged and aortic pressure (coronary perfusion pressure) is permitted to fall to very low levels, blood flow ceases at a pressure significantly greater than zero (Bellamy, 1978). This phenomenon, which has been attributed to extravascular pressure and is independent of coronary venous pressure, has been termed a "vascular waterfall" because the flow over a waterfall is independent of the distance from the edge of the falls to the stream below (Downey and Kirk, 1975; Permutt and Riley, 1963; Bellamy and Lowensohn, 1980). Despite considerable work on this phenomenon, the mechanism remains controversial. To what extent vasomotor activity and possibly coronary venous pressure are contributing factors and to what extent venous capacitance is involved is not altogether clear. Furthermore, the physiological role of this so-called vascular waterfall in the regulation of CBF is unknown.

Neural Factors

Sympathetic Nerves

The fact that stimulation of the sympathetic nerves to the heart elicits changes in CBF has been known for many years, but whether activation of the cardiac sympathetic nerves induced constriction or dilation of the coronary resistance vessels was controversial. The principal reason for the controversy is that early studies could not differentiate between a direct effect on the coronary vessels from one that was secondary to the inotropic and chronotropic effects of such stimulation on the myocardium. Before the discovery of alpha- and beta-adrenergic blocking agents, experiments in which these myocardial effects could be dissociated from direct coronary effects by studying the coronary vascular response to sympathetic nerve stimulation or intracoronary catecholamine administration were accomplished in the potassium-arrested heart, the fibrillating heart or the beating heart in late diastole when extravascular compression was virtually absent (Berne, 1958; Berne et al., 1965). Conclusions reached from these early studies were that the primary effect of stellate ganglion stimulation or the intracoronary administration of epinephrine or norepinephrine was vasoconstriction and that the vasodilation observed with these interventions was secondary to stimulation of the myocardium (β_1 receptors) resulting in a release of vasodilator metabolites. Hence, the coronary vessels contained alpha receptors, a conclusion later supported by the observation of coronary vasoconstriction after administration of the agonist, phenylephrine (Mark et al., 1972), or with stellate ganglion stimulation after beta-adrenergic receptor blockade (Feigl, 1967). Evidence for beta receptors on the coronary vessels (β_2 receptors) was obtained by administration of the beta agonist, isoproterenol, in the potassium-arrested heart (Klocke et al., 1965) and by relaxation of potassium-contracted helical strips of coronary arteries after the administration of catecholamines (Zuberbuhler and Bohr, 1965). Subsequent studies in conscious dogs showed that epinephrine elicited coronary dilation, whereas after beta-adrenergic receptor blockade coronary constriction was observed (Pitt et al., 1967). Although it was firmly established that the coronary vessels contained alpha and beta receptors their functional significance was not fully appreciated.

Recently, however, several reports have appeared that indicate the existence of tonic sympathetic constriction and a competition between metabolic vasodilation and neural vasoconstriction in the coronary vascular bed. Stimulation of the carotid sinus nerve in unanesthetized dogs produced a decrease in coronary resistance at rest and during exercise that was not blocked by atropine or propranolol (hence not via beta receptor stimulation), but was abolished by alpha-adrenergic receptor blockade, indicating tonic vasoconstrictor activity (Vatner et al., 1970). Competition between neural and metabolic effects on coronary resistance was demonstrated by intracoronary norepinephrine adminstration or by bilateral carotid artery occlusion that produced a decrease in coronary sinus blood pO_2 and a small increment in oxygen delivery to the heart that was changed to a lesser decrease in coronary sinus blood pO_2 and a larger oxygen delivery to the heart after alpha-adrenergic receptor blockage (Mohrman and Feigl, 1978). In the conscious dog the coronary dilation observed with exercise was partly attenuated by alpha-adrenergic receptor blockade (Murray and Vatner, 1979) and bilateral carotid occlusion elicited an increase in vascular resistance in the right coronary artery, which could be almost abolished by alpha-adrenergic receptor blockade (Murray and Vatner, 1981). Even with rather severe hypotension produced by hemorrhage, alpha-constriction tone was present in dogs and could be unmasked by alpha-adrenergic receptor blockade (Smith et al., 1981). Hence it is apparent that despite the disadvantage of coronary constrictor activity under conditions of myocardial stress, metabolically induced vasodilation can be opposed by alpha-adrenergic activity. In general, however, metabolic mechanisms supervene in most instances of myocardial hypoxia whether brought about by reduced supply or increased demand of oxygen. For example, dogs conditioned to respond to a noxious stimulus showed an initial, transient decrease in CBF followed by a prolonged increase when exposed to the stimulus (Billman and Randall, 1981). One can comprehend the opposing effects of the neural and metabolic effects on CBF if the neural effects are limited to the larger coronary vessels. If this is indeed the case, then even if the coronary arterioles are maximally dilated, flow to the myocardial tissue could be reduced by upstream constriction of the cognate arteries. Further studies are needed to clarify the nature of this neural-metabolic interaction.

With respect to the beta-adrenergic receptors, the consensus is that the myocardium contains β_1 receptors which, when stimulated, have a positive inotropic and chronotropic effect. These receptors can be activated by beta receptor agonists (e.g., isoproterenol) or by direct or reflex neural stimulation when interfering responses such as alpha-mediated constriction and acetylcholine-induced dilation are blocked by alpha-adrenergic blocking agents and atropine, respectively. With the use of an alpha-adrenergic blocker in conjunction with practolol, a β_1 receptor blocker, stellate ganglion stimulation elicited only a small transient increase in CBF that was reduced but not abolished by propranolol (McRaven et al., 1971). These observations suggest, at best, a minimal physiological role for coronary β_2 receptors in the regulation of CBF.

Parasympathetic Nerves

As in the case of the cardiac sympathetic nerves, there existed complete confusion about the effects of vagus nerve stimulation on CBF. The reasons were the same, namely an inability to separate the direct effects on the coronary vessels from those secondary to the negative inotropic and chronotropic effects on the myocardium. When these interfering variables were eliminated by stimulation of the vagi in fibrillating hearts or empty paced hearts (Berne et al., 1965) or in paced hearts after beta-adrenergic receptor blockade (Feigl, 1969), a small increase in CBF was observed that could be blocked with atropine. A vagally induced decrease in coronary resistance was also demonstrated reflexly by stimulation of the chemoreceptors during β_1-adrenergic receptor blockade in dogs with cardiac pacing and constant flow perfusion (Hackett et al., 1972). Recently it was shown in the isolated perfused guinea pig heart that acetylcholine administration probably elicits a sizable fraction of the observed coronary dilation by the release of adenosine possibly from the endothelial cells, (Schrader et al., 1981). To what extent vagal dilation occurs under physiological conditions is not known, but judging from the small effects elicited experimentally it is doubtful if the vagus nerves are significantly involved in normal adjustments of CBF.

Metabolic Factors

It is well established that an excellent correlation exists between myocardial oxygen consumption and CBF with a wide variety of stimuli. What has puzzled investigators for years is the nature of the link between cardiac metabolic activity and the contractile state of the coronary vascular smooth muscle. Many substances have been suggested but few have stood the test of time. A few of the more viable candidates are considered.

Oxygen

Although a reduction in oxygen delivery to the myocardium, whether accomplished by a reduction in CBF, hypoxemia or the administration of cyanide, results in a decrease in coronary resistance; it has not been possible to exclude the release of a vasodilator metabolite from the hypoxic myocardium. In fact, there is no evidence for an "oxygen sensor," whereas there is considerable evidence that an inadequate oxygen supply for the needs of the myocardium results in the release of a messenger that induces resistance vessel relaxation. Were a reduction in oxygen tension per se an arteriolar dilator, then one would expect prompt restoration of CBF after 10–30 sec occlusions of the left coronary artery, because the coronary venous blood is bright red during a large part of the period of reactive hyperemia observed upon release of the brief coronary occlusion. Actually, the duration of the reactive hyperemia is greater for the long occlusions than for the short ones, although the vascular smooth muscle of the arterioles is exposed to high oxygen tensions in both cases. Hence, it appears that hypoxia does not operate directly but elicits vasodilation by another mechanism.

Carbon Dioxide and pH

Carbon dioxide has been known to have a dilator effect on the coronary vessels but in the heart-lung preparation the effect was small, as was the effect of the associated reduction in pH (Hilton and Eichholtz, 1925). Recent studies have revived the concept that CO_2 may produce significant decreases in coronary resistance (Case et al., 1978). It is difficult to reconcile these recent observations with the earlier studies, and further evaluation of the importance of CO_2 in determining CBF is needed. With respect to pH, only minor increments inflow have been attributable to H^+ and very recent experiments showed no effect of prevention of a decrease in pH during reactive hypermia on coronary resistance (Steinhart and Nixon, 1981).

Potassium

Since the report of Dawes in 1941, potassium has been considered to be a potential mediator of metabolic vasodilation. Previously, Katz and Lindner (1938) had shown that low doses of K^+ produced moderate coronary dilation, whereas large doses produced vasoconstriction. However, studies on open chest dogs given intracoronary KCℓ revealed only slight vasodilation, and enhanced cardiac work (increased afterload or catecholamine administration) failed to show K^+ release from the active myocardium (Driscol and Berne, 1957). However, these were steady state conditions, and when coronary venous blood was assayed for potassium immediately after abrupt increases in heart rate or after 15-sec coronary occlusions a moderate but transient increase of CBF was observed (Murray and Vatners, 1979). Therefore, it is possible that the initial increase in CBF with enhanced oxygen demand or reduced supply is caused by potassium release from the myocardium.

Adenosine

In 1929 Drury and Szent-Györgyi described many of the properties of adenosine, and particularly noted its dilator effect on the coronary vessels. Three years later Rigler (1932) proposed that adenosine might play a role in the regulation of muscle blood flow, but he provided no experimental proof in support of his idea. The subject lay dormant until the late 1950s when, during our efforts to discover the link between CBF and myocardial metabolism, we decided to investigate the possibility that adenosine could serve as mediator.

For adenosine to play a key role in the metabolic regulation of CBF, certain criteria must be met: 1) It must be a potent dilator of the coronary resistance vessels. 2) There must be an endogenous source of the nucleoside. 3) Adenosine should have access to arterioles and be present under basal physiological conditions. 4) The concentration reached in the interstitial fluid (ISF) must be capable of eliciting vasodilation, and there should be a close relationship between the ISF concentration and CBF. 5) The time course of oxygen deficit (either decreased oxygen supply or increased oxygen demand) should parallel the increment in CBF. 6) The physiological effect at different concentrations of adenosine should be mimicked by exogenous administration of the nucleoside. 7) Agents that potentiate or attentuate the action of administered adenosine should elicit a similar effect on endogenously liberated mediator. 8) A direct cause-and-effect relationship should be established under all physiological and pathophysiological conditions between change in CBF and adenosine release. Most of these criteria are met by adenosine but it is currently impossible to measure ISF concentrations. There is a controversy regarding the effects of potentiators and attenuators on endogenously released adenosine, and a direct cause-and-effect relationship has not been firmly established.

The initial experiments on the isolated perfused cat heart and the heart of the open chest dog revealed only the release of inosine and hypoxanthine when subjected to anoxia or hypoxia (Berne, 1963). However, subsequent studies that employed better techniques revealed that adenosine was released by the hypoxic heart and the amount released closely paralleled the degree of hypoxia as well as the increase in coronary flow (Katori and Berne, 1966; Rubio et al., 1974). Adenosine was also found in the normal heart (Rubio and Berne, 1969; Olsson, 1970) and during reactive hyperemia (Rubio et al., 1969; Olsson et al., 1978) in which condition there were good correlations between the duration of the reactive hyperemia and the levels of adenosine in the myocardium (Olsson et al., 1978).

All of the studies mentioned above dealt with situations in which there was a limitation of oxygen supply to the heart. However, under physiologic conditions, an increase in CBF occurs in response to an increase in oxygen demand by the heart, and more recent studies have addressed this aspect of

CBF regulation by adenosine. Increased cardiac work produced in the rat (Foley et al., 1978) and in the dog (McKenzie et al., 1980a) by constriction of the thoracic aorta resulted in highly significant elevations of myocardial adenosine release from the heart. Furthermore, stellate ganglion stimulation in the open chest dog resulted in adenosine release from the heart (Miller et al., 1979). Similar observations were made in the conscious dog subjected to treadmill exercise. In one study there was about a threefold increase in the release of adenosine from the heart with moderate exercise (Watkinson et al., 1979) and in another study samples of myocardium obtained immediately after cessation of exercise also showed a threefold increase with moderate exercise (McKenzie et al., 1980b). The effects of treadmill exercise, excitement (repeated loud noise) and eating on CBF, myocardial oxygen consumption, mean arterial blood pressure, heart rate and adenosine release from the heart of the conscious dog are shown in Table 1. In none of the experiments in which cardiac work was increased in the anesthetized or the conscious state was there any indication (such as lactate formation) that the heart was hypoxic. Therefore, it is apparent that stimuli that increase myocardial metabolic activity and CBF show a concomitant increase in adenosine formation and release, and that there is a significant correlation between CBF and adenosine function and release (Miller et al., 1979; McKenzie et al., 1980b). These results, in conjunction with the observation (Thompson et al., 1980) that myocardial adenosine levels change in a single cardiac cycle (high in systole, low in diastole) strongly support the concept that adenosine plays an important role in the regulation of CBF.

Table 1. Hemodynamic and metabolic effects of experimental maneuvers in the conscious dog.

Effect	Control	Treadmill Exercise 10% Grade		Excitement	Eating
		2 mph	4 mph		
CBF (ml/min/100 g)	95 ± 3	138 ± 7*	163 ± 10*	158 ± 11*	155 ± 12*
MVO_2 (ml/min/100 g)	10.4 ± 1.3	20.0 ± 1.8*	24.0 ± 0.8*	21.1 ± 1.8*	20.3 ± 2.4*
MABP (mm Hg)	92. ± 8	113 ± 8*	116 ± 7*	118 ± 11*	117 ± 7*
HR (beats/min)	125 ± 15	209 ± 11*	242 ± 11*	186 ± 8*	196 ± 17*
ADO (pmos/ml)	91 ± 9	169 ± 28*	223 ± 28*	285 ± 56*	204 ± 39*

Values are means ±SEM. CBF = coronary blood flow, MVO_2 = myocardial oxygen consumption, MABP = mean arterial blood pressure, HR = heart rate, ADO = adenosine. The adenosine is expressed in terms of picomoles per millimeter of pericardial infusate. In these experiments 25 ml of Krebs-Henseleit solution were introduced into the pericardial sac via a previously placed catheter where it remained for 4.5 min of each control and experimental period. It was then removed and analyzed for adenosine and its degradative products. Earlier control experiments (Miller et al., 1979) showed that the pericardial concentration of adenosine was a reliable index of the myocardial concentration under control and experimental conditions.
*Denotes significant changes from control. $P < 0.05$, n = 4.

There are adenosine receptors on the coronary resistance vessels (Olsson et al., 1976; Schrader et al., 1977) and presumably adenosine formed from adenosine monophosphate (AMP) at the myocardial cell margins by the enzyme 5'-nucleotidase is released into the ISF where it contacts the coronary resistance vessels (Rubio et al., 1973). This source of adenosine has recently been questioned because adenosine can also arise intracellularly from S-adenosylhomocysteine (SAH) by the action of SAH hydrolase (Schrader and Schütz, 1979; 1980). To what extent this occurs in the regulation of CBF is not known because it is not clear how free adenosine can escape being metabolized by adenosine deaminase and adenosine kinase in the cell cytoplasm and be transported out of the myocardial cell intact. Most of the adenosine found in the normal heart is apparently bound to protein and is inaccessible to adenosine deaminase (Olsson et al., 1981). The protein that tightly binds adenosine is the same enzyme that cleaves SAH to adenosine and homocysteine, namely SAH hydrolase (Hershfield and Kredich, 1978). A serious problem created by the large amount of protein-bound (and probably inactive) adenosine is that it constitutes a high background and makes it difficult to accurately quantify small increases in tissue adenosine levels.

How adenosine causes relaxation of coronary vascular smooth muscle is not known. Only at pharmacological doses (10^{-3} M) does adenosine induce increases in the cyclic AMP levels (Herlihy et al., 1976). Therefore, it is unlikely that this mechanism is involved in physiological adjustments of coronary vascular resistance. Based on some indirect experiments (De Gubareff and Sleator, 1965; Schrader et al., 1977; Berne, 1975) it seems that adenosine probably acts by interfering with calcium uptake or the accessibility of the vascular smooth muscle contractile machinery to calcium, but direct evidence in support of this concept is still lacking.

Assuming that adenosine is primarily formed by the action of 5'-nucleotidase on AMP, the control of adenosine production is most likely achieved by regulation of the 5'-nucleotidase activity in vivo as well as to some extent by the levels of the substrate, AMP. In vitro experiments on cardiac 5'-nucleotidase indicate that the enzyme is about 100-fold more active in vitro than in vivo and that it is inhibited in vivo by ATP, ADP and phosphocreatine (PCr) (Rubio et al., 1979). Because ATP and ADP show little change with increases in cardiac activity whereas PCr decreases, it is conceivable that the reduction in PCr leads to less inhibition of 5'-nucleotidase. However, of greater importance is the fact that free magnesium strongly reverses the inhibition of 5'-nucleotidase by PCr. Hence, it is postulated that in vivo, increased myocardial metabolic activity is associated with a slight increase in AMP (breakdown from ATP), a decrease in PCr and liberation of some Mg^{2+} that was chelated to ATP and was released when undetectable reductions in ATP occurred during the enhanced cardiac activity. This mechanism is only speculative and will require considerably more work to test its validity.

Other Factors

None of the additional possible mediators of metabolic coronary vasodilation fulfill the criteria for the messenger between parenchymal tissue and arteriolar vascular smooth muscle. Increases in plasma osmolarity have not been observed in the heart, there is no evidence that calcium is directly involved in CBF regulation and the prostaglandins, although they exhibit striking vasoactive properties, do not appear to function as physiological regulators of CBF; they may, however, be responsible for vascular resistance changes that occur in pathophysiological conditions.

Summary

The coronary circulation is influenced by mechanical, neural and metabolic factors. Other than the perfusion pressure (arterial pressure), the most important mechanical factor is the extravascular compression created by contraction of the left ventricle. Of the neural factors, sympathetic constrictor activity is of primary importance. Coronary constriction (alpha) activity of the cardiac sympathetic nerves exists during basal conditions and can be enhanced by direct or reflex activation during different physiological and pathophysiological states, to the point where it competes with vasodilator responses to increased rates of cardiac metabolism. Positive inotropic and chronotropic effects on the heart that secondarily augment CBF result from β_1 activation. However, β_2 (direct effect on the coronary vessels) and vagal activation exert minor direct effects on CBF. Metabolic factors are most important in the regulation of CBF and the chief metabolic mediator is adenosine. Other factors such as potassium, CO_2 and pH contribute to unknown degrees in the adjustments of CBF to the needs of the myocardium.

Acknowledgment

The research of the authors referred to in this chapter was supported by Grant HL 10384 of the United States Public Health Service.

References

Anrep, G. V., Davis, J. C. and Volhard, E. 1931. The effect of pulse pressure on coronary blood flow. J Physiol (Lond) 73:405–425

Baggar, H. 1977. Distribution of coronary blood flow in the left ventricular wall of dogs evaluated by the uptake of Xe-133. Acta Physiol Scand 99:421-431

Bellamy, R. F. 1978. Diastolic coronary artery pressure-flow relations in the dog. Circ Res 43:92–101

Bellamy, R. F. and Lowensohn, H. S. 1980. Effect of systole on coronary pressure-flow relations in the right ventricle of the dog. Am J Physiol 238:H481–H486

Belloni, F. L. 1979. The local control of coronary blood flow. Cardiovasc Res 13:63–85

Berne, R. M. 1958. Effect of epinephrine and norepinephrine on coronary circulation. Circ Res 6:644–655

Berne, R. M. 1963. Cardiac nucleotides in hypoxia: Possible role in regulation of coronary blood flow. Am J Physiol 204:317–322

Berne, R. M. 1964. Regulation of coronary blood flow. Physiol Res 44:1–29

Berne, R. M. 1974. The coronary circulation. In *The Mammalian Myocardium*, eds. G. A. Langer and A. Brady, p. 251. New York: John Wiley and Sons, Inc.

Berne, R. M. 1975. Myocardial blood flow: Metabolic determinants. In *The Peripheral Circulations*, ed. R. Zelis, p. 117. New York: Grune and Stratton, Inc.

Berne, R. M., DeGeest, H. and Levy, M. N. 1965. Influence of the cardiac nerves on coronary resistance. Am J Physiol 208:763–769

Berne, R. M. and Rubio, R. 1979. Coronary circulation. In *Handbook of Physiology—Section 2, The Cardiovascular System* I, eds. R. M. Berne and N. Sperelakis, p. 873, Bethesda: American Physiological Society

Billman, G. E. and Randall, D. C. 1981. Mechanisms mediating the coronary vascular response to behavioral stress in the dog. Circ Res 48:214–223

Buckberg, G. D., Kattus, A. A., Jr. 1973. Factors determining the distribution and adequacy of left ventricular myocardial blood flow. Adv Exp Med Biol 39:95–113

Case, R. B., Felix, A., Wachter, M., Kyriakidis, G. and Castellana, F. 1978. Relative effect of CO_2 on canine coronary vascular resistance. Circ Res 42:410–418

Cutarelli, R. and Levy, M. N. 1963. Intraventricular pressure and the distribution of coronary blood flow. Circ Res 12:322–327

Dawes, G. S. 1941. The vaso-dilator action of potassium. J Physiol (Lond) 99:224–238

De Gubareff, T. and Sleator, W., Jr. 1965. Effects of caffeine on mammalian atrial muscle, and its interaction with adenosine and calcium. J Pharmacol Exp Ther 148:202–214

Domenech, R. J., Hoffman, J. I. E., Noble, M. I. M., Saunders, K. B., Henson, J. R. and Subijanto, S. 1969. Total and regional coronary blood flow measured by radioactive microspheres in conscious and anesthetized dogs. Circ Res 25:581–596

Downey, J. M. and Kirk, E. S. 1975. Inhibition of coronary blood flow by a vascular waterfall mechanism. Circ Res 36:753–760

Driscol, T. E. and Berne, R. M. 1957. Role of potassium in regulation of coronary blood flow. Proc Soc Exp Biol Med 96:505–508

Driscol, T. E., Moir, T. W. and Eckstein, R. W. 1964. Vascular effects of changes in perfusion pressure in the nonischemic and ischemic heart. Circ Res (Suppl I) 15:94–102

Drury, A. N. and Szent-Györgyi, A. 1929. The physiological activity of adenine compounds with special reference to their action upon the mammalian heart. J Physiol (Lond) 68:213–237

Eikens, E. and Wilcken, D. E. L. 1974. Reactive hyperemia in the dog heart. Effects of temporarily restricting arterial inflow and of coronary occlusions lasting one and two cardiac cycles. Circ Res 35:702–712

Feigl, E. O. 1967. Sympathetic control of coronary circulation. Circ Res 20:262–271

Feigl, E. O. 1969. Parasympathetic control of coronary blood flow in dogs. Circ Res 25:509–519

Foley, D. H., Herlihy, J. T., Thompson, C. I., Rubio, R. and Berne, R. M. 1978. Increased adenosine formation by rat myocardium with acute aortic contriction. J Mol Cell Cardiol 10:293–300

Gregg, D. E. 1963. Physiology of the coronary circulation. Circulation 27:1128–1137

Hackett, J. G., Abboud, F. M., Mark, A. L., Schmid, P. G. and Heistad, D. D. 1972. Coronary vascular responses to stimulation of chemoreceptors and baroreceptors. Evidence for reflex activation of vagal cholinergic innervation. Circ Res 31:8–17

Herlihy, J. T., Bockman, E. L., Berne, R. M. and Rubio, R. 1976. Adenosine relaxation of isolated vascular smooth muscle. Am J Physiol 230:1239–1243

Hershfield, M. S. and Kredich, N. M. 1978. S-Adenosylhomocysteine hydrolase is an adenosine-binding protein: A target for adenosine toxicity. Science 202:757–760

Hilton, R. and Eichholtz, F. 1925. The influence of chemical factors on the coronary circulation. J Physiol 59:413–525

Katori, M. and Berne, R. M. 1966. Release of adenosine from anoxic hearts: Relationship to coronary flow. Circ Res 19:420–425

Katz, L. N. and Lindner, E. 1938. The action of excess Na, Ca and K on the coronary vessels. Am J Physiol 124:155–160

Klocke, F. J., Kaiser, G. A., Ross, J., Jr. and Braunwald, E. 1965. An intrinsic adrenergic vasodilator mechanism in the coronary vascular bed of the dog. Circ Res 16:376–382

Mark, A. L., Abboud, F. M., Schmid, P. G., Heistad, D. D. and Mayer, H. E. 1972. Differences in direct effects of adrenergic stimuli on coronary, cutaneous, and muscular vessels. J Clin Invest 51:279–287

McKenzie, J. E., McCoy, F. P. and Bockman, E. L. 1980a. Myocardial adenosine and coronary resistance during increased cardiac performance. Am J Physiol 239:H509–515

McKenzie, J. E., Steffen, R. P., West, E. J. and Haddy, F. J. 1980b. Myocardial adenosine content and coronary vascular resistance in the exercising dog. Fed Proc 39 (Abs): 1002

McRaven, D. R., Mark, A. L., Abboud, F. M. and Mayer, H. E. 1971. Responses of coronary vessels to adrenergic stimuli. J Clin Invest 50:773–778

Miller, W. L., Belardinelli, L., Bacchus, A., Foley, D. H., Rubio, R. and Berne, R. M. 1979. Canine myocardial adenosine and lactate production, oxygen consumption and coronary blood flow during stellate ganglia stimulation. Circ Res 45:708–718

Mohrman, D. E. and Feigl, E. O. 1978. Competition between sympathetic vasodilation in the canine coronary circulation. Circ Res 42:79–86

Murray, P. A. and Vatner, S. F. 1979. αAdrenoceptor attenuation of the coronary vascular response to severe exercise in the conscious dog. Circ Res 45:654–660

Murray, P. A. and Vatner, S. F. 1981. Autonomic vs. autoregulatory factors in the right coronary response to bilateral carotid occlusion in the conscious dog. Fed Proc 40(Abs):563

Olsson, R. A. 1970. Changes in content of purine nucleoside in canine myocardium during coronary occlusion. Circ Res 26: 301–306

Olsson, R. A., Davis, C. J., Khouri, E. M. and Patterson, R. E. 1976. Evidence for an adenosine receptor on the surface of dog coronary myocytes. Circ Res 39:93–98

Olsson, R. A., Saito, D., Nixon, D. G. and Vomacka, R. B. 1981. Compartmentation of the cardiac adenosine pool. Fed Proc 40 (Abs):564

Olsson, R. A., Snow, J. A. and Gentry, M. K. 1978. Adenosine metabolism in canine myocardial reactive hyperemia. Circ Res 42:358–362

Permutt, S. and Riley, R. L. 1963. Hemodynamics of collapsible vessels with tone: Vascular waterfall. J Appl Physiol 18:924–932

Pitt, B., Elliott, E. C. and Gregg, D. E. 1967. Adrenergic receptor activity in the coronary arteries of the unanesthetized dog. Circ Res 21:75–84

Rigler, R. 1932. Über die Ursache der vermehrten Durchblutung des Muskels während der Arbeit. Arch Exp Pathop Pharmacol 167:54–56

Rodbard, S. 1971. The burden of the resistance vessels. Circ Res 28–29 (Suppl I):I-51–I-58

Rubio, R., Belardinelli, L., Thompson, C. I. and Berne, R. M. 1979. Cardiac adenosine: Electrophysiological effects, possible significance in cell function, and mechanisms controlling its release. In *Physiological and Regulatory Functions of Adenosine and Adenine Nucleotides*, eds. H. P. Baer and G. I. Drummond, p. 167. New York: Raven Press

Rubio, R. and Berne, R. M. 1969. Release of adenosine by the normal myocardium in dogs and its relationship to the regulation of coronary resistance. Circ Res 25:407–415

Rubio, R. and Berne, R. M. 1975. Regulation of coronary blood flow. In *Progress in Cardiovascular Diseases, 18*, p. 105. New York: Grune and Stratton, Inc.

Rubio, R. and Berne, R. M. 1978. Myocardium. In *Peripheral Circulation*, ed. P. C. Johnson, p. 231. New York: John Wiley and Sons, Inc.

Rubio, R., Berne, R. M. and Dobson, J. G., Jr. 1973. Sites of adenosine production in cardiac and skeletal muscle. Am J Physiol 225:938–953

Rubio, R., Berne, R. M. and Katori, M. 1969. Release of adenosine in reactive hyperemia of the dog heart. Am J Physiol 216:56–62

Rubio, R., Wiedmeier, V. T. and Berne, R. M. 1974. Relationship between coronary flow and adenosine production and release. J Mol Cell Cardiol 6:561–566

Sabiston, D. C., Jr. and Gregg, D. E. 1957. Effect of cardiac contraction on coronary flow. Circulation 15:14–20

Schrader, J., Nees, S. and Gerlach, E. 1977. Evidence for a cell surface adenosine receptor on coronary myocytes and atrial muscle cells: Studies with an adenosine derivative of high molecular weight. Pflügers Arch 369:251–257

Schrader, J. and Schütz, W. 1979. Sites of adenosine production in the hypoxic heart. Fed Proc 38(Abs):1037

Schrader, J. and Schütz, W. 1980. Effect of L-homocysteine on the release of adenosine formed by the hypoxic heart. Proc Int Union Physiol Sci 14(Abs):688

Schrader, J., Thompson, C. I., Hiendlmayer, G. and Gerlach, E. 1981. Role of purines in acetylcholine-induced coronary vasodilation. Fed Proc 40(Abs):564

Schwartz, G. G., McHale, P. A. and Greenfield, J. C., Jr. 1981. Coronary vasodilation following a single ventricular extrastimulus in the conscious dog. Fed Proc 40(Abs):566

Smith, E. E., Jones, C. E. and Young, P. J. 1981. Neural limitation to coronary blood flow during hemorrhagic hypotension. Fed Proc 40(Abs):563

Steinhart, C. R. and Nixon, D. G. 1981. Role of acidosis in myocardial reactive hyperemia. Fed Proc 40(Abs):565

Thompson, C. I., Rubio, R. and Berne, R. M. 1980. Changes in adenosine and glycogen phosphorylase activity during the cardiac cycle. Am J Physiol 238:H389–398

Tillmanns, H., Ikeda, S., Hansen, H., Sarma, J. S. M., Fauvel, J. M. and Bing, R. J. 1974. Microcirculation in the ventricle of the dog and turtle. Circ Res 34:561–569

Vatner, S. F., Franklin, D., Van Citters, R. L and Braunwald, E. 1970. Effects of carotid sinus nerve stimulation on the coronary circulation of the conscious dog. Circ Res 27:11–21

Watkinson, W. P., Foley, D. H., Rubio, R. and Berne, R. M. 1979. Myocardial adenosine formation with increased cardiac performance in the dog. Am J. Physiol 236:H13–H21

Zuberbuhler, R. C. and Bohr, D. F. 1965. Responses of coronary smooth muscle to catecholamines. Circ Res 16:431–440

Discussion

Dr. Berne: You demonstrate that cyclic AMP increases might result in a decrease in contraction or relaxation. This is in agreement with work of others who have shown this correlation. What about the study of cyclic GMP in this situation?

Dr. Butler: We have not done any work on the cyclic AMP-dependent phosphorylation of the light chain kinase, and I know of no reported effects of cGMP on this system. The majority of the work on phosphorylation of the light chain kinase comes from Dr. Adelstein's laboratory at the National Institutes of Health. The attractiveness of the hypothesis is that an increase in cyclic AMP would tend to result in relaxation, however, this could be overcome by an increase in the calcium concentration in the cell.

Dr. Berne: We were wondering about the role of cyclic AMP on the effect of adenosine because the brain slides of adenosine result in moderate increase in cyclic AMP in the tissue. Dr. Herley in our laboratory, using coronary arteries, was unable to show with physiological concentrations of adenosine any changes in cyclic AMP; only at pharmacologic levels.

Dr. Butler: The effects of adenosine may be mediated directly through changes in intracellular calcium levels. There is certainly a possibility that there is a regulatory system not dependent on calcium that could have a direct effect on the contractile proteins.

Dr. Berne: How do you explain the catch phenomenon?

Dr. Butler: The classical catch muscle is the anterior byssus retractor muscle (ABRM) of *Mytilus edulis*. This muscle has a very high economy of force maintenance. Its crossbridge cycle must be very slow. I consider this muscle to be simply a part of a continuum of crossbridge cycle rates between mammalian smooth and striated muscle. The ABRM and mammalian smooth muscles seem to have a mechanism by which they can vary crossbridge cycle rates under almost identical mechanical conditions.

Dr. Berne: Dr. Cox, have you studied small versus large coronary arteries in the aspect of the various mechanical components that you had mentioned?

Dr. Cox: No. I don't know of anyone who has done any direct mechanical studies on small coronary arteries other than those we have talked about. Bohr and Archida, about 10–15 years ago, isolated small branches of coronary arteries from the heart. But I don't know anyone who has really done any kind of direct extensive studies of mechanics of such vessels.

Dr. Berne: When you did your studies on the actin and myosin content of smooth muscle, did you isolate the smooth muscle from the rest of the vessel wall? Gary Owens from Seattle just recently did a seminar up at our place and, if I remember correctly, in these spontaneously hypertensive rats, he didn't find a difference in the actin/myosin ratio as opposed to controls.

Dr. Cox: Well, as a matter of fact, I just talked to him in Atlanta where he presented information on hypertrophy of smooth muscle cells. In our conversation he indicated that he found an elevated actin content but he did not study myosin. He found this in all types of hypertension, experimental as well as spontaneous. Further, he definitely said that actin was elevated in proportion to the increase in cell volume so that the amount of actin per unit cell volume was unchanged.

Dr. Aiken: In the first cross-sectional picture you showed of an artery, the internal elastic lamina looked very similar to a coiled spring. Could you expand? And at what pressure does the artery get fully extended?

Dr. Cox: Yes. That particular slide was made from a specimen that was not pressure fixed. That is, it was fixed at 0 mm Hg. At physiological pressures, the internal elastic lamina is straight. It is not curved and undulated as shown in the slide. That is a characteristic of a collapsed artery.

Dr. Winbury: You showed a slide on the relation of the diameter of the vessels. Now, I am thinking in very simple terms. Was it normalized? Because I am thinking in terms of the smaller diameter versus a larger diameter and how it affects resistance. Furthermore, how does the waterfall phenomenon fit in with some of these concepts?

Dr. Cox: Yes, it was normalized. It was normalized by dividing by the resting diameter in order to allow for the differences in different arterial sites. In vitro, of course, there is no waterfall, so I am not sure if I can really answer that question.

Dr. Wolf: Dr. Cox, you mentioned that you looked at hypertensive and aging arteries. Have you looked at atherosclerotic arteries? And, although it is an intimal process, is there any difference in the smooth muscles and how they respond to active contraction?

Dr. Cox: Yes, as a matter of fact, we did a series of experiments in collaboration with Dr. David Detweiler at the Vet School in which we restudied experimental hyperlipemia in the racing greyhound. There was a reduction in the maximal values of active force development, which suggests that there must have been some kind of degenerative process. This particular animal was unusual in that the kind of lesion that we found with hyperlipemia was not a medial lesion but an intimal one. The size of the intima in some of these affected segments was as large as the medial thickness and we couldn't tell whether this enlarged intima was simply interfering with the contractile response of the medial smooth muscle, or if in fact there had been a change in the smooth muscle per se. It was just an entirely different structure. It is like turning an artery inside out, with the adventitia inside, but I can't really answer that question. From the mechanical point of view there is a big difference in this experimental model of "atherosclerosis."

Unidentified: Your slides show that the different properties in passive stress-strain curves occurring from the different arteries were related to recruitment of collagen. I was wondering if you had repeated any of those experiments or generated the curves after treating the vessel with collagenase or elastase.

Dr. Cox: Yes, I did. The effects of collagenase are surprisingly small. You can remove about 50% of collagen from the wall and produce only a fairly small effect. So you can't completely explain it by simply a shift up and down the curve based on the relative amount of collagen. Obviously, what you have done is interfere in some way with the interconnection between collagen and elastin, which is an important determinant of mechanics and which really wasn't incorporated in the simplistic model. So, the next level of complexity would be to incorporate interactions between the elements of the connective tissue matrix, which certainly is an order of magnitude or more in complexity.

Dr. Dillon: Dr. Butler showed a calcium dependency. Dr. Cox, were the passive strain characteristics you measured varied with the level of calcium in your bath?

Dr. Cox: That is an interesting question. I was going to say no, but I am not so sure now. I used to be sure that it didn't have any effect. When I first started doing this kind of experiment, I employed chemical factors to relax the muscle, like papaverine and inhibitors of metabolism like cyanide, and iodoacetate. One means of inhibition that is used quite a bit now is a zero calcium with EDTA solution to chelate all the calcium out of the bath to inhibit the smooth muscle. The changes that I have seen in some cases suggest to me that something may be going on, other than simply related to the smooth muscle component. The answer to your question is that maybe there is an effect of calcium on passive mechanics.

Dr. Dillon: When I was working with Dick Murphy in Charlottesville, we found that the shortening velocity varied with the time of the stimulation. You showed some substantial changes in the isobaric shortening rates. I was wondering how long the tissue was stimulated before you did those experiments and whether you could see any variation due to the thickness of the tissue, because when you use potassium you can have different activations of the tissue.

Dr. Cox: Well, they weren't shortening rates; they were shortening extents. In fact, there is a correlation. Arterial smooth muscles, which shorten to a greater extent, also seem to shorten more rapidly. This doesn't relate to thickness because the renal artery, which is fairly thick compared to the coronary artery, exhibits this sort of behavior. I don't think diffusion of potassium is the answer to these differences. I think it is an intrinsic characteristic of the ATPase.

Dr. Nanarday: Is there any relationship between the diameter of the coronary arteries and to their responsiveness to the sympathetic stimulation? My question is specifically for the people who work in nitroglycerin factories. When they go back home they have a myocardial infarction. This is due to the increased sensitivity.

Dr. Cox: I think you are talking about acute versus chronic effects. I don't think I can answer that. As far as the acute effect is concerned, there is a difference in diameter. However, there is a pressure dependence that is related to the characteristics of smooth muscle and the degree of overlap between thick and thin filaments. That determines the total shortening capacity. In terms of a long term chronic effect, I don't think that there is any information that could answer that kind of question.

Dr. Walinsky: Dr. Cox, in the pressure range that we will be dealing with clinically, that is, a distal coronary pressure of approximately 89–90 during systole down to 20–40 during diastole, what difference in diameter sizes were you demonstrating there in terms of millimeters?

Dr. Cox: Well, the sizes that I demonstrated were from 3–2 mm; this of course is in a dog. With activation, do you mean?

Dr. Walinsky: Well, with regard to passive changes, what would the difference in diameter be, say, with an intraluminal pressure ranging from 80 going down to 40 mm Hg?

Dr. Cox: Well, it could certainly be 1½–2 mm. Of course, you would have to scale that up for a human patient.

Dr. Wiedeman: Dr. Berne, has there been any comparison between the increase in coronary blood flow when using a vasodilator (a direct vasodilator) and when using an alpha-adrenergic blocker? Is there a difference between the degree of increase in blood flow?

Dr. Berne: If you administer an alpha-adrenergic receptor blocker, under basal conditions, the increase is relatively small. In contrast, a vasodilator such as adenosine elicits a large increase in coronary blood flow and the response is dose-dependent. The vasodilator dose range of adenosine is about 10^{-8}–10^{-4} M with the greatest inflection of the dose-response curve at 10^{-6} M, a physiological concentration. At 10^{-4} M, the vessels become maximally dilated.

Dr. Bentavoglio: Can you comment on the mechanism of action of dipyridamole as a coronary vasodilator?

Dr. Berne: Dipyridamole is a very potent coronary dilator and works by preventing the destruction of adenosine. Adenosine uptake by cultured cardiac cells is inhibited by dipyridamole, but its release is not. Because interstitial fluid does not contain enzymes that metabolize (inactive) adenosine, the concentration of the nucleoside increases, and hence, produces greater coronary dilation.

Dr. Aiken: You commented on dipyridamole and how it affects the transport of adenosine and therefore produces vaodilation. What about the adenosine deaminase to which you referred? Does that enzyme have an affect on vascular resistance?

Dr. Berne: That is a good point. The problem with adenosine deaminase is that it is such a large molecule that it cannot reach the interstitial space where it can deaminate adenosine to inactive inosine. Recently, there have been some studies of low molecular weight active subunits of adenosine deaminase that can cross the capillary membrane and attenuate reactive hyperemia in the heart (Olsson, personal communication) and block hypoxia-induced dilation of the pial vessels of the brain (Kontos and Wei, 1981, Fed Proc 40:454).

Dr. Gould: If you look at the A-V differences in oxygen across the vascular bed during reactive hyperemia, the A-V differences narrow rather dramatically, indicating that there is plenty of oxygen available to the myocardium and that myocardial pO_2 has gone up as well. And yet, the reactive hyperemia persists for some period of time. If adenosine is the oxygen-stimulated mediator, how do we explain the fact that flow persists at very high levels far longer and higher than the oxygen demands would indicate? Could you explain that?

Dr. Berne: Although low tissue pO_2 results in enhanced adenosine formation, this is not the only mechanism involved in adenosine production. Increased metabolic activity of the heart without impairment of oxygen supply also elicits greater adenosine release from the parenchymal tissue. For example, the experiments I showed in which cardiac work was increased by exercise, excitement or feeding in the unanesthetized normal dog produced marked increases in coronary blood flow and in adenosine release from the heart without changes in the coronary venous blood oxygen levels. Hence, there is ample oxygen available and we believe that adenosine release is linked to cardiac metabolic activity and not only to oxygen availability. In vivo, 5'-nucleotidase is inhibited (it is 100 times more active in the test tube than in intact tissue) by ATP, ADP and phosphocreatine. On the basis of in vitro studies, we believe, that with increased cardiac activity, ATP and ADP do not undergo detectable changes in concentration but phosphocreatine decreases, which leads to some disinhibition of 5'-nucleotidase. In addition, there may be release of magnesium (chelated to ATP), which can strongly reverse the phosphocreatine inhibition of 5'-nucleotidase. Finally, some increase in AMP (substrate for 5'-nucleotidase) can occur, and hense these three mechanisms, decreased phosphocreatine, increased free magnesium and increased AMP, may act in concert to disinhibit 5'-nucleotidase and lead to enhanced adenosine production.

Dr. Gould: I am wondering why adenosine did not decrease reactive hyperemia more than 40%. Could you elucidate the argument a little bit?
Dr. Berne: Certainly. I do not claim that adenosine is the sole mediator of vasodilation in active or reactive hyperemia. As you may recall from the slide depicting Dr. Olsson's data on reactive hyperemia, there was good correlation between the duration of reactive hyperemia, the magnitude of the postocclusion blood flow and the concentration of adenosine in the tissues. However, factors other than adenosine are certainly operating in the regulation of coronary blood flow based on the observation that only about 40% of the reactive hyperemia can be abolished by adenosine deaminase. As I mentioned earlier, there are problems with the deaminase experiments. The enzyme is a large molecule and even the smaller subunits may not reach all of the interstitial fluid in concentrations high enough to inactivate all of the released adenosine. To what extent other factors, such as potassium, hydrogen ion and a myogenic mechanism, contribute remains to be determined.
Unidentified: Dr. Berne, it would be logical that adenosine would be produced in a ratio somewhat similar to the metabolic demands of the tissue. Have you found in isolated strips that the adenosine ratio is higher at the beginning and falls off later along the lines of the metabolic changes measured by Dr. Butler?
Dr. Berne: In isolated strips of vascular smooth muscle, the adenosine concentration is quite low, and its release could only be demonstrated during hypoxia by isotope dilution techniques. Furthermore, just on a quantitative basis alone, there is not enough adenosine precursor in vascular smooth muscle to account for the amounts released during an inadequate oxygen supply or increased cardiac metabolic activity.
Dr. Euler: Dr. Berne, adenosine is rapidly metabolized in the bloodstream. Of course, that has been one of the problems with collecting it and measuring it. Some recent data by Dr. Carl Jones' lab in Texas has indicated that the adenosine metabolite, inosine, is a potent coronary vasodilator. Would you comment on that?
Dr. Berne: We have looked at a possible role for inosine as a mediator of vasodilation, as have a number of other investigators. We find that only in huge concentrations does inosine induce vasodilation, and this may be due to contamination of inosine with small amounts of adenosine.
Dr. Wendling: Dr. Berne, how does adenosine act on vascular smooth muscle to produce relaxation? Does it act mainly on cyclic AMP or possibly on a calcium pool? Why are larger concentrations of adenosine required to produce an increase in cyclic AMP in vascular smooth muscle than are required to produce relaxation of this tissue?
Dr. Berne: I do not think it is cyclic AMP because in vitro it requires pharmacological doses of adenosine to elevate cyclic AMP in strips of vascular smooth muscle. Primarily, on indirect evidence, we believe that

adenosine interferes with calcium uptake or its accessibility to the contractile machinery. In isolated atria with the sodium channels blocked by partial potassium depolarization or by tetrodotoxin, and with the tissue stimulated in the presence of norepinephrine, a typical calcium inward current is produced; this response can be abolished by adenosine and restored by the addition of adenosine deaminase. Furthermore, the contractions, produced by caffeine in skeletal muscle by releasing calcium, can be markedly attenuated by the addition of adenosine. We tried to demonstrate a direct effect by studying ^{45}Ca fluxes in cultured vascular smooth muscle cells and vascular strips without much success. So far, only the uptake of Ca^{2+} that is enhanced by high potassium can be reversed by adenosine.

Section II

Drug Effects on Coronary Vessels

Martin M. Winbury, *Chairperson*

Proximal and Distal Coronary Arteries

Martin M. Winbury

Introduction

This presentation will consider the differences between the function and the response of the large coronary arteries and the smaller resistance vessels. With the development of potent coronary dilators such as dipyridamole and the use of cineangiography over the past several decades, the differences between the two types of coronary vessels have been appreciated.

Nitroglycerin, the standard antianginal agent, does not have a marked effect on the rate of coronary blood flow in animals or man, but does produce a distinct widening of the large epicardial arteries, which can be visualized by cineangiographic techniques. On the other hand, dipyridamole, which produces a marked increase in the rate of coronary blood flow, has little effect on the large coronary vessels. Accordingly, it was recognized that there are major differences in the response of the large arteries and the arterial resistance vessels. Various studies that have emphasized these differences and show the relative importance of the large vessels particularly in the response to drugs and under disease circumstances are described below.

The large coronary arteries (proximal) have as their primary function the conducting and distributing of blood flow throughout the wall of the myocardium. This is a low resistance system, which normally is not involved in blood flow regulation. There is some vasomotion but certainly not to the same extent as the resistance vessels. Under normal circumstances the vasomotion of the large vessels is of minor significance. However, under disease states, this vasomotion can produce significant changes in blood flow, for example during spasm, and can be influenced by drugs. The small resistance vessels, primarily arterioles, are involved in regional blood flow regulation. These arterioles (distal) exert fine regulation of blood flow through the process of autoregulation. Finally, there are the precapillary sphincters, which are involved in the nutrient circulation via the capillaries and which govern the exchange between the blood and the tissues.

Distribution Through Left Ventricular Wall

The anatomy through the left ventricular wall illustrates well the function of the small and large arterial vessels (Fig. 1). There are the large superficial epicardial vessels, the conductive and penetrating vessels and the collateral vessels, which may or may not be present under normal circumstances. The conductive or penetrating vessels have as their function the blood flow distribution throughout the left ventricular wall (epicardium and endocardium). The collateral vessels permits retrograde blood flow between a normal region and a region made ischemic as a result of an occlusion in the large superficial epicardial artery.

When obstructive atherosclerotic plaques develop in the large superficial arteries, the region distal to the stenosis responds by relaxation of the arterioles in order to maintain blood flow as illustrated in Figure 2. But at a certain point the vasodilator reserve of the region is exhausted, and blood flow is then dependent upon the resistance of the large vessel stenosis. Normally, the reserve of the deeper endocardial region is lower than that of the more superficial epicardial region. Furthermore, open capillary density is greater in the deeper region than in the more superficial region. Accordingly, arteriolar reserve capacity and capillary reserve capacity is lower in the deeper endocardial regions.

The effect of stenosis on the response to nitrates and potent vasodilator drugs is illustrated schematically in Figure 2 (Lichtlen et al., 1974). The poststenotic region, A, has a lower oxygen tension (pO_2) than the normal region, B, as a result of a deficiency in blood flow, Q_4. Autoregulation produces compensatory arteriolar vasodilation; thus R_4 is lower than R_3. The collateral vessel between Regions B and A permits blood flow, Q_C, to supplement that which passes through the stenosis. The blood supply to Region A is adequate under basal conditions, but when there is stress and a greater amount of blood flow is required there is an insufficiency in Region A.

Nitrates, illustrated in the middle panel, produce a widening of the large vessels and the collaterals with an improvement of blood flow (Q_4) to Region A as a result of increased blood flow through the collateral, Q_C, and possibly increased flow through the stenosed vessel (see Chapters 10 and 12). Total regional flow remains unchanged or may decrease slightly. Because of the

Proximal and Distal Coronary Arteries   65

Fig. 1. Blood supply through the left ventricular wall. The superficial and penetrating arteries are large arteries and serve to distribute the blood flow to the epicardial (A) and endocardial (B) regions. The collateral vessels permit blood flow between Regions I and II if there is a block in the superficial epicardial artery. These are all part of the large artery system. The microcirculation in the insert shows the arteriolar and capillary circulation. Arteriolar tone is lower and open capillary dimensions greater in the endocardium (B) than in the epicardium (A). Thus endocardial vasodilator reserve and open capillary reserve are more limited than epicardium.

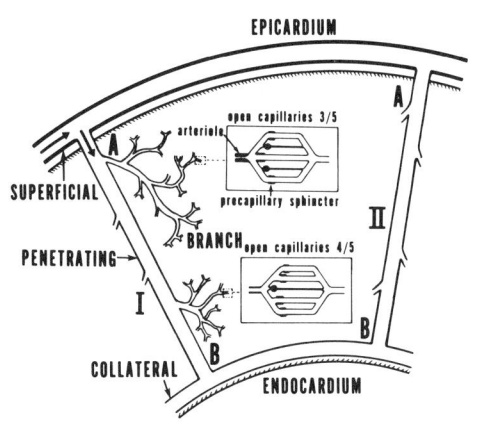

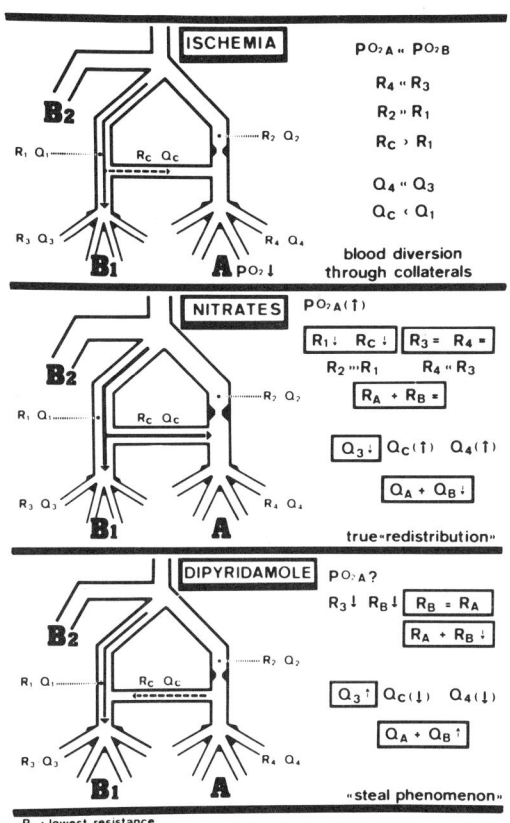

Fig. 2. Schematic diagram of effect of nitrate and dipyridamole on normal (B) and ischemic (A) region. Regional tissue blood flow (Q_4) and oxygen tension (pO_2) are lower in Region A because of the stenosis (R_2). Normally collateral blood flood (Q_c) goes from Region B to Region A because R_4 is less than R_3, but with dipyridamole this is not the case due to a marked decrease in R_3. The resistance of the normal large artery is represented by R_1.

improved balance between supply and demand in Region A the pO_2 is elevated. This is known as "redistribution" of blood flow to the ischemic region.

Dipyridamole, a highly effective coronary dilator, produces the primary effect on the resistance vessels of Region B_1. Thus, R_3 is diminished and Q_3 increases markedly. This occurs at the expense of circulation to Region A, which means that Q_4 and Q_C are markedly decreased. This is known as "coronary steal" or inappropriate blood flow distribution. Additionally, dipyridamole may reduce the luminal area by the stenosis, thereby causing an increased severity of the stenosis and conceivably a decrease in Q_2 (see Chapters 10 and 12).

This comparison of the nitrates and dipyridamole illustrates on a theoretical basis the difference between agents that cause relaxation of the tone of the large vessels and collaterals and those that produce arteriolar dilation.

Physiological and Biochemical Characteristics

The basic physiological and biochemical characteristics of the large and small vessels are given in Table 1. There are fundamental differences that are related to function, namely, that the large vessels are conducting vessels concerned with blood flow distribution, whereas the arterioles are resistance vessels and concerned with blood flow rate. Some of these functions are inherent to the blood vessel per se and others to the surrounding tissue. Although the small

Table 1. Physiological and Biochemical Characteristics.

Characteristic	Large	Small
Autoregulation	No	Yes
Reactive Hyperemia	Slight Constriction	Dilation
Ischemia	Constriction	Dilation
Passive Distension	Yes	Yes then Autoregulation
Total Resistance (%)	5–20	95–80
Adenosine	Constriction	Dilation
Hypoxia	No △	Dilation
KCN	No △	Dilation
Mitochondria	10/unit	23/unit
Succinic Dehydrogenase Activity	1	2.6

vessels are more sensitive to hypoxia than the large vessels in vitro, autoregulation is probably associated with tissue metabolism and oxygen tension with release of adenosine from the tissues into the extracellular fluid surrounding the arterioles. We can now discuss in more detail some of these properties.

Autoregulation permits blood flow to be maintained at a level consistent with regional tissue requirements. As increase in metabolism is accompanied by a like increase in the rate of blood flow. When coronary perfusion pressure is diminished, arteriolar resistance decreases to maintain a constant blood flow over the physiological pressure range. This is also an example of autoregulation. However, the large vessels show an increase in resistance as perfusion pressure is decreased; this is an example of passive distensibility. When there is an abrupt increase or decrease in perfusion pressure the large vessels and small vessels show an initial passive distensibility change, but in the small vessels this is followed by autoregulation (Winbury et al., 1969). Thus, during ischemia there is vasodilation of arterioles but an increase in resistance of the large vessels.

During reactive hyperemia immediately after coronary occlusion, the arterioles are markedly dilated and blood flow is increased three to four fold, whereas the resistance of the large vessels is increased slightly.

Under basal conditions the resistance of the large superficial vessels in the dog heart accounts for approximately 5% of the total resistance. However, during maximal arteriolar dilation resulting from administration of potent coronary dilators or during reactive hyperemia when blood flow is increased severalfold, the large vessels can account for as much as 20–25% of the total resistance. Under these circumstances, changes in the resistance of the large vessels can influence blood flow because the small vessels are maximally dilated.

The response to hypoxia has been studied in the intact animal, the fibrillating heart and large and small isolated coronary arteries (Kamitani et al., 1977). Hypoxia was produced by having the animal respired with less than 20% oxygen, perfusing the tissue with blood or salt solution at a lower oxygen tension or using a bath medium at a lower oxygen tension. All of these conditions produced vasodilation or a reduction in tone of the smaller vessels with little or no change in tone of the larger vessels. A similar change was observed when the isolated fibrillating heart was perfused with a solution containing KCN, which produces cytotoxic anoxia. These changes are consistent with the response to adenosine in the intact animal, namely, a marked decrease in total or small vessel resistance with no change or an increase in resistance of the larger vessels. Isolated coronary arteries show a greater sensitivity to adenosine for vessels <0.5 mm in diameter compared with those 2 mm in diameter.

Table 2. Effects of Coronary Drugs.

Coronary Drugs			RL and RT (5 min)		
	ABP	Q	RL	RT	RL/RT
TNG	0	0	−	+	−
DIP	−	+++	+	−−−	+++
PAP	0	+	+	−	+
CHR	0	+++	++	−−−	+++
PREN	−	++	+	−	+
LIDO	−	+	+	−	++
VER	−	+	+	−	++
NIF	−	++	0+	−−	++
AMINO	−	+	+	−	+

Key: TNG, nitroglycerin; DIP, dipyridamole; PAP, papaverine; CHR, chromonar; PREN, prenylamine; LIDO, lidoflazine; VER, verapamil; NIF, nifedipine; AMINO, aminophylline; ABP, blood pressure; Q, coronary blood flow; RL, large artery resistance; RT, total resistance; −, decrease; +, increase.

Variable Flow (Winbury et al., 1969). Similar pattern in fibrillating heart for TNG, DIP, PAP, PREN and VER (Kamitani et al., 1977).

Finally, there are the biochemical differences based on mitochondrial content, with a greater concentration in the small vessels and a higher succinic dehydrogenase activity in the small vessels (Kamitani et al., 1977). This leads to the conclusion that the small vessels are more sensitive to hypoxia and more aerobic dependent.

Segmental Coronary Effects

The differential response between large coronary arteries and small coronary arteries was studied in the intact animal by perfusion at aortic pressure and measuring blood flow, or at constant flow and measuring pressure changes (Cohen and Kirk, 1973; Fam and McGregor, 1968, Forman and Kirk, 1980; Takeda et al., 1977; Winbury et al., 1969). The pressure gradient was measured between the aorta and a 0.5-mm branch of the superficial coronary artery for *large* vessel resistance and the gradient between the aorta and right atrium for *total* resistance. In some cases *small* vessel resistance was based on the peripheral coronary pressure.

Coronary Drugs

Tables 2 and 3 summarize the findings on several drugs. Organic nitrates invariably produced a prolonged decrease in large vessel resistance and only a transient decrease in total or small vessel resistance. In the variable blood flow studies, nitroglycerin was injected intravenously (Table 1), and when perfusion pressure was permitted to fall total resistance showed an initial decline for approximately 30 sec and was then increased for as long as 10 min. Other agents that caused some decrease in large vessel resistance include isoproterenol and nitroprusside. However, with these two agents the effect was not selective or greater for the large vessels. Accordingly, when one considers the ratio of large vessel resistance/total resistance, the nitrates invariably produced a decrease, but the other two agents produced no change.

In contrast to the selective effect of the nitrates on large vessel resistance, other agents studied had the primary dilator action on small vessels, reducing total resistance or small vessel resistance. Included among these compounds were dipyridamole, papaverine, chromonar, prenylamine, lidoflazine, verapamil, nifedipine, aminophylline and perhexiline. This group of compounds is diversified in action and includes conventional vasodilators, calcium entry blockers, phosphodiesterase inhibitors, and inhibitors of adenosine uptake.

It has been well established that ergonovine produces spasm of the large coronary arteries in those patients with variant forms of angina pectoris. Yet ergonovine administered directly into the coronary artery produced no change in large vessel resistance (RL) and a small increase in total resistance, (RT) (Forman and Kirk, 1980). On the other hand, angiotensin caused a like increase in both large vessel and total resistance (Cohen and Kirk, 1973).

Table 3. Coronary Drugs on RL and RT.

Coronary drug	RL	RT
TNG	— —	—
NP	—	—
PER	0	—
VER	+	—
NIF	+	—
ERGO	0	+
ANGIO	++	++

Key: NP, nitroprusside; PER, perhexiline; ERGO, ergonovine; ANGIO, angiotensin; other abbreviations defined in footnote to Table 2.
Constant flow (Forman and Kirk, 1980; Cohen and Kirk, 1973.)

Adenosine Nitrates

A point of interest is the effect of adding nitrate groups to the ribose of adenosine. Adenosine and adenosine mononitrate, intravenously, produce a decrease in RT with no change in RL. In contrast, addition of two or three nitrates to adenosine results in activity on the large vessels similar to other organic nitrates. Thus, there is a shift from arteriolar dilator action to large vessel dilator action as the nitrate groups are added (Winbury et al., 1974).

Catecholamines and Sympathetic Stimulation

The effects of the catecholamines and sympathetic stimulation before and after beta-adrenoceptor blockade with propranolol was studied by Murthy et al. (1973). Before propranolol, isoproterenol reduced RL, but norepinephrine, epinephrine and sympathetic stimulation had variable effects. RT was consistently decreased and coronary blood flow elevated by all of these interventions. Propranolol blocked completely all of the effects of isoproterenol. After propranolol, norepinephrine, epinephrine and sympathetic stimulation produced an increase in RL and RT, probably associated with an unopposed alpha-adrenoceptor effect. The response to sympathetic stimulation after propranolol suggests that both the large and small vessels are innervated.

Beta-adrenoceptor blockade by propranolol increased the resistance of the large and small vessels having a greater effect on RT (Winbury et al., 1969). Thus, the ratio of RL/RT was diminished. Alpha-adrenoceptor blockade produced by phenoxybenzamine caused a decrease in resistance with a greater effect on RT producing an increase in the ratio of RL/RT (Malindzak et al., 1978). It would appear that adrenergic blockade has a greater effect on small vessels. However, because propranolol blocks both B_1 and B_2, it is not possible to determine if this is a direct effect or an indirect effect via the influence on myocardial contractility. The latter is probably more important. It seems unlikely that metabolism would affect the large vessel and under these circumstances one could conclude that there are both alpha- and beta-adrenoceptors present and that there is both alpha- and beta-background tone.

Ischemia on Response to Drugs

The effect of ischemia on the response to nitrates, adenosine and other drugs was studied at constant flow (Cohen and Kirk, 1973) or variable flow (Csik et al., 1976) intracoronary injections. Under both circumstances, the flow was diminished about 35% in one case by reducing the pump perfusion rate and in the other by producing a critical stenosis. In either case, reactive hyperemia was diminished to a considerable extent. The most significant point is that the selective large vessel vasodilator effect of the nitrates was unaffected during ischemia. The decrease in small vessel resistance (RS) produced by nitroglycerin, adenosine or dipyridamole was markedly attenuated or eliminated. In a similar study, maximal arteriolar dilation was produced by chromonar, which of itself produced a slight increase in RL. Under these circumstances, nitroglycerin was still able to produce a selective decrease in RL (Winbury et al., 1969). However, there was no decrease in RS with adenosine, nitroglycerin or reactive hyperemia, indicating that vasodilator reserve was exhausted.

Isolated Coronary Arteries

Comparison of the response of large (2-mm) and small (0.5-mm) canine coronary arteries in Table 4 established that the large arteries are more sensitive to the vasodilator action of nitrates than the smaller arteries. On the other hand, the small vessels are more sensitive to adenosine, chromonar and prenylamine. Papaverine, dipyridamole and verapamil produce equal effects on the large and small vessels (Kamitani et al., 1977; Schnaar and Sparks, 1972).

Table 4. Isolated Coronary Arteries and Coronary Drugs.

Coronary drug	Large (2 mm)	Small (0.5 mm)
TNG	---	--
PETRIN	---	--
NANO$_2$	---	--
AD	--	---
PAP	--	--
CHR	0	--
PREN	0	--
DIP	--	--
VER	---	---
PROP	---	---

Key: PETRIN, pentrinitrol; AD, adenosine; PROP, propranolol; other abbreviations defined in footnote to Table 2.
K^+ contraction (Schnaar and Sparks, 1972; Kamitani et al., 1977)

72 Section II Drug Effects on Coronary Vessels

Hypoxia induced by lowered oxygen tension in bath medium or by the addition of KCN caused relaxation of small vessels and had no effect on large vessels (Kamitani et al., 1977). It should be pointed out that it was necessary to produce K^+ depolarization of these isolated vessels in order to induce a tone, otherwise the vasodilator would not show an effect.

Action Potential of Isolated Coronary Arteries

The selective response of isolated coronary arteries of different sizes is also demonstrated for action potentials, induced by electrical stimulation of vessels treated with tetraethylammonium, in Table 5 from the studies of Harder et al., (1979). Nitroglycerin at a concentration of $10^{-5}\,M$ abolished the overshoot of large arteries but had no effect on small arteries. Adenosine, on the other hand, abolished the action potential of the small arteries at $10^{-5}\,M$ but was without effect on the large arteries. Finally, verapamil abolished the overshoot of both size vessels at $10^{-5}\,M$. Thus, it can be concluded that the large arteries are more sensitive to nitroglycerin, the small ones to adenosine, and that calcium is involved in the action potential. This tends to confirm the previous information from isolated coronary arteries or segmental resistance studies.

Large Coronary Artery Diameter

The diameter of the large coronary artery of the conscious dog was measured by means of an ultrasonic dimension gauge chronically implanted around the left circumflex coronary artery (Vatner et al., 1980). Total coronary resistance was calculated from arterial pressure and coronary blood flow.

Table 5. Action Potential of Isolated Coronary Arteries.

Coronary drug	Large (> 1.0 mm)	Small (< 0.5 mm)
TNG	Abolish 10^{-5}	No Effect 10^{-5}
AD	No Effect 10^{-4}	Abolish 10^{-5}
AD + DEAMIN		Recovery
VER	Abolish 10^{-5}	Abolish 10^{-5}

Key: TNG, nitroglycerin; AD, adenosine; DEAMIN, deaminase; VER, verapamil.

Methoxamine at a dose of 50 µg/kg/min induced a sustained reduction in the left circumflex cross-sectional area by 27% while arterial pressure increased by 65%. Mean coronary blood flow was unchanged. The calculated large vessel resistance increased by 108% and total coronary resistance by 92%. In contrast, nitroglycerin at a dose of 25 µg/kg induced a prolonged increase in large coronary diameter, reaching a maximum of 5 min after an initial transient decrease. Cross-sectional area of the left circumflex coronary artery increased 11%, and large vessel resistance was reduced by 18%. Total coronary resistance fell initially but was elevated by 11% at 5 min. It was concluded that the large vessels demonstrate passive distensibility changes initially but then show substantial active changes (Vatner et al., 1980). The alpha-adrenergic stimulation of methoxamine is sufficient to overcome the increased distending pressure and reduce diameter, and the vasodilation produced by nitroglycerin overcomes the passive reduction in diameter resulting from reduced perfusion pressure.

Nifedipine produced no significant change in large coronary diameter under basal conditions (Hintze et al., 1980a). However, if an increase in tone was produced by methoxamine, nifedipine then caused large coronary artery dilation (Hintze et al., 1980b). Total resistance was reduced by nifedipine under basal conditions as well as after vasoconstriction produced by methoxamine.

Isoproterenol increased left circumflex diameter by 17% and reduced total resistance by 42%. After cardioselective beta-adrenoceptor blockade with atenolol and maintaining constant heart rate, the changes produced by isoproterenol were +6 and −11%, respectively. Propranolol blocked completely the effects of isoproterenol. Both of these β-blocking agents caused a slight (7–8%) reduction in coronary diameter and slight (12–13%) increase in total coronary resistance (Macho and Vatner, 1981).

Acetylocholine increased left circumflex diameter by 20% and decreased total resistance by 62%. Atropine blocked all of these changes (Cox et al., 1981).

Left Coronary Spasm by K^+ Sephadex Gel

The previous studies by Vatner and co-workers demonstrated that methoxamine could produce a decrease in the diameter of the large coronary arteries of the conscious dog. On the other hand, other investigators reported that ergotamine, which can produce angiographic documented coronary spasm in patients with Prinzmetal's variant angina, was unable to produce any change in large coronary artery resistance (Forman and Kirk, 1980). Application of a Sephadex gel containing K^+ directly on the vessel produced a decrease in the diameter of the left circumflex coronary artery of 18–21% measured either cineangiographically or with ultrasonic gauges (Perez et al., 1980; 1981). Intracoronary artery infusion of norepinephrine, tyramine or serotonin, or electrical stimulation of the vessel or application of Na^+ gel, did not produce a marked reduction in diameter of the large coronary artery (Perez et al., 1980). This reduction in diameter produced by the K^+ containing gel was accompanied by a 38% reduction in coronary blood flow in the regions subserved by that vessel. Nitroglycerin partially reversed the decrease in diameter, whereas nifedipine or Bay K5552 produced complete reversal (Perez et al., 1981).

Role of Cholesterol and Atherosclerosis

A recent series of studies on isolated canine coronary arteries demonstrated that addition of cholesterol to the isolated organ bath at a concentration of 10^{-10} M produced an increase in tone (Yokoyama et al., 1978; Yokoyama and Henry, 1979a). LDL, but not VLDL, IDL, HDL or albumin, had a similar effect (Henry et al., 1978). This increase in tone produced by cholesterol or LDL was blocked by verapamil but not by propranolol, phentolamine or 6-OH dopamine (Henry et al., 1978; Yokoyama et al., 1978). Thus, the coronary construction is Ca^{2+} dependent, and adrenergic mechanisms are not critical. Other investigations by the same group (Yokoyama and Henry, 1979b) indicated that the immediate precursor of cholesterol, mevalonic acid, also produced contraction, but acetate had no effect. Mevalonate was incorporated into the arterial cholesterol but not into the acetate. Probucol or exogenous cholesterol prevented the mevalonic contraction or incorporation into the arterial steroid (Yokoyama and Henry, 1979b). It has been concluded that the cholesterol acquisition into the membrane affects the contractile properties of the vascular smooth muscle.

Cholesterol or LDL also sensitizes the isolated canine coronary artery to the constrictor effect of Ca^{2+} or ergonovine (Fisher et al., 1980a, b; Yokoyama and Henry, 1979a). Mevalonate also increases the sensitivity, and this is prevented by probucal.

In another study, rabbits were fed a cholesterol-containing diet to produce atherosclerosis (Henry and Yokoyama, 1980). The aortae from these atherosclerotic rabbits show supersensitivity to ergonovine and serotonin, but not to phenylephrine. Prazosin or phentolamine produces only partial blockage of ergonovine in the atherosclerotic aorta, and cyproheptadine blocks ergonovine to a greater extent in the atherosclerotic than in the control aorta. The combination of the prazosin and cyproheptadine block completely the response to ergonovine in the atherosclerotic aorta. Thus the supersensitivity to ergonovine is predominantely serotoninergic, but alpha-adrenergic mechanisms are involved to some extent.

This last group of studies indicates another effect of the deposition of cholesterol in the vessel wall. Not only is there the development of atherosclerotic plaques and the production of vessel stenosis, but there is increased sensitivity to vasoconstrictor agents.

This may be of significance in explanation of the coronary spasm produced by ergonovine in some but not all of the coronary patients.

Summary

The large coronary arteries respond differently to various drugs and physiological interventions than the small coronary arteries typified by arterioles. The large arteries are selectively dilated by organic nitrates in vivo while the arterioles are dilated by a number of vasodilators that have little effect on the large vessels. The small arteries and arterioles are selectively dilated during ischemia and hypoxia and are involved in coronary autoregulation. Blood flow regulation normally is controlled by the arterioles but during maximal arteriolar dilation the larger vessels may contribute as much as 25% to total resistance and participate in blood flow control.

The exquisite sensitivity of the large vessels to organic nitrate has been demonstrated not only by the selective vasodilation in vivo and in vitro but by abolition of the action potential of the large but not small isolated coronary artery. Adenosine has a more selective effect on small coronary arteries.

Cholesterol and the immediate precursor mevalonate increase the tone of large isolated coronary arteries. This is associated with the LDL fraction of the lipoproteins. Contractions induced by Ca^{2+} or K^+ are enhanced by cholesterol, mevalonate or LDL. Probucol blocks the response to mevalonate and mevalonate's incorporation into arterial cholesterol. Atheroscerlotic rabbit aortae have increased sensitivity to ergonovine as compared to normal aortae.

References

Cohen, M. V. and Kirk, E. S. 1973. Differential response of large and small coronary arteries to nitroglycerin and angiotensin. Circ Res 33:445–453

Cox, D., Hintze, T. and Vatner, S.F. 1981. Effects of acetylcholamine on large coronary vessels in conscious dogs. Fed Proc 40:707

Csik, V., Szekeres, L. and Udvary, E. 1976. Drug induced augmentation of coronary flow in vessels with maximum ischemic dilation. Arch Int Pharmacodyn Ther 224:66–76

Fam, W. M. and McGregor, M. 1968. Effect of nitroglycerin and dipyridamole on regional coronary resistance. Circ Res 649–659

Fisher, S., Lucas, C. and Henry, P. D. 1980a. Increased sensitivity to isolated canine coronary arteries to ergonovine after exposure to mevalonate. Clin Res 28:235

Fisher, S., Lucas, C. and Henry, P. D. 1980b. Increased sensitivity of isolated canine coronary arteries to Ca^{++} after stimulation of sterol synthesis in vitro. Clin Res 28:169.

Forman, R. and Kirk, E. S. 1980. Comparative effects of vasodilator drugs on large and small coronary resistance vessels in the dog. Cardiovasc Res 14:601–605

Harder, D. R., Belardinelli, L., Sperelakis, N., Rubio, R. and Berne, R. M. 1979. Differential effects of adenosine and nitroglycerin on the action potentials of large and small coronary arteries. Circ Res 44:176–182

Henry, P. D., Witztum, J. L. and Yokoyama, M. 1978. Vasoconstrictor effect of low density lipoprotein on canine coronary artery. Circulation 58:78

Henry, P. D. and Yokoyama, M. 1980. Supersensitivity of atherosclerotic rabbit aorta to ergonovine mediation by a serotonergic mechanism. J Clin Invest 66:306–313

Hintze, T. H., Macho, P. and Vatner, S. F. 1980a. Effects of nifedipine on large and small coronary blood vessels in conscious dogs. Clin Res 28:613

Hintze, T., Macho, P. and Vatner, S. F. 1980b. Effects of nifedine on large and small coronary vessels in the presence and absence of coronary vasoconstriction in conscious dogs. Circulation 62:III-253

Kamitani, T., Nakano, K., Mori, J., Katsuki, S. and Honda, F. 1977. Local specificity in responses of canine coronary vessels to oxygen deficiency and antianginal drugs. Arch Int Pharmacodyn Ther 225:257–274

Lichtlen, P., Halter, J. and Gattiker, K. 1974. The effect of isosorbidinitrate on coronary flow, coronary resistance, and left ventricular resistance in patients with coronary artery disease. Basic Res Cardiol 69:402–421

Macho, P. and Vatner, S. F. 1981. Beta adrenergic control of large coronary vessels in conscious dogs. Am J Cardiol 47:472

Malindzak, G. S. Jr., Kosinski, E. J., Green, H. D. and Yarborough, G. W. 1978. The effects of adrenergic stimulation on conductive and resistive segments of the coronary vascular bed. J Pharmacol Exp Ther 206:248–258

Murthy, V. S., Howe, B. B. and Winbury, M. M. 1973. Response of canine surface epicardial vessels to sympathetic stimulation. Pharmacologist 15:115

Perez, J. E., Lucas, C. and Henry P. D. 1980. Experimental coronary artery spasm in dogs; relief by nifedipine and nitroglycerin. Circulation 62:III-253

Perez, J. E., Lucas, C. and Henry, P. D. 1981. Experimental coronary artery spasm in intact dog; angiographic characterization, recording of flow, and response to dihydropyridines. Am J Cardiol 47:449

Schnaar, R. L. and Sparks, H. V. 1972. Response of large and small coronary arteries to nitroglycerine, $NaNO_2$, and adenosine. Am J Physiol 223:223–228

Takeda, K., Nakagawa, Y., Katano, Y. and Imai, S. 1977. Effects of coronary vasodilators on large and small coronary arteries of dogs. Jpn Heart J 18:92–101

Vatner, S. F., Pagani, M., Manders, W. T. and Pasipoularides, A. D. 1980. Alpha adrenergic vasoconstriction and nitroglycerin vasodilation of large coronary arteries in the conscious dog. J Clin Invest 65:5–14

Winbury, M. M., Howe, B. W. and Hefner, M. A. 1969. Effect of nitrates and other coronary dilators on large and small coronary vessels: An hypothesis for the mechanism of action of nitrates. J. Pharmacol Exp Ther 168:70–95

Winbury, M. M., Wilkes, S. B. and Howe, B. B. 1974. Myocardial and coronary actions of adenosine and adenosine nitrates. J Carbohydrates Nucleosides Nucleotides 1:369–373

Yokoyama, M., Witztum, J. L. Sobel, B. E. and Henry, P. D. 1978. Direct vasoconstrictor effects of cholesterol on canine arteries. Clin Res 26:280

Yokoyama, M. and Henry P.D. 1979a. Sensitization of isolated canine coronary arteries to calcium ions after exposure to cholesterol. Circ Res 45:479–486

Yokoyama, M. and Henry, P. D. 1979b. Coronary contraction mediated by stimulation of the biosynthesis of sterol in vitro. Clin Res 27:217A.

Blood-Blood Vessel Wall Interaction

James W. Aiken

Introduction

The inner surface of the blood vessel wall is repeatedly exposed to a battery of procoagulant substances and activated platelets yet because of its nonthrombogenic properties, the endothelium maintains blood flow even under some severe pathological conditions. The endothelial cell surface repels platelets by electrostatic forces, contains enzymes that may either form anticoagulant substances such as heparin or destroy (or bind) prothrombotic agents such as ADP and thrombin. Prostacyclin, the most potent inhibitor of platelet aggregation, is synthesized from arachidonic acid stored in the phospholipids of endothelial cells, and its formation can be induced by a variety of hormonal (thrombin, angiotensin) or mechanical (stretch) stimuli. Recently, a great deal of effort has gone into exploring the mode of action of protacyclin, its role in protecting against excessive intravascular platelet aggregation and the means to exploit this property of the blood vessel wall for therapeutic purposes.

When the endothelial surface of an artery is damaged, as it must occasionally be under normal conditions of blood flow and most certainly under pathological conditions, blood platelets adhere to the injured surface and release substances that initiate the normal repair process. The extent of the platelet thrombus formed can be influenced by many interacting factors. Ideally, the adjoining normal endothelium should limit adhesion and aggregation to the damaged region. However, in the narrowed lumen of an atherosclerotic vessel, where endothelium may be absent or lack some of its nonthrombogenic properties and where the stimulus for platelet aggregation is more severe because of abnormally high mechanical cell-to-surface interactions and shear forces, platelet aggregation and thrombus formation may result in occlusion of the vessel (Folts et al., 1976). Much is known about these interactions between platelets and the surfaces of cells grown in culture and platelet aggregation in vitro, but in vivo these interactions are difficult to study. Use of our knowledge of platelet function in vitro, however, has been a fruitful springboard for studying platelet-vessel wall interactions in vivo and, more specifically to this study, the role of endogenous prostacyclin in the control of coronary artery thrombosis.

Platelets aggregate in two phases. Primary aggregation, which can be initiated by chemical stimuli such as adenosine 5′-diphosphate (ADP),

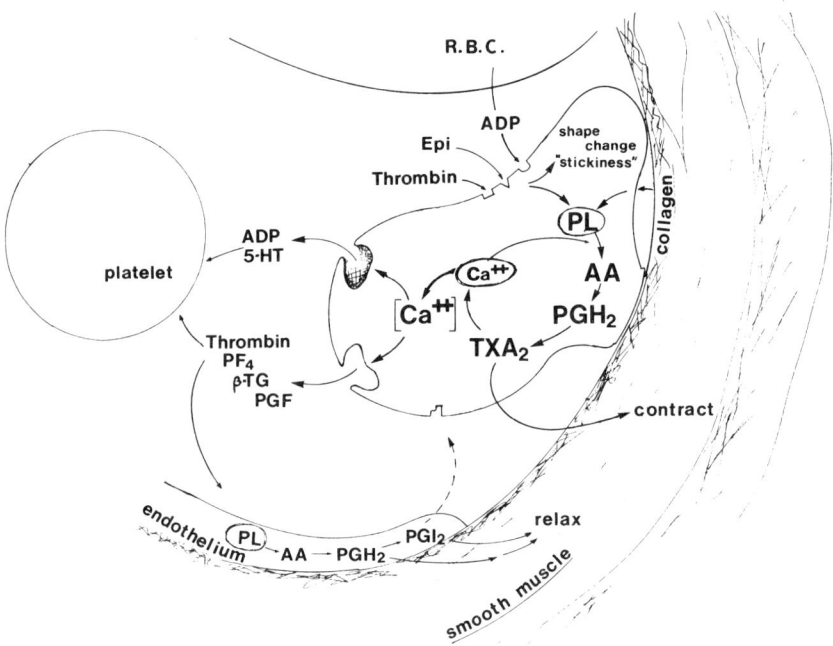

Fig. 1. Schematic representation of a platelet adhering to the exposed collagen surface of the vessel wall at a point where the endothelium has been lost. The picture illustrates the aggregatory response. Stimulation can occur via the collagen, ADP, epinephrine (epi) or thrombin-binding sites resulting in activation of phospholipases that free arachidonic acid (AA) from phospholipids (PL). Cyclooxygenase activity converts AA to PGH_2 and TXA_2 synthetase activity forms TXA_2, which stimulates Ca^{2+} release from storage sites, and perhaps also contraction of vascular smooth muscle. Increased cytoplasmic Ca^{2+} concentration causes further activation of phospholipase, release from the platelets of the contents of the dense granules (ADP and 5-hydroxytryptamine, 5-HT) and the alpha granules (thrombin, platelet factor 4, beta thromboglobulin, platelet growth factor and others). Released substances trigger many events including activation of other platelets causing aggregation, and stimulation of adjoining endothelium to make prostacyclin (PGI_2), which may cause vasodilation or prevent platelet thrombus from spreading.

thrombin or epinephrine, is followed by a secondary phase that involves the activation of thromboxane (TXA_2) synthesis in the platelet and the release of additional ADP and other factors from platelet storage granules (Fig. 1), resulting in recruitment of more platelets to aggregate. Only the secondary phase is prevented by substances that inhibit the formation of TXA_2 (Gorman et al., 1977) but both primary and secondary aggregation can be blocked by substances that elevate platelet adenosine 3′, 5′-cyclic monophosphate (cyclic AMP), such as adenosine or prostacyclin (Mills and Smith, 1971; Gorman, 1979). In vivo, the initial step may be adhesion of platelets to collagen exposed by damage to the endothelium (Fig. 1) but the relative contribution of each endogenous stimulatory or inhibitory substance to the control of intravascular platelet aggregation and thrombosis is difficult to evaluate. However, from an empirical point of view, certain in vivo models of experimental thrombosis can be used to demonstrate differences in efficacy between substances that inhibit only the second phase of aggregation and those, such as prostacyclin, that block both the primary and secondary phases. For example, in dogs with partially obstructed coronary arteries, complete blockage of the artery with platelet aggregates can be prevented more effectively with i.v. infusions of prostacyclin than with aspirin-like drugs that block platelet TXA_2 formation at the cyclooxygenase step (Aiken et al., 1979a; 1980).

Cyclooxygenase inhibitors prevent the synthesis of TXA_2 in platelets by blocking the conversion of arachidonic acid into the common prostaglandin (PG) endoperoxide intermediate, PGH_2. But, of course, the snythesis of prostacyclin, which likewise is formed in blood vessels from PGH_2 (Moncada et al., 1976), is also blocked by cyclooxygenase inhibitors (Fig. 1). Thus, using cyclooxygenase inhibitors to control thrombosis has the potential disadvantage of blocking not only the formation of the proaggregatory substance TXA_2 but also the antiaggregatory substance prostacyclin. Selective inhibition of the conversion of PGH_2 to TXA_2, without interfering with the formation of prostacyclin, might have some advantages over inhibition of the cyclooxygenase if, indeed, there is sufficient continuous basal prostacyclin production in vivo to exert a tonic antiaggregatory effect, or if inhibition of TXA_2 synthesis results in some amplification of the endogenous prostacyclin synthesis or activity. Certainly there is a "reciprocal regulation" of adenylate cyclase activity and platelet aggregation by TXA_2 and prostacyclin demonstrable in vitro (Gorman, 1979), and the removal of TXA_2 might, therefore, be expected to amplify in vivo the endogenous prostacyclin effects. Furthermore, one might expect that inhibition of the TXA_2 synthetase would shunt the prostaglandin precursor PGH_2 toward the formation of prostacyclin. This diversion of PHG_2 away from TXA_2 synthesis toward prostacyclin could occur either generally, throughout the circulation, or only locally at the site of a vascular lesion (the so-called "steal hypothesis;" see Bunting et al., 1976). One way to test these hypotheses is to compare the antiaggregatory efficacy of cyclooxygenase inhibitors and a selective TXA_2-synthesis inhibitor (Miyamoto et al., 1980) in an experimental model of platelet-dependent coronary artery thrombosis. This was done recently in our laboratory (Aiken et al., 1981) and the results indicated that TXA_2-synthesis inhibition is distinguishable from and more effective than cyclooxygenase inhibition for preventing coronary arterial thrombosis. Furthermore, defining the mode of action of a TXA_2 synthetase inhibitor gave us some insight into blood-blood vessel wall interactions.

Methods and Materials

Adult mongrel dogs (25–35 kg) of either sex were anesthetized with 35 mg/kg of sodium pentobarbital. The circumflex coronary artery was then dissected free from the surrounding myocardium for a distance of 20 mm, tying side branches when necessary. An electromagnetic flow probe (Carolina Medical Electronics, King, NC) was placed on the proximal portion of the circumflex coronary artery; a snare ligature was placed on the distal end of the artery to determine zero flow and to produce reactive hyperemic responses by occluding the vessel for 20 sec. Phasic and mean aortic blood pressure were monitored via a catheter in the left carotid artery; the left cephalic vein was cannulated for administration of drugs. All parameters were recorded on a polygraph with curvilinear writing pens (Grass Model 7D, Quincy, MA).

Platelet Aggregation in the Dog Coronary Artery

To monitor platelet aggregation in vivo, a technique originally described by Folts and colleagues (1976) was used with some modifications (Aiken et al., 1979a and b). The circumflex coronary artery was partially obstructed with a plastic (Lexan) cylinder so that intravascular platelet aggregation could be monitored as a gradual reduction in blood flow as platelets occluded the narrowed lumen at the obstructed site. The vessel lumen was reduced 90–95% (Gallagher et al., 1978). In our experiments the initial level of obstruction reduced mean circumflex blood flow by 26 ± 7%. Under these conditions reactive hyperemia was abolished; any further reduction in lumen size at the site of the obstructive cylinder could be recorded as a reduction in blood flow.

With the plastic cyclinder in place around the artery, blood flow was not maintained but instead gradually declined over a 2—4 min period until the vessel was almost completely blocked. Sometimes flow was suddenly restored spontaneously but usually flow declined to zero. When flow approached zero, gentle sliding of the obstructor back and forth a few millimeters along the vessel restored coronary blood flow. This sequence of events, the gradual decline in blood flow followed by shaking the obstructor to restore flow, can be repeated for several hours. It was originally suggested by Folts et al. (1976) that the cyclical declines in blood flow were due to platelet adhesion and aggregation in the narrowed lumen. We have confirmed by electron microscopy that the vessel becomes plugged with platelets. There is substantial pharmacological evidence to support the conclusion that the stopping of blood flow is due to platelet aggregation because pharmacological prevention of the cyclical declines in blood flow correlates with inhibition of platelet aggregation but not with the vascular effects of the drugs (Aiken et al., 1979 a, b; Hemker et al., 1980). Because the cyclical declines in coronary blood flow appear to be a rather selective indicator of the adhesion and aggregation of platelets at the obstructed site, this technique behaves as in vivo assay for antiaggregatory substances (Hemker et al., 1980; Shebuski and Aiken, 1980).

One change from the original technique described by Folts et al. (1976) that has allowed quantitation of aggregation was obtaining a consistent rate of aggregation (as indicated by the slope of the decline in circumflex blood flow) that almost always proceeds to complete blockage of the artery. Hence, blood flow must be restored by shaking the platelet thrombus loose every 2–4 min. These conditions were obtained by intentionally damaging the vessel endothelium, simply by rolling the artery with forceps so that the endothelial surface rubbed against itself. Then the obstructor was positioned over the damaged site. Thus, when drug intervention changed the aggregability of the platelets there was a clear-cut change in the pattern of the cyclical declines in flow. To quantitate the effect of drugs administered in vivo on the cyclical declines in coronary blood flow, a rating system (0, 1, 2, and 3) was devised (Aiken and Shebuski, 1980). A rating of 0 indicates the drug had no effect on the rate of aggregation; a score of 1 indicates a flattening in the slope of the decline in flow, but flow still declined to 0; a score of 2 indicates the platelet aggregates are being shed spontaneously without having to manually dislodge them, and when aggregation has been completely blocked so that blood flow is maintained at a constant level a maximum rating of 3 is given. Blind evaluation by two different investigators gave better than 95% agreement.

Substances Used

The TXA_2-synthesis inhibitor used in this study was (E)-2-methyl-3 [4-(3-pyridinylmethyl)phenyl]-2-propenoic acid, sodium salt, synthesized at The Upjohn Company. The hydrochloride salt of this compound is OKY-1555, characterized by Miyamoto et al. (1980) as a selective thromboxane-synthesis inhibitor. Prostacyclin (PGI_2), aspirin and ibuprofen were also synthesized at

The Upjohn Company. Other substances used were: nitroglycerin (Eli Lilly, Indianapolis, IN), indomethacin (Merck, West Point, PA) and thrombin (3000 units/mg) (Sigma Chemical Co., St. Louis, MO).

Efficacy of Cyclooxygenase Inhibitors Compared to TXA_2 Synthetase Inhibitors

Intravenous injection of the TXA_2 synthetase inhibitor (MPPA) at 1 mg/kg caused an immediate inhibition of platelet aggregation, which was detected as a prevention of blockage of the partially obstructed coronary artery of the dog. This dose produced effects in vivo consistent with selective inhibition of TXA_2 synthesis. First, when MPPA blocked aggregation the vasodepressor effects of an i.v. injection of arachidonic acid, which has been shown in dogs to be due to the formation of prostacyclin (Mullane et al., 1979), was not blocked. This indicated, indirectly, that conversion of exogenous arachidonic acid to prostacyclin was not reduced by MPPA. Cyclooxygenase inhibitors (aspirin, ibuprofen or indomethacin) always completely blocked the vasodepressor effects of arachidonic acid. Second, when blood samples were drawn from the carotid artery and platelet-rich plasma was prepared and exposed to arachidonic acid in vitro, the generation of TXA_2-like activity was reduced by MPPA treatment with a concurrent increase in the formation of PGE_2-like activity. Again, indomethacin treatment blocked the formation of both the TXA_2 and the PGE_2-like activity formed in platelets exposed to arachidonic acid. These results in vivo were consistent with the original conclusion from in vitro studies by Miyamoto et al. (1980) that MPPA is a selective thromboxane-synthesis inhibitor. Furthermore, our data indicate that coronary artery thrombosis in the dog can be prevented with this thromboxane-synthesis inhibitor.

Inhibition of either the cyclooxygenase or TXA_2 synthetase would prevent formation of TXA_2 in platelets, and therefore block the second phase of platelet aggregation. However, in vivo there were some striking differences between the effects of cyclooxygenase inhibitors and those of MPPA. First, under the standardized obstruction used in these experiments, cyclooxygenase inhibitors prevented blockage of the coronary artery with platelet aggregates in only 50–58% of the dogs. This was observed with either aspirin at a low dose (2 mg/kg) or at a high dose (20 mg/kg) with ibuprofen (10 mg/kg) or indomethacin (2 mg/kg). In contrast, MPPA inhibited platelet aggregation in 36 out of 40 dogs. In this respect, the efficacy of MPPA (90%) resembled that of i.v. prostacyclin (97%).

The second difference observed between MPPA and cyclooxygenase inhibitors was that the effectiveness of cyclooxygenase inhibitors was dependent on the degree of obstruction of the coronary artery, whereas the efficacy of MPPA was independent of the degree of obstruction. After inhibition of aggregation with a cyclooxygenase inhibitor, either aspirin, indomethacin or ibuprofen, aggregation in the coronary artery could be restored by increasing the degree of obstruction. In previous studies with indomethacin and aspirin (Aiken et al., 1980) we demonstrated that, after restoring aggregation by increasing the level of obstruction, platelets from the dog, studied in vitro, were still incapable of forming any TXA_2-like material when exposed to arachidonic acid. In contrast to cyclooxygenase inhibitors, inhibition of platelet aggregation by MPPA prevented obstruction of the coronary artery in the dog in spite of repeated increases in the level of obstruction, even to the point that coronary flow was reduced to less than 5 ml/min. Thus, the effectiveness of the TXA_2 synthetase inhibitor appeared to be independent of the degree of obstruction. In this regard, the activity of MPPA again resembled that of i.v. infusions of prostacyclin, which were effective regardless of the degree of obstruction.

Efficacy of TXA_2 Synthetase Inhibitor Depends on Prostacyclin

The circumflex coronary artery was usually obstructed so that mean coronary blood flow was reduced by approximately 30%. However, by obstructing the artery further we could accentuate the differences in efficacy between a TXA_2

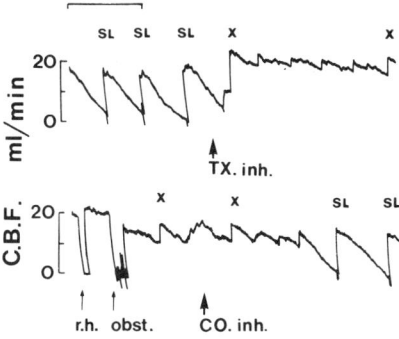

Fig. 2. Continuous record of circumflex blood flow (C.B.F.) in an anesthetized dog with a standard (see "Methods and Materials") partially obstructed circumflex coronary artery. Thrombi were shaken loose (SL) or came loose spontaneously (X) from the obstructed site causing periodic restorations in coronary blood flow. At the first arrow a TXA_2 synthetase inhibitor (TX inh.), MPPA 1 mg/kg, was given intravenously. At the next two arrows the reactive hypermia (r.h.) was checked and the degree of mechanical obstruction was increased by squeezing a silk thread into the lumen of the obstructor with the artery (obst.). Platelet aggregation could not be restored by increasing the degree of obstruction but was restored by giving a cyclooxygenase inhibitor (Co. inh.), ibuprofen (10 mg/kg), intravenously. The horizontal bracket at the top shows 5 min.

synthetase inhibitor and cyclooxygenase inhibitors. Figure 2 illustrates an experiment in which the initial degree of obstruction was greater than that usually used. The mean coronary flow after obstruction was reduced approximately 70% (60 ml/min before obstruction to about 18 ml/min after obstruction). Even under these conditions of severe obstruction, i.v. injection of MPPA blocked aggregation (Fig. 2, top). In those dogs with severely obstructed coronary arteries in which platelet aggregation has been prevented by MPPA, subsequent intravenous injection of a cyclooxygenase inhibitor actually produced a proaggregatory effect (Fig. 2, bottom). This reversal of the effects of MPPA could not have been due to MPPA's effects wearing off because subsequent injections of MPPA were no longer effective after cyclooxygenase inhibition, and pretreatment of severely obstructed animals with indomethacin prevented the effects of MPPA. Observations similar to the one illustrated in Figure 2 were made in 12 dogs with severely obstructed arteries in which either indomethacin, aspirin or ibuprofen was given after MPPA.

Reciprocal Control of Aggregation by TXA_2 and Prostacyclin

Previous experiments with cyclooxygenase inhibitors, of a nonquantitative nature, suggested that when platelets cannot make TXA_2 an enhanced sensitivity to prostacyclin would occur (Aiken et al., 1980). Therefore, experiments were designed to quantitate the change in sensitivity to prostacyclin that might occur in vivo in platelets that could not synthesize TXA_2. Such an experiment could not readily be done using MPPA to block TXA_2 synthesis because no aggregation was detectable in vivo after MPPA (except under special conditions reported below). But, by restoring aggregation after cyclooxygenase inhibition by increasing the level of obstruction, it was possible to assess the antiaggregatory activity of exogenous prostacyclin in vivo before and after blocking platelet TXA_2 synthesis with a cyclooxygenase inhibitor. When this was done, there was a striking increase in the sensitivity of platelets to prostacyclin. Before ibuprofen an antiaggregatory score of 2 to 3 (see "Methods and Materials") was obtained with a prostacyclin infusion rate of about 60 ng/kg/min. After ibuprofen only 2.5 ng/kg/min of prostacyclin was required to achieve complete inhibition. This was equivalent to about a 30-fold increase in sensitivity to prostacyclin. Similar results were obtained using either aspirin (10 mg/kg, i.v.) or indomethacin (2 mg/kg, i.v.). Interestingly, there was no enhancement of the depressor activity of prostacyclin in these experiments.

Platelet Provides Precursor for Prostacyclin

The results above suggested that an increase in sensitivity of the platelets to prostacyclin might contribute to the antithrombotic effect of MPPA, but they still did not rule out the possibility that the TXA_2-synthesis inhibitor might also elevate prostacyclin synthesis. If MPPA acted by elevating the concentration of circulating prostacyclin, one would expect a concomitant elevation in platelet cyclic AMP levels. Exogenous prostacyclin infused intravenously at rates sufficient to inhibit or block aggregation in the partially obstructed coronary arteries of the dog always increased in the level of intracellular platelet cyclic AMP. However, MPPA had no significant effect on platelet cyclic AMP levels (24.0 ± 2.5 before and 21.6 ± 2.8 pmols/10^9 platelets, after MPPA; n = 6), even though aggregation was completely inhibited. Furthermore, i.v. infusions of prostacyclin sufficient to block platelet aggregation always lowered blood pressure 10–30 mm Hg whereas MPPA blocked aggregation with no concomitant change in blood pressure. Thus, it was unlikely that MPPA blocked aggregation by elevating the circulating prostacyclin concentration.

Although circulating prostacyclin levels were not elevated by MPPA, it was possible that local synthesis of prostacyclin by the blood vessel at the site of the obstructor contributed to the antiaggregatory activity of MPPA. Previous studies (Aiken et al., 1979a) showed that topical application of prostacyclin onto the obstructed site could prevent blockage of the artery without lowering blood pressure or elevating cyclic AMP levels in the circulating platelets. To test this hypothesis we severely obstructed coronary arteries, as we had done in the experiment in Figure 2, and then treated the dog with MPPA (Fig. 3,

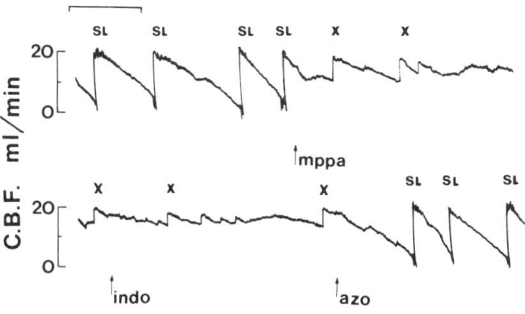

Fig. 3. Continuous record of circumflex blood flow (C.B.F.) in an anesthetized dog with a severely obstructed circumflex coronary artery. Thrombi were shaken loose (SL) periodically to restore blood flow or came loose spontaneously (X). At the first arrow a TXA_2 synthetase inhibitor (MPPA) was given i.v.; at the second arrow indomethacin (indo) was dripped topically in a volume 200 μl on the obstructed site; at the third arrow 9,11-azorpostadienoic acid (azo) was dripped topically on the obstructed site in a volume of 100 μl. The prostacyclin synthetase inhibitor (azo) reversed the effects of MPPA. The horizontal bracket at the top shows 5 min.

top), which inhibited aggregation. Topical application of 2 mg of indomethacin directly to the obstructed site of the artery did not change the pattern of coronary flow. However, topical application of 9,11-azoprostadienoic acid (azo; a prostacyclin synthetase inhibitor, Gorman et al., 1977) resulted in an immediate return of aggregation (Fig. 3, bottom). The dose of indomethacin used topically (2 mg) was sufficient to block the antiaggregatory effects of topically applied arachidonic acid (1 mg) and the dose of azo (1 mg) was enough to block the antiaggregatory activity of topically applied PGH_2 (20 μg). Neither antagonist prevented the antiaggregatory effect of topically applied prostacyclin (1−10 μg).

These data supported the conclusion that local synthesis of prostacyclin was responsible for preventing blockage of the coronary arteries after MPPA. Furthermore, the poor effectiveness of topical indomethacin compared to the complete effectiveness of i.v. indomethacin (see above) for reversing the effects of MPPA suggested that the PGH_2 used to synthesize prostacyclin was not generated in the blood vessel but locally in the blood. The PGH_2 then must have been taken up by the artery and converted into prostacyclin.

The ability to reverse the effects of MPPA with topical prostacyclin-synthesis inhibitors made it possible to test the change in sensitivity to prostacyclin of dog platelets after blocking TXA_2 synthesis but without the use of a cyclooxygenase inhibitor. When this was done, a similar 30-fold increase in sensitivity of the platelets to prostacyclin was observed (four experiments). This result confirmed the hypothesis that the enhanced responsiveness of the platelets was due to the absence of TXA_2.

Discussion and Conclusions

This study (Aiken et al, 1981) demonstrates first, that a TXA_2-synthesis inhibitor (MPAA) prevents blockage of partially obstructed coronary arteries with platelets. Second, MPPA is more effective than drugs that reduce platelet aggregation by inhibiting the prostaglandin cyclooxygenase and its efficacy is similar to that of intravenously administered prostacyclin. Third, the greater efficacy of a TXA_2 synthetase inhibitor compared to cyclooxygenase inhibitors depends on several interacting factors; most importantly, endogenous prostacyclin biosynthesis in the vessel wall is not blocked, and hence, prostacyclin can contribute to the antiaggregatory activity. Also, the conditions in the narrowed lumen of the coronary artery at the obstructed site, which normally act as a stimulus for thrombus formation, induces the synthesis of PGH_2 that, when it cannot be converted to TXA_2, apparently is diverted into the vascular prostacyclin synthetase pathway (Fig. 4). And finally, when platelets cannot form TXA_2, much less prostacyclin is needed to prevent blockage of the coronary arteries. Thus, a basal level of prostacyclin production, which normally may not be sufficient to affect platelet aggregability, might exert antiaggregatory effects after a TXA_2 synthetase inhibitor.

Platelet aggregability can be regulated by a type of reciprocal relationship between TXA_2 and prostacyclin (Gorman, 1979). With platelets studied in vitro, the antiaggregatory and biochemical effects of prostacyclin are attenuated by adding TXA_2 to platelet-rich plasma and vice versa. However, demonstration of the importance of this relationship in vivo has not previously been possible. One suggestion that such a relationship exists in vivo comes from the observation of O'Grady and Moncada (1978) that low doses of aspirin prolong bleeding time more effectively than high doses of aspirin. Because low doses of aspirin are suspected of having a preferential effect on platelet cyclooxygenase compared to the vascular enzyme (Baenziger et. al., 1979), these studies suggested that selective blockade of TXA_2 snythesis might shift the "set point" of this reciprocal relationship in the direction of increased prostacyclin-like effects. The 30-fold shift to the left in the dose-response relationship for preventing blockage of the coronary arteries with prostacyclin, which occurs after inhibiting TXA_2 formation in platelets with either cyclooxygenase inhibitors or MPPA, suggests that the reciprocal control of platelet aggregation by TXA_2 and prostacyclin may be particularly relevant to the pathological state mimicked by the partially obstructed coronary arteries in dogs. After blocking the formation of TXA_2 with MPPA, the primary stimuli for aggregation at the obstructed site (turbulent flow, shear forces, ADP, etc.) are still there but the TXA_2-mediated events (calcium mobilization, platelet-release reaction, etc.; Gorman, 1979) are presumably gone (Fig. 4). In the absence of TXA_2 synthesis, prostacyclin becomes much more effective, probably because less cyclic AMP is needed to maintain a low cytoplasmic calcium concentration.

We have reported previously that, under the control conditions of these experiments, there is no evidence to support the hypothesis that local prostacyclin production is sufficient to affect the blockage of the coronary artery at the site of the obstructor (Aiken et. al., 1979b). However, this situation is strikingly altered by selectively blocking TXA_2 synthesis with MPPA (Fig. 4). After MPPA, local biosynthesis of prostacyclin was responsibile for the high efficacy of the drug for preventing blockage of the coronary artery. Several observations point to the mechanism involved; first, topically applied prostacyclin synthetase inhibitors reversed the effects of MPPA but a similar reversal usually could not be produced with a cyclooxygenase inhibitor applied topically (indomethacin). This suggested that most of the precursor (PGH_2) for prostacyclin synthesis was not formed in the blood vessel wall per se. However, cyclooxygenase inhibitors readily reversed the effects of MPPA when given intravenously, supporting the hypothesis that

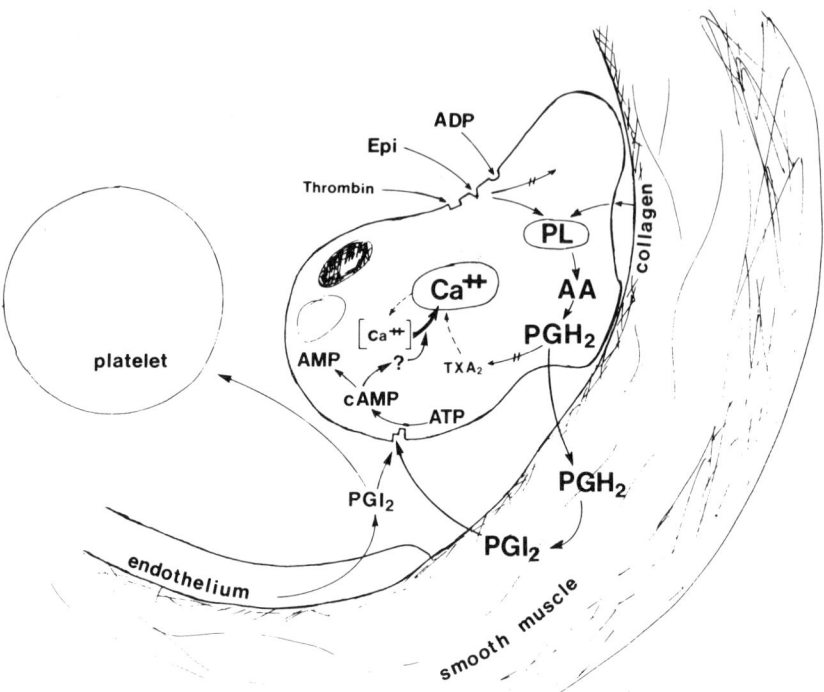

Fig. 4. Schematic representation of a platelet adhering to the vessel wall in Figure 1 but depicting what occurs in the presence of a TXA_2 synthetase inhibitor. Stimulatory substances still activate phospholipases but the PGH_2 not converted to TXA_2 is taken up by the blood vessel wall and converted by prostacyclin (PGI_2) synthetase to PGI_2. PGI_2 activates platelet adenylate cyclase, increasing the conversion to ATP to cyclic AMP, which through some unknown mechanism reduces cytoplasmic Ca^{2+} concentration by increasing its uptake into intracellular binding sites. Hence, dense and alpha granules do not release contents and other platelets are not activated. Also, because TXA_2 is not promoting Ca^{2+} release the platelet is much more sensitive to the basal production of PGI_2 from the endothelium.

the PGH_2 was formed in the blood and then taken up by the artery and converted to prostacyclin. These observations fit well with the localization of the biosynthetic enzymes in arteries for producing prostacyclin. The cyclooxygenase is found in the highest concentration in endothelial cells (Smith and Bell, 1978), which in our experiments have likely been rubbed off for the most part. However, prostacyclin synthetase is found uniformly throughout the smooth muscle (W. L. Smith, personal communication) so there would still be plenty at the obstructed site ready to convert PGH_2 into prostacyclin if there was a source of this precursor.

From our study we cannot say precisely where the PGH_2 used for local prostacyclin biosynthesis comes from. However, the results are consistent with the hypothesis of Gryglewski and colleagues (1976) and the results of Marcus et al. (1980) that the vessel wall may "steal" the precursor from the juxtaposed platelets in the narrowed lumen at the obstructed site. If the PGH_2 used for prostacyclin synthesis after MPPA comes from the platelets, one would predict that any drug that blocked platelet cyclooxygenase would prevent or reverse that portion of the activity of a TXA_2 synthetase inhibitor that depends on endogenous prostacyclin activity. And indeed, cyclooxygenase inhibitors given intravenously, readily produced this effect in animals with severely obstructed vessels. In our studies, we found no difference in the efficacy of low versus high doses of aspirin, or aspirin versus ibuprofen or indomethacin for preventing coronary artery thrombosis. This, however, does not rule out the possibility that these agents might show some preferential inhibition of platelet versus blood vessel cyclooxygenase at certain doses. In our experiments, the inhibition of just the platelet cyclooxygenase would be expected to block not only TXA_2 synthesis but also most of the relevant prostacyclin synthesis if, indeed, the precursor for prostacyclin synthesis also was platelet derived. Thus, all cyclooxygenase inhibitors would behave similarly in our experiments.

This raises some important questions concerning the use of low doses of aspirin to obtain selective inhibition of TXA_2 production. On the one hand, if the PGH_2 used for prostacyclin synthesis at a lesion in the vasculature comes from platelets, low doses of aspirin, in spite of selectively blocking platelet versus vessel wall cyclooxygenase, would locally inhibit both TXA_2 and prostacyclin synthesis. On the other hand, if the vessel wall still makes some prostacyclin from arachidonic acid, a relatively small change in the balance of the platelet TXA_2 to vascular prostacyclin, in favor of prostacyclin, would magnify the effects of the prostacyclin due to the 30-fold enhanced sensitivity of platelets that occurs after inhibiting TXA_2 synthesis. It is notable in our experiments that only a partial inhibition of platelet TXA_2 with MPPA was sufficient to prevent blockage of the coronary artery. The comparative usefulness of low doses of aspirin or selective TXA_2 synthetase inhibitors for preventing thrombosis will have to be resolved by appropriate clinical trials.

References

Aiken, J. W., Gorman, R. R. and Shebuski, R. J. 1979a. Prevention of blockage of partially obstructed coronary arteries with prostacyclin correlates with inhibition of platelet aggregation. Prostaglandins 17:483–494

Aiken, J. W., Gorman, R. R. and Shebuski, R. J. 1979b. Prostacyclin prevents blockage of partially obstructed coronary arteries. In *Prostacyclin*, eds. J. R. Vane and S. Bergstrom, pp. 311–321. New York: Raven Press

Aiken, J. W., Shebuski, R. J. and Gorman, R. R. 1980. Blockage of partially obstructed coronary arteries with platelet thrombi: Comparison between its prevention with cyclooxygenase inhibitors versus prostacyclin. In *Advances in Prostaglandin Thromboxane Research,* Vol. 7, eds. B. Samuelsson and R. Paoletti, pp. 635–639. New York: Raven Press

Aiken, J. W. and Shebuski, R. J. 1980. Comparison in anesthetized dogs of the antiaggregatory and hemodynamic effects of prostacyclin and a chemically stable prostacyclin analog, 6a-carba-PGI$_2$ (carbacyclin). Prostaglandins 19: 629–643

Aiken, J. W., Shebuski, R. J., Miller, O. V. and Gorman, R. R. 1981. Endogenous prostacyclin contributes to the efficacy of a thromboxane synthetase inhibitor for preventing coronary artery thrombosis. J Pharmacol Exp Ther 219:299–308

Baenziger, N. L., Becherer, P. R. and Majerus, P. W. 1979. Characterization of prostacyclin synthesis in cultured human arterial smooth muscle cells, venous endothelial cells, and skin fibroblasts. Cell 16:907–974

Bunting, S., Gryglewski, R., Moncada, S. and Vane, J. R. 1976. Arterial walls generate from prostaglandin endoperoxides a substance (prostaglandin X) which relaxes strips of mesenteric and coeliac arteries and inhibits platelet aggregation. Prostaglandins 12:897–913

Feuerstein, N. and Ramwell, P. W. 1981. OKY-1581, a potential selective thromboxane synthetase inhibitor. Eur J Pharmacol 69:533–534

Folts, J. D., Crowell, E. D. and Rowe, G. G. 1976. Platelet aggregation in partially obstructed vessels and its elimination with aspirin. Circulation 54:365–370

Gallagher, K. P., Folts, J. D. and Rowe, G. G. 1978. Comparison of coronary arteriograms with direct measurements of stenosed coronary arteries in dogs. Am Heart J 95:338–347

Gorman, R. R., 1979. Modulation of human platelet function by prostacyclin and thromboxane A$_2$. Fed Proc 38: 79–88

Gorman, R. R., Bundy, G. L., Peterson, D. C. Sun, F. F., Miller, O. V. and Fitzpatrick, F. A. 1977. Inhibition of human platelet thromboxane synthetase by 9,11-azoprosta-5,13-dienoic acid. Proc Nat Acad Sci USA 74:4007–4011

Gryglewski, R. J., Bunting, S., Moncada, S., Flower, R. J. and Vane, J. R. 1976. Arterial walls are protected against deposition of platelet thrombi by a substance (prostaglandin X) which they make from prostaglandin endoperoxides. Prostaglandins 12:685–713

Hemker, D. P., Shebuski, R. J. and Aiken, J. W. 1980. Release of a prostacyclin-like substance into the circulation of dogs by intravenous adenosine 5′-diphosphate. J Pharmacol Exp Ther 212: 246–252

Marcus, A. J., Weksler, B. B., Jaffe, E. A. and Broekman, M. J. 1980. Synthesis of prostacyclin from platelet-derived endoperoxides by cultured human endothelial cells. J Clin Invest 66:979–986

Mills, D. C. B. and Smith, J. B. 1971. The influence on platelet aggregation of drugs that affect the accumulation of cAMP in platelets. Biochem J 121:185–196

Miyamoto, T., Taniguchi, K., Tanouchi, T. and Hirata, F. 1980. Selective inhibitor of thromboxane synthetase: Pyrdine and its derivatives. In *Advances in Prostaglandin Thromboxane Research,* Vol. 6, eds. B. Samuelsson and R. Paoletti, pp. 443–445. New York: Raven Press

Moncada, S., Gryglewski, R. J., Bunting, S. and Vane, J. R. 1976. An enzyme isolated from arteries transforms prostaglandin endoperoxides to an unstable substance that inhibits platelet aggregation. Nature 263:663–665.

Mullane, S., Moncada, S. and Vane, J.R. 1979. Formation and disappearance of prostacyclin in the circulation. In *Prostacyclin,* eds. J. R. Vane and S. Bergstrom, p. 221. New York: Raven Press

O'Grady, J. O. and Moncada, S. 1978. Aspirin: A paradoxical effect on bleeding time. Lancet 2:780

Shebuski, R. J. and Aiken, J. W. 1980. Angiotensin II stimulation of renal prostaglandin synthesis elevates circulating prostacyclin in the dog. Cardiovas Pharmacol 2:667–677

Smith, W. L. and Bell, T. G. 1978. Immunohistochemical localization of the prostaglandin-forming cyclooxygenase in renal cortex. Am J Physiol 235(5): F451–F457

Calcium Entry Blocking Agents: Actions and Utility in Ischemic Heart Disease

James L. Perhach, Jr., William Diamantis, Joseph P. Buckley, R. Duane Sofia and Bhagavan S. Jandhyala

Introduction

The advent or discovery that chemical entities were available that had the capacity to interfere with the movement of calcium across membranes led to a classification of these molecules as calcium antagonists (Fleckenstein, 1977). Although this nomenclature will probably last longer than the compounds, the ubiquitous nature of calcium and the fact that these compounds do not exhibit the classic agonist/antagonist interaction makes the term calcium antagonist inappropriate. More specific, but still permitting an overall general classification, are the terms calcium influx blockers as well as calcium entry blocking agents. The latter was the result of a consensus agreement at a recent symposium (Vanhoutte and Bohr, 1981) and allows for the inclusion of an agent that would affect either the receptor-operated channel or the voltage-operated channel. The most specific term to be applied or utilized is that of calcium slow-channel blocking agent. This terminology indicates that a significant component of the drug's action is through interference of calcium flux in the slow channel.

To qualify for inclusion as a slow-channel blocking agent, the action of the drug must, obviously, be on the slow channel, which carries the inward current during the action potential with little or no effect on the fast sodium channel. Because vascular smooth muscle is virtually devoid of the fast sodium channels the potential for these drugs to influence ischemic disorders is greatly enhanced. However, it must be recognized that in cardiac muscle the slow channel for inward current is not specific for calcium. An inhibitor of the slow inward current in cardiac tissue may interfere with slow sodium as well as the slow sodium-calcium channel.

It is quite likely that as the evidence continues to evolve, it will be found that calcium entry blocking agents do not act by any single mechanism, rather there are a number of sites at which they are interacting, both intra- and extracellularly, to modify the excitation-contraction coupling process.

Compounds

The evaluation of the concept of interference with calcium flux that was initiated in the late 1960s has resulted in the inclusion of a large number of compounds being proposed as candidates possessing this activity. Among the first agents to be classified as belonging to the class of calcium entry blocking agents were nifedipine and verapamil. Also often included are lidoflazine, flunarizine and cinarizine as well as perhexiline. More recent additions to the list include bepridil and diltiazem. This chemically heterogeneous group of compounds is shown in Figure 1. The compounds include a pyrrolidine (bepridil), a benzothiazepine (diltiazem), a dihydroperidine (nifedipine), a piperidine (perhexiline) and a benzoacetonitrile (verapamil). The list does not include any inorganic ions such as Mn^{2+}, Ni^{2+}, Co^{2+} or La^{3+}, although they qualify as inhibitors of calcium influx.

Table 1. Action of Calcium Entry Blockng Agents on a Variety of Smooth Muscle Preparations.

Preparation	Stimulus	Agent	$IC_{50}(M)$	Reference
Dog Coronary	TEA	Bepridil	5×10^{-6}	Harder & Sperelakis (1981)
Guinea Pig	Ach	Bepridil	6×10^{-6}	Diamantis (1980)
Ileum		Diltiazem	$\sim 10^{-6}$	Triggle & Swamy (1980)
		Nifedipine	5×10^{-9}	
Pig Coronary	K^+	Diltiazem	2×10^{-7}	Triggle & Swamy (1980)
		Nifedipine	5×10^{-9}	
		Verapamil	2×10^{-7}	
Rabbit Aorta	NE	Verapamil	$\sim 10^{-4}$	Triggle & Swamy (1980)
	K^+	Verapamil	2.7×10^{-8}	
Rat Aorta	NE	Verapamil	>10	Triggle & Swamy (1980)
	K^+	Verapamil	$\sim 10^{-6}$	
Rat Uterus	5-HT	Bepridil	$>10^{-6}$	Diamantis (1980)
	A-II	Verapamil	5×10^{-7}	Triggle & Swamy (1980)

Key: TEA, tetraethylammonium A_2; Ach, acetylcholine; NE, norepinephrine; 5-HT, 5-hydroxytryptamine; A-II, angiotensin II.

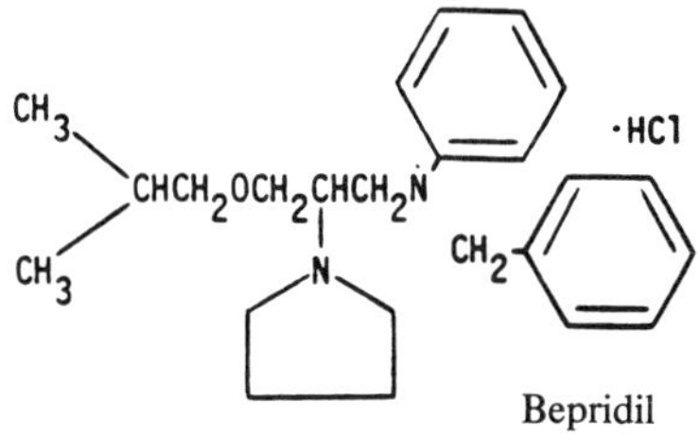

Bepridil

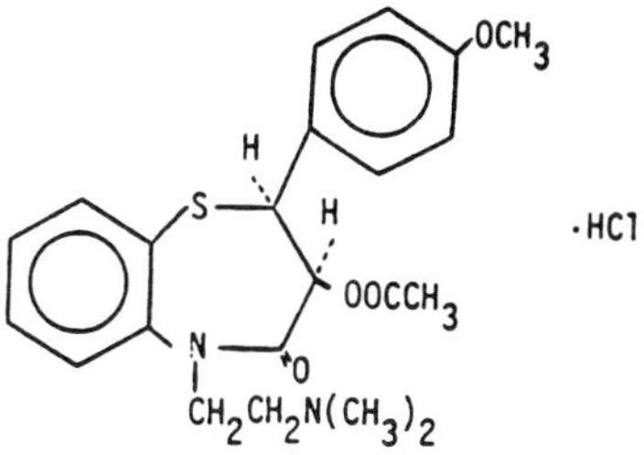

Diltiazem

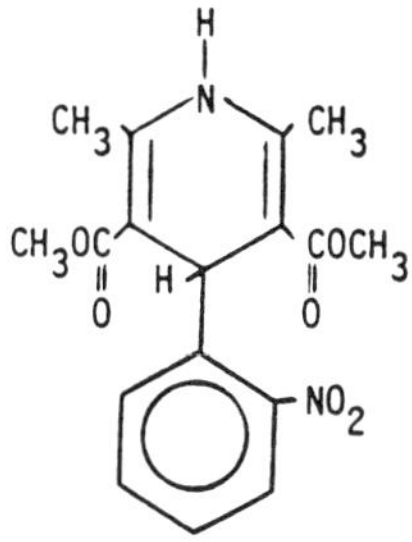

Nifedipine

Perhexiline

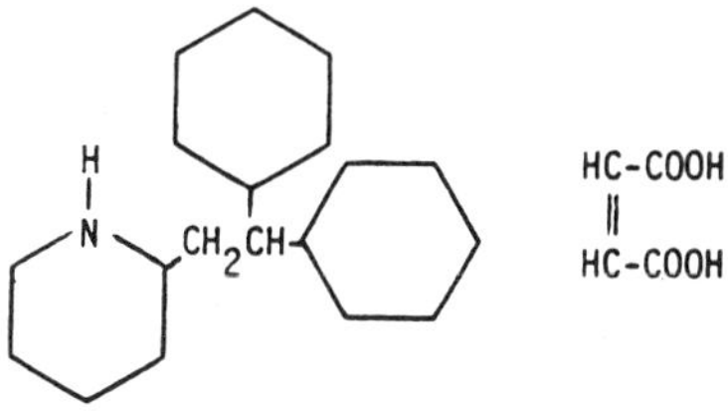

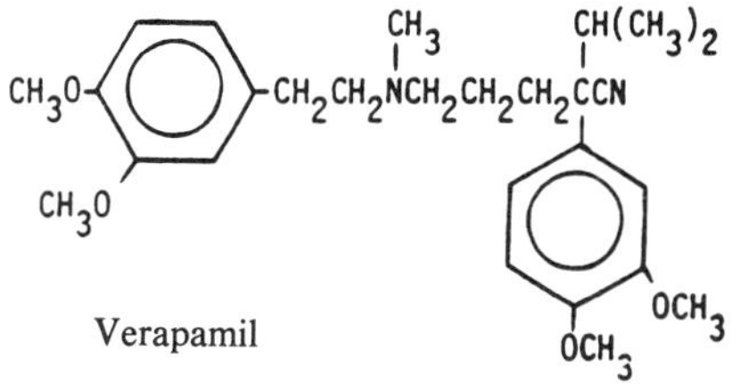

Verapamil

Fig. 1. Chemical structure of a selected group of calcium entry blocking agents.

In Vitro Assessment

The evidence that calcium entry blocking agents act on the slow inward calcium channel comes from a variety of sources. The selectivity of action is also supported from data that indicate that these agents have little or no effect on the fast sodium channel. A recent report by Vogel et. al. (1979) showed that neither bepridil nor verapamil had significant influence on the rate of rise (V_{max}) of the normal action potential, but were capable of abolishing the slow action potentials in isolated perfused guinea pig hearts.

The actions of this class of agents on a variety of vascular smooth muscle preparation are shown in Table 1. These agents have varying degrees of potency including little to no activity against norepinephrine in rat and rabbit aortae. The in vitro order of potency in vascular tissue is generally agreed to be

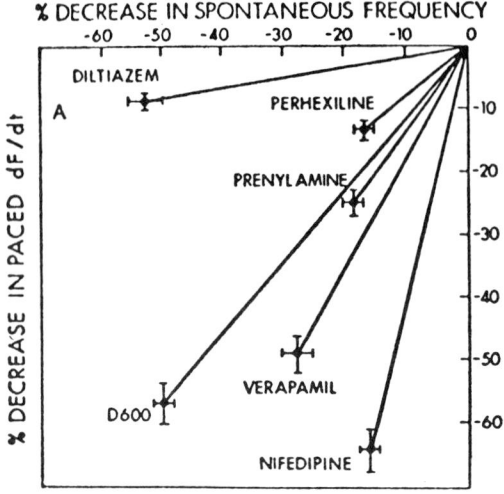

Fig. 2. Responses of first derivative of force development (dF/dt) during electrical pacing and of spontaneous rate (frequency) of isolated guinea pig atria to selected vasodilators, all administered to produce a drug concentration of 10^{-6} M (From Henry, 1980; reproduced with permission.)

nifedipine, verapamil, diltiazem and bepridil in descending order of potency. Similar potency differences occur in the ileum, which may partially explain the reduction in the incidence of constipation seen clinically for bepridil and diltiazem. Other smooth muscle such as the uterus does not appear to be influenced by some agents, while verapamil still retains a high level of activity.

Additional evidence of an action on the slow inward calcium current comes from electrophysiologic evidence in cardiac tissue. These actions on calcium events have recently been summarized by Triggle and Swamy (1980). Recently, Mras and Sperelakis (1981) have shown that bepridil concentrations of 10^{-8}–$10^{-5}M$ depressed the amplitude and duration of the plateau and blocked the spike component of the action potential in cultured rat aortic smooth muscle cells. The uncoupling of the excitation-contraction process by these agents displays a frequency-dependent inhibition, which may suggest selectivity for the open channel.

The comparative cardiac effects of calcium entry blocking agents on guinea pig atria have been studied by monitoring force development in a paced preparation and changes in spontaneous rate. The results of administering a drug concentration of 10^{-6} M of a variety of these agents are displayed in Figure 2. These data were obtained from a recent publication by Henry (1980). Diltiazem acted primarily on frequency and nifedipine on the changes in force during the electical pacing, while verapamil influenced both rate and frequency.

The ability of these agents to influence events in other cardiac tissue has also been well demonstrated. Nifedipine has been shown to inhibit the contractile response in cat papillary muscle at $5 \times 10^{-7} M$ while verapamil exhibited equal molar potency in the guinea pig papillary muscle (Triggle and Swamy, 1980). Similar results would be anticipated with bepridil and diltiazem. However, it is also suggestive with these agents that they exert a concentration-dependent effect on the slow-channel current and at higher concentrations may influence the fast sodium channel.

In Vivo Evaluation

Although the delineation of the in vitro effect of these agents is necessary for us to understand the cellular basis of activity of the compounds, it is the expression of these factors in the intact organism that is the most clinically relevant information. Because it is virtually impossible in the constraints of a manuscript to cover all these agents, data related to the calcium entry blocking agent that we have the most experience with, bepridil, is used as the agent representative of the hemodynamic effects of these agents. Nifedipine must be excluded because of its intrinsic reflex tachycardia properties.

Anesthetized Animals

The data shown in Figure 3 are from separate groups of mongrel dogs that had been treated with placebo or bepridil, 10 mg/kg, orally for 14 days. Before receipt of the dose on Day 15 the animals were anesthetized. The parameters shown are the effects found 12–14 hours after the last dose. The data indicate that the slow-channel blocker, bepridil, resulted in a significant increase in coronary blood flow with a concomitant decrease in coronary vascular resistance. A marked increase in myocardial oxygen utilization also occurred. This enhanced coronary flow occurred without any changes in myocardial contractility. Neither renal nor mesenteric blood flows were altered by chronic treatment with bepridil, while acute administration of bepridil produces transient reductions in these flows (Cosnier et al., 1977). Mean blood pressure and heart rate were reduced in the treated animals. Ventricular function curves in response to volume loading in both treated and placebo animals revealed that the myocardium of the bepridil-treated group performed more efficiently.

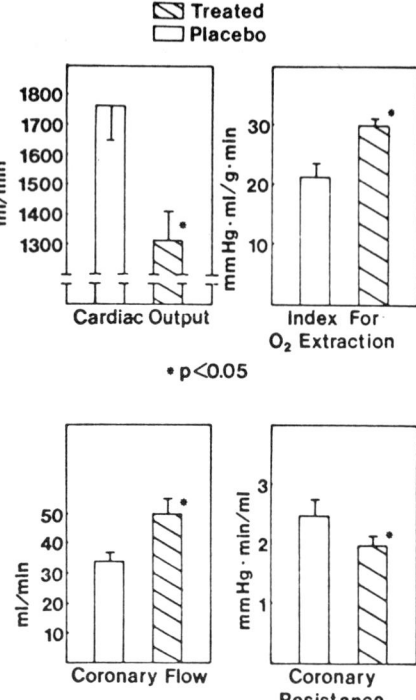

Fig. 3. Effect of bepridil (10 mg/kg, orally, twice a day for 14 days) on cardiac output, coronary blood flow and resistance and index for O_2 contraction in anesthetized dogs.

The actions of these agents do not intimately involve alpha or beta receptors. This was found in vivo as well as in the in vitro work with bepridil (Labrid et al., 1979) and diltiazem (Flaim et al., 1980) that beta receptors are not involved in the classical concepts of these drugs.

Conscious Animals

In order to determine the potential of anesthesia on the hemodynamic parameters the effects of repeat administration of the slow-channel blocker, bepridil, were evaluated in surgically prepared, chronically instrumented mongrel dogs. The animals were equipped with aortic flow probes and arterial pressure catheters. The results of treating the animals with bepridil at a dose level of 10 mg/kg, twice daily, are shown in Figure 4. Compared to the control (Day 1, before treatment), bepridil, even when measured 12–14 hours after the treatment, i.e., Days 2 and 5, resulted in a decrease in myocardial oxygen

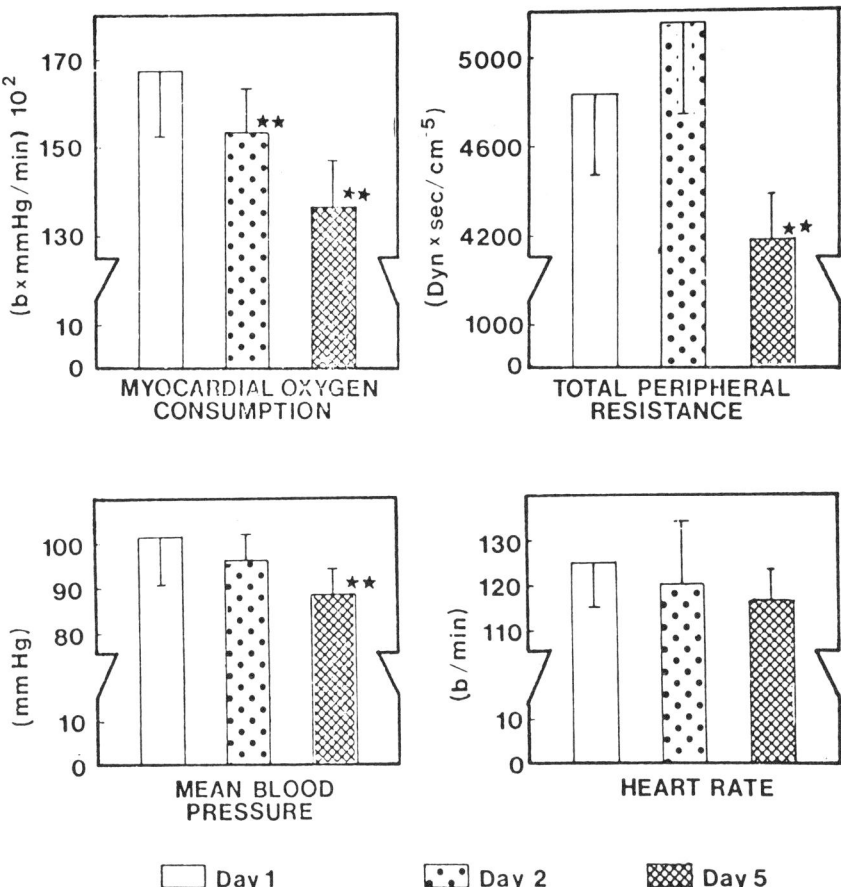

Fig. 4. Effect of bepridil (10 mg/kg, orally, twice a day for 5 days) on blood pressure, heart rate, myocardial oxygen consumption and total peripheral resistance in conscious dogs.

consumption. By the 5th day of the experiment total peripheral resistance and mean blood pressure were reduced while heart rate in the conscious animals was unchanged. Cardiac output was also not affected. Calculation of left ventricular stroke work and left ventricular minute work showed that both were reliably decreased by Day 5 of the experiment (i.e., after 4 days of treatment).

The data represented here as well as the existing data with the other calcium entry blocking agents indicate that they have the potential to alleviate myocardial ischemia by improving oxygen supply and reducing its demand.

Other Pharmacologic Properties

The activity of these agents on influencing the action of bradykinin has received considerable attention. The role of bradykinin in mediating the pain in response to myocardia ischemia is yet to be resolved. Evaluation of bepridil against bradykinin-induced contractions in the guinea pig ileum showed that it was significantly more potent than nitroglycerin, propranolol and papaverine. The results of this experiment are shown in Table 2.

Antagonism of bronchospasm has also been reported. Bepridil has been shown to be effective against bradykinin-induced bronchospasm in the guinea pig (Diamantis, unpublished data). Similar observations have been made for verapamil and its methoxy analog (O'Donnell and Diamond, 1980). This potential involvement in calcium-mediated release relative to involvement in bronchospasm was recently supported by a report that indicated that nifedipine was capable of protecting against exercise-induced bronchospasm in humans (Cerrina et al., 1981).

Activity of these agents in platelet aggregation, a topic of controversy in ischemic disorders, has received recent attention. While diltiazem, nifedipine and verapamil have been reported to be reasonably potent inhibitors of platelet aggregation in vivo in animals, (Riberio et al., 1980; Dimantis, 1980) the results with human platelets using diltiazem, nifedipine and verapamil do not provide complete support (Margolis et al., 1980). Bepridil resembles the action of nitroglycerin in that there is little effect on inhibition of platelet aggregation in vivo in rat platelets (Diamantis, 1980).

Potential Clinical Utility

All compounds are well absorbed after oral administration, with diltiazem and verapamil having the most rapid distribution time (Braunwald et al., 1980) while bepridil and perhexiline have the longest elimination half-life (Henry, 1980; Weliky, 1980).

The use of these agents in the treatment of ischemic heart disease both of the vasospastic and other types is well documented throughout the literature. Utility as an antihypertensive agent has been indicated for verapamil (Midtbo and Hals, 1980) and nifedipine, but usually in combination with a diuretic. The evidence for diltiazem and bepridil is yet to be established. In addition, supraventricular arrhythmias seem to be an obvious indication for these agents, but use beyond this indication remains to be established.

Table 2. The in Vitro IC_{50} Values for Antibradykinin Activity of Agents Used in Treatment of Ischemic Disorders.

Drug	IC_{50}		Relative Activity (Phenylbutazone Na = 1) Based on	
	µg/ml	M	µg	M
Bepridil	0.52	1.24×10^{-6}	163	207
Papaverine HC1	3.1	8.25×10^{-6}	29	33
Propranolol HC1	14.0	4.75×10^{-5}	6	5.7
Nitroglycerin	31.0	1.37×10^{-4}	3	2
Phenylbutazone Na	85.0	2.57×10^{-4}	1	1

The broad area of cardiac preservation holds a high degree of potential for these agents. Reduction of infarct size in animals has been achieved (Faria et al., 1980) and can be expected from the others. In addition, protection against ventricular fibrillation in reperfusion arrhythmias has been shown for bepridil (Marshall and Muir, 1981).

Retardation of cardiomyopathy is also suggested from the literature (Hanrath et al., 1980) as is utility in myocardial preservation during cardiac surgery. Other vasospastic disorders that have been speculated to have some relief from these types of agents include migraine, cerebral vasospasm, irritable bowel syndrome and the previously mentioned bronchospasm.

References

Braunwald, E., Stone, P. H., Antman, E. M. and Muller, J. E. 1980. Calcium channel blocking agents in the treatment of cardiovascular disorders. Part II: Hemodynamic effects and clinical applications. Ann Intern Med 93:886–904

Cerrina, J., Denjean, A., Alexandre, G., Lockhart, A. and Duroux, P. 1981. Inhibition of exercise-induced asthma by a calcium antagonist nifedipine. Am Rev Resp Dis 123:156–160

Cosnier, D., Duchene-Marullaz, P., Rispat, G. and Streichenberger, G. 1977. Cardiovascular pharmacology of bepridil. Arch Int Pharmacodyn Ther 255:133–151

Diamantis, W. 1980. Data on file at Carter-Wallace, Inc., Cranbury, NJ 08512

Faria, D. B., Cheung, W. and Maroko, P. R. 1980. Beneficial effects of W2799M on the extent of ischemic myocardial damage. Circulation 62:(Suppl. III)240

Flaim, S. F., Flaim, K. E. and Zelis, R. 1980. Diltiazem: Lack of myocardial β-adrenergic receptor-binding capacity. Pharmacology 21:306–13

Fleckenstein. A. 1977. Specific pharmacology of calcium in myocardium cardiac pacemakers and vascular smooth muscle. Ann Rev Pharmacol Toxicol 17:149–166

Hanrath, P., Mathey, D., Kremer, P., Sonntag, F., and Bleifeld, W. 1980. Effect of verapamil on left ventricular isovolumic relaxation time and regional left ventricular filling in hypertrophic cardiomyopathy. Am J Cardiol 45:1258–1264

Harder, D. R. and Sperelakis, N. 1981. Bepridil blockade of Ca^{2+}-dependent action potentials in vascular smooth muscle of dog coronary artery. J Cardiovasc Pharmacol 3:906–914

Henry, P.D., 1980. Comparative pharmacology of calcium antagonists: Nifedipine, verapamil and diltiazem. Am J Cardiol 46:1047–1058

Labrid, C., Grosset, A., Dureng, G., Minronneau, J., and Duchene-Marullaz, P. 1979. Some membrane interactions with bepridil, a new antianginal agent. J Pharmacol Exp Ther 211:546–554

Marshall, R. J. and Muir, A. W. 1981. The antiarrhythmic, hemodynamic and metabolic effects of a new antianginal agent, bepridil, in the early stages of acute myocardial infarction. Br J Pharmacol 72:114

Margolis, B., Lucas, C. and Henry, P. D. 1980. Effects of Ca^{++} antagonists on platelet aggregation and secretion. Circulation 62:(Suppl III)191

Midtbo, K. and Hals, O. 1980. Verapamil in the treatment of hypertension. Curr Ther Res 27:830-838

Mra, S. and Sperelakis, N. 1981. Bepridil (CERM-1978) blockade of action potentials in cultured rat aortic smooth muscle cells. Eur J Pharmacol 71:13-19

O'Donnell, M. and Diamond, L. 1980. Effects of calcium antagonist (verapamil) on active bronchial and passive cutaneous anaphylaxis. Fed Proc 39:1016

Riberio, L., Brandon, T. A., Horak, J. K., Solis, R. T. and Miller, R. R. 1980. Inhibition of platelet aggregation by verapamil: Further rationale for the use of calcium antagonists in coronary artery disease. Circulation 62:(Supp. III)293

Triggle, D. J. and Swamy, V. C., 1980. Pharmacology of agents that affect calcium. Chest 78:1(Suppl)174–179

Vanhoutte, P.M. and Bohr, D. F. 1981. Calcium influx blockers. Fed Proc in press.

Vogel, S., Crampton, R. and Sperelakis, N. 1979. Blockade of myocardial slow channels by bepridil (CERM 1978). J Pharmacol Exp Ther 210:378–385

Weliky, I. 1980. Data on file at Carter-Wallace, Inc., Cranbury, NJ 08512

Effects of Pharmacologic Agents on Isolated Human Coronary Arteries

*Robert Ginsburg, Michael R. Bristow,
John S. Schroeder, Edward B. Stinson
and Donald C. Harrison*

Introduction

From clinical studies in our institution (Ricci et al., 1970; Schroeder et al., 1977; McLaughlin et al., 1977; Orlick et al., 1978; Ginsburg and Schroeder, 1980; Rosenthal et al., 1980) and from the work of others, it has become apparent that the human epicardial coronary artery is not just a passive conduit through which blood flows, but rather is a highly dynamic, reactive vascular structure that is subject to functional alterations by a variety of influences. To gain a better insight into the pathophysiologic processes involved in coronary spasm, we studied the pharmacologic responses of human coronary vascular smooth muscle using isolated ring segments of human coronary arteries derived from both normal and diseased hearts. Although these types of in vitro studies can provide interesting and useful data, extrapolation to intact systems must be made with caution, because these studies focus on only a single aspect of the many variables that exist in vivo. Even with this reservation, we believe that our observations, as presented in this symposium, have increased the understanding of the pharmacologic mechanisms involved in human coronary arterial smooth muscle contraction and have provided us with valuable insights into the potential pathophysiologic processes involved in coronary artery spasm.

General Methodology

The cardiac transplant program at Stanford Medical Center provides us with coronary arteries from normal and diseased hearts. To date, we have performed pharmacologic studies on over 1000 coronary artery segments from 43 human hearts.

The human coronary arteries were studied using a specially designed 12-chamber muscle bath, employing classic pharmacologic techniques. The right, left and circumflex epicardial coronary arteries were removed from the heart, cleaned of all adherent fat and connective tissue and sectioned into 5-mm wide ring segments. The segments were mounted and placed under 1.2 g tension and allowed to equilibrate for 60–90 min in Tyrode's solution with 2 mM calcium chloride. This solution contained an ionized calcium measured by ion-specific electrode of 1.26 mM, which is similar to that of human serum. The bath was kept at 36°C, pH 7.40–7.45, and each bath was aerated with 95% O_2, 5% CO_2.

The coronary arteries were obtained immediately upon removal of the recipient heart from the transplant patient. Bovine, porcine and canine coronary arteries were also studied in an attempt to characterize species differences; this material was obtained from other laboratories or from slaughter houses.

Basic Pharmacologic Characteristics of Human Coronary Artery—Basal Tone

Basal tone, by our definition, is the tension generated by the resting coronary segment. Human coronary ring segments exhibit basal tone. This tone is calcium dependent, and can be observed in innervated as well as denervated coronary arteries and in atherosclerotic ring segments. Only in severely diseased segments with marked calcification is basal tone not consistently found.

Inhibition of specific receptors with adrenergic, histaminic or muscarinic blocking agents does not affect basal tone. Of the various endogenous vasoactive substances that act through a receptor mechanism, prostaglandins appear to be the only class of compounds that influence basal tone. Prostacyclin, which is a potent relaxer of coronary arteries (Kulkarni et al., 1976), is produced by the endothelial cells of the artery. The addition to the bath of prostaglandin (PG) synthetase inhibitors, such as indomethiacin or ibuprofen, causes contraction of the coronary segment from its basal state, probably by inhibiting the synthesis of prostacyclin production. The importance of prostaglandins in regulating tone has been shown by Kalsner (1975) in bovine coronary arteries and we have demonstrated similar findings in human tissue.

Recently, Bevan (1979) proposed that transient contractile responses of isolated vascular smooth muscle to norepinephrine correlated well with basal tone. If there is such a correlation, then the human coronary artery is another example, as transient contractile responses are seen in response to norepinephrine. These transient responses are due to the release of intracellular calcium stores, but whether or not this mechanism is crucial for the regulation of tone is as yet unknown (see below).

Spontaneous and Induced Phasic, Rhythmic Myogenic Activity

Human coronary ring segments demonstrate spontaneous, rhythmic periods of contraction and relaxation (Ross et al., 1980). This rhythmic activity has been described previously in veins and arteries from a variety of vascular beds and animal species (Johansson and Bohr, 1966). The physiologic role of such spontaneous activity is presently unknown.

In human coronary arteries, this cyclic activity is usually uniform, with cycle lengths between 60 and 80 sec. Various agonists can induce this rhythmicity and change the amplitude and cycle length. Not all segments have spontaneous rhythmicity, and there is presently no one characteristic that

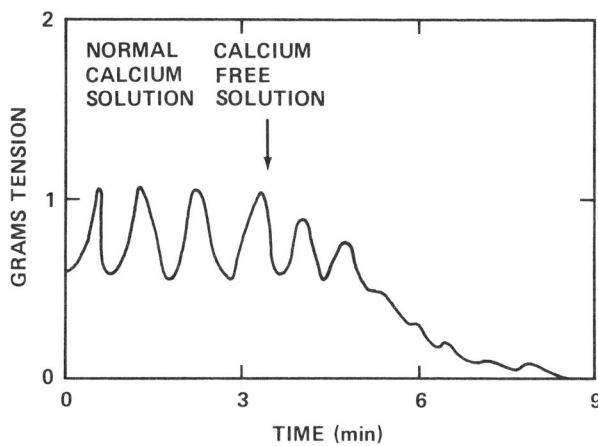

Fig. 1. Recording from one human coronary ring segment demonstrating resting tone and spontaneous rhythmicity in normal and Ca^{2+}-free solution.

identifies which arteries will or will not demonstrate this type of activity. This rhythmic activity and basal tone and their dependency on calcium is shown in Figure 1.

Phasic, rhythmic contraction has been observed in human coronary segments from the three major vessels. This phenomenon must induce synchronous contraction of many cells of the ring segment and thus demonstrates single-unit organization in vascular smooth muscle. In order for this synchronization to occur, communication between smooth muscle cells is necessary. Electron micrograms have revealed nexus or gap junctions between smooth muscle cells of arteries. These have been described in other types of vascular smooth muscle cells (Bevan and Yung, 1974) and are thought to be the pathway for electrical activity. Electrophysiological studies imply that action potentials generated from a pacemaker focus are propagated along the coronary segment through these nexus, which permit synchronization of electrical and mechanical activities.

Rhythmic activity is affected by environmental factors and various vasoactive substances. Changing the pH of the bathing fluid to a more alkaline state increases cyclic amplitude but not frequency. An acid pH causes cessation of all activity. Cold and hypoxia also decrease rhythmic activity. Vasoactive substances that induce activity in quiescent ring segments include norepinephrine, acetylcholine, histamine, PGE_2 (in high doses), ergonovine or potassium. Nitroglycerin, lidocaine, D-600 or diltiazem cause cessation of rhythmic activity.

Previous neural innervation is not necessary for rhythmic activity, as there is no difference between denervated or innervated ring segments. Rhythmic activity is unaffected by alpha- or beta-adrenergic, muscarinic or histaminic blocking agents. This spontaneous rhythmicity occurs in normal or diseased coronary arteries but cyclic pattern and frequency in atherosclerotic segments is usually quite irregular. This may be due to a degenerative process involving the nexus.

The functional importance of action potentials, pacemaker foci and conduction pathways on the resulting rhythmic activity is presently unknown. However, we do know that coronary artery segments can exhibit this activity and secondarily can generate large forces on contraction. It is interesting to speculate that the clinical phenomenon of focal coronary artery spasm might involve a triggering of electromechanical activity by this spontaneous rhythmicity in the artery.

Agonist-induced Vascular Smooth Muscle Contraction

Brodie (1963) originally separated agonist-mediated contractile responses into two types, one operating at a faster rate than the other. Subsequently, Bohr (1963) demonstrated that the dual effects of calcium on membrane excitation and its coupling to contraction could be seen in a single contractile response to an agonist. He separated the epinephrine-induced contraction into two components, a phasic or fast component and a tonic or slow component. In a later study, Sitrin and Bohr (1971) demonstrated that the fast component utilized cellular bound calcium, and that the rate-limiting factor for the release of this bound calcim was the excitability of the cell membrane. Furthermore, these investigators, as well as others (Karaki et al., 1979), showed that the slow component was dependent upon extracellular calcium because this part of the response was inhibited in a calcium-free solution and increased as the concentration of calcium was raised towards physiological levels. The slow component of the norepinephrine response was also accompanied by an increase in ^{45}Ca uptake.

The human coronary artery responds to stimulation by an agonist with a similar biphasic response. This biphasic response has been previously studied in detail by many investigators in rabbit aorta and rabbit ear artery. The initial rapid phase of contraction is felt to be partially due to the release of tightly bound or intracellular calcium. Whether this intracellular calcium comes from sites located in sinks on the inner surface of the plasma membrane, from the sacroplasmic reticulum or from the mitochondria is still unknown. The slow, tonic phase of contraction, the other portion of the biphasic response, is felt to be due mainly to the influx of freely exchangeable or extracellular calcium through the calcium slow channels located in the cell membrane.

The biphasic response is found only in certain vascular beds (Steinsland et al., 1973; Bevan and Waterson, 1971; Bevan et al., 1973). It has been a consistent observation in our coronary artery studies, and probably reflects differences in calcium stores and mechanisms for release compared with other vascular tissue. The initial phasic response of the human coronary ring segment is a rapid contraction and can, depending on the agonist, account for 70% of the overall maximal tension generated. If the same response is elicited in a calcium-free solution, rapid contraction can be shown to generate up to 20–50% of the maximal tension produced by the same segment in a physiologic (1.26mM) calcium solution. These responses suggest that the release of intracellular calcium contributes significantly to overall contraction of human coronary vascular smooth muscle.

The characteristics of the slow, tonic phase in human coronary arteries are similar to those seen in other animal models. This phase is presumably due to the influx of extracellular freely exchangeable calcium. In our studies in calcium-free solutions no tonic response can be observed during an agonist challenge.

Species Differences

We have compared the characteristics of coronary arteries from the dog, pig and cow using the same techniques employed for human coronary studies. Dose-response curves to a variety of agonists were compared, receptor distribution was analyzed and basal tone and rhythmic vasoactivity were evaluated.

Our results have shown a marked difference in sensitivity of the contractile response to various agonists among animal models. No animal has all the features found in man. These differences have been quite impressive and suggest that care should be taken when selecting a species for study in an in vitro setting. For example, in the canine coronary artery, Van Breeman (Van Breemen and Siegel, 1980) has shown an influx of extracellular Ca^{2+} and no release of intracellular calcium in response to norepinephrine. This is in contradistinction to the rabbit, pig or human coronary artery, which utilizes both intracellular and extracellular calcium pools in response to norepinephrine stimulation.

Norepinephrine

The exposure of the human coronary artery ring segment to phenylephrine or norepinephrine in the presence of propranolol results in contraction of the segment. The maximal tension that a segment generates in response to these drugs is usually less than to other agonists we have studied. However, the sensitivity to these drugs ($ED_{50} = 10^{-7} M$) is similar to that found in other animal species. Unlike the canine coronary artery, the human coronary artery mobilizes two pools of calcium for contraction upon exposure to norepinephrine. There is both the influx of extracellular calcium and the release of intracellular calcium as demonstrated in Figure 2.

The contribution of the adrenergic nervous system to coronary vasoregulation has been intensively investigated. Studies in the intact dog have shown that coronary blood flow can be influenced markedly by stimulation or blockade of the alpha-adrenergic receptors that supply the large coronary

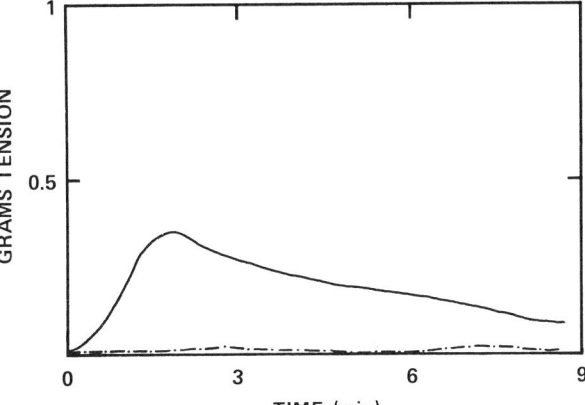

Fig. 2. Recording from one human coronary ring segment (solid line) and one canine coronary segment (dotted line) after exposure to 10^{-5} M norepinephrine in a Ca^{2+}-free solution. Notice that only the human coronary contracts under these conditions.

arteries. Because of this, much emphasis has been placed on the neurogenic influence on the coronary circulation (Mohrman and Feigl, 1978). Clinically, Ricci et al. (1979) described altered adrenergic activity in patients with coronary spasm. They demonstrated that phentolamine administration could reverse coronary spasm and decrease coronary vascular resistance. The mechanism of action of phentolamine, however, is not completely known. Although it is an alpha antagonist in vitro, it may have direct smooth muscle effects. Studies with long acting alpha blockers such as phenoxybenzamine have not demonstrated uniform effectiveness in the treatment of spasm and, therefore, the role of the adrenergic system in mediating coronary spasm is subject to question.

Thus, although sympathetic nerves, norepinephrine and alpha-adrenergic stimulation may play a role in the contraction of the human coronary artery, data from muscle bath studies suggest that this is not the sole mechanism nor the most important, either in normal physiologic processes or in pathophysiologic states such as vasospasm.

Acetylcholine

In the human coronary ring segment, acetylcholine stimulation results in contraction. Its potency lies between norepinephrine and histamine. Acetylcholine receptor density also changes along the length of the vessel. Of interest is the marked variability of response in animal models, the dog having essentially no response to acetylcholine.

Methacholine has been used in human studies to provoke coronary spasm (Yasue et al., 1974). It has been postulated that methacholine acts by the indirect stimulation of the sympathetic nervous system, thereby provoking spasm through alpha-adrenergic receptors. However, at least in vitro, this mechanism is not necessary because acetylcholine (and presumably methacholine) causes contraction of the coronary segment. Acetylcholine and carbachol both act through specific membrane receptors.

Histamine

The sympathetic nerves, cardiac muscle and coronary arteries are rich in mast cells and histamine. Histamine has been shown to be released into the circulation during sudden withdrawal of sympathetic tone and after direct stimulation of sympathetic nerves and spinal nerve roots (McGrath and Shepherd, 1976). Histamine, therefore, has a regulatory role in adrenergic neurotransmission. Histamine, along with acetylcholine, angiotension, prostaglandins and norepinephrine, has the potential to alter the neurotransmitter by acting on sympathetic nerve endings. In the tissue bath histamine causes a potentiation of norepinephrine effects in vascular smooth muscle (Bevan et al., 1975). Thus, the potential exists for histamine to play a role in coronary vasoregulation.

In human coronary segments histamine is not very potent ($ED_{50}=1 \times 10^{-5}$ M), but it does generate one of the greatest contractile responses in terms of grams tension of the agonists studied. We previously reported (Ginsburg et al., 1980) that this contraction is mediated by an H_1-receptor subtype. Also, histamine always induces rhythmic, myogenic activity. Receptor distribution analysis has demonstrated a greater density of H_1 receptors proximally than distally along the length of the coronary arteries.

Prostaglandins

Prostaglandins have been previously studied using in vitro preparations, including human coronary arteries (Kulkarni et al., 1976). Our data indicate that prostaglandins are significant mediators of basal tone. PGE_1, PGE_2 and PGF_{2a} can cause contraction of the human coronary artery. PGI_2 has been classified as a potent coronary smooth muscle relaxant. However, in the human coronary segment, PGI_2 gives a biphasic response. At low doses PGI_2

is a potent relaxer, but at higher concentrations ($> 10^{-6} M$) PGI_2 produces a contractile response that is similar to all other vasoconstrictors studied. Therefore, a prostaglandin known to be produced in the vessel wall of the human coronary artery can cause contraction or relaxation.

Prostaglandins are formed by the enzymatic oxygenation of certain polyunsaturated fatty acids. A prostaglandin precursor such as arachodonic acid is acted upon by the enzyme cyclooxygenase, resulting in the formation of the cyclic endoperoxides (PGH_2). In the rabbit aorta and in porcine and human coronary arteries, PGH_2 is a potent vasoconstrictor, and acts primarily on the intracellular Ca^{2+} pool, while in the bovine coronary artery, PGH_2 causes relaxation (Needleman and Isakson, 1980), again emphasizing that species differences do exist and that generalizations cannot be made about human pharmacology strictly from animal experiments.

Ergonovine

While not an endogenously produced substance, ergonovine has made an important contribution to the diagnosis of coronary spasm. At present ergonovine is the most consistent provoker of coronary spasm in the clinical setting. Although ergonovine and other ergot alkaloids are known stimulators of smooth muscle contractions (Muller et al., 1974), they have not as yet been intensively investigated in coronary artery smooth muscle. From studies in the human coronary, ergonovine operates partially through an alpha-adrenergic receptor in the smooth muscle cell membrane. Rabbit studies have suggested that ergonovine operates more specifically through a serotonin-type receptor. Interestingly, although ergonovine does constrict the human coronary artery, the maximal tension generated is one of the least of all the agonists studied to date. Ergonovine's action in vivo, especially in provoking coronary spasm, may not be a result of direct stimulation of a specific receptor, but may be indirect through the release of other mediators. Clearly, understanding the pharmacologic mechanism of action of ergonovine may help in understanding the pathophysiology of spasm.

Calcium Entry Blocking Agents

Fleckenstein (1977) and others have previously examined the pharmacology of calcium entry blocking drugs in vascular smooth muscle. The calcium blockers are now clinically important in the treatment of arrhythmias, coronary spasm, exertional angina pectoris and cardiomyopathies.

The human coronary artery has at least two membrane channels for calcium. One is a voltage sensitive pathway and the other is a receptor-operated channel. The voltage-sensitive pathway can be activated by depolarization with high concentrations of potassium and is exquisitely sensitive to calcium entry blockers such as D-600, diltiazem, nifedipine and verapamil. Administration of these blockers eliminates basal tone and myogenic rhythmicity—physiologic phenomena operating through the voltage-sensitive pathway. The receptor-operated pathway is blocked by calcium antagonists only at high concentrations when the calcium antagonists' activity is probably "nonspecific" in nature. Also, the release of intracellular calcium is not inhibited by these channel blockers. The observation that calcium blockers only affect the voltage-sensitive pathway is an important clue in understanding potential mechanisms involved in spasm (see Fig. 3).

Some calcium entry blockers exhibit selectivity in the human heart. That is, some block calcium entry preferentially in the coronary artery compared to the myocardium. Diltiazem is 10 times more active on the coronary bed than on cardiac muscle. D-600, nifedipine and verapamil are not selective, and block calcium entry at equimolar concentrations in the coronary arteries as well as

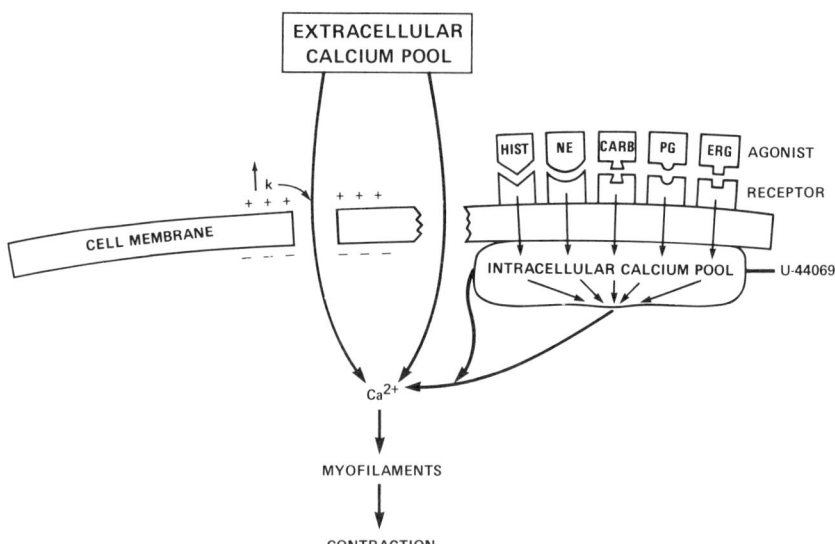

Fig. 3. Schematic diagram of single human epicardial coronary artery smooth muscle cell. Shown are the extracellular and intracellular Ca^{2+} pools utilized in contraction. These pools are activated by a variety of vasoactive agents (HIST, histamine, NE, norepinephrine; CARB, carbachol; PG, prostaglandins; ERG, ergonovine; K, potassium; U-44069, PGH_2 analog).

myocardium. This difference has clinical significance when employing these agents in patients with left ventricular dysfunction.

In the human coronary artery, calcium entry blockers eliminate basal tone. They also cause relaxation of segments that are contracted by potassium or their vasoactive agents. Relaxation is a slow process, but at high doses these blockers cause complete relaxation of the segments. It appears that these blocking agents act solely through the voltage-sensitive pathway when producing vascular relaxation.

Nitroglycerin

Although nitrates have had clinical importance for over 100 years, their mechanism of action is not fully understood. In the human coronary segment, nitroglycerin causes immediate relaxation of the segments. This relaxation is only 20–40% of that attained by calcium entry blockers, although it occurs more rapidly. The responses of nitrates and calcium entry blockers are additive in the muscle bath and this is also appreciated clinically in patients taking these drugs.

Nitrates are not calcium entry blockers, and are in a different pharmacologic class. Nitrates act intracellularly and appear to remove or inactivate a portion of calcium utilized in contraction. Whether or not this involves cyclic GMP is not clear.

Atherosclerosis

Coronary artery spasm usually occurs in areas of atherosclerosis. Recent work on dog coronary arteries has shown that cholesterol sensitizes coronary vascular smooth muscle to the effects of external calcium by a nonadrenergic mechanism (Yoloyama and Henry, 1979). Thus it is postulated that cholesterol may alter the contractile properties of the muscle for the cell membrane. Rabbits fed high cholesterol diets have been shown to have increased sensitivity to ergonovine and serotonin, but not to norepinephrine. These animal studies plus clinical studies demonstrated altered pharmacologic responses in areas of atherosclerosis.

In our studies on human coronary segments, all atherosclerotic segments were able to generate tension and displayed an increased sensitivity to histamine compared to normal segments. There was no change in sensitivity to carbachol, calcium or norepinephrine, however. Thus, it appears that atherosclerosis can affect membrane receptors and that increased sensitivity to specific vasoactive agonists can occur. The role of this supersensitivity in the pathophysiology of coronary spasm is presently unclear.

Summary

The human coronary artery studied in vitro has enabled us to characterize responses to a variety of agonists, examine contractile responses, identify receptor subtypes and distribution and delineate species differences. Whether or not these observations have direct correlates in the in vitro setting is unknown, but these types of pharmacologic studies allow us to study a single organ in detail without the influence of local mediators or blood-borne agents. Our studies have characterized the responses to endogenous vasoactive agents and other cardioactive drugs, such as calcium entry blockers. Two operational calcium membrane channels have been identified, as well as the functional calcium pools utilized in contraction. Understanding these properties will hopefully place us one step closer to understanding the pathophysiologic and pathopharmacologic phenomena involved in coronary artery spasm, and vascular supersensitivity in areas of atherosclerosis.

References

Bevan, J. A. 1979. Transient responses of rabbit cerebral blood vessels to norepinephrine. Circ Res 45:566-572

Bevan, J. A., Dickles, S. P., and Lee, T. J. 1975. Histamine potentiation of nerve and drug induced responses of a rabbit cerebral artery. Circ Res 36:647-653

Bevan, J. A., Garstka, J., Su, C., and Su, H. 1973. The binodal basis of the contractile response of the rabbit ear artery to norepinephrine and other agonists. Eur J Pharmacol 22:47-53

Bevan, J. A., and Waterson, J. G. 1971. The biphasic constrictor response of the rabbit ear artery. Circ Res 28:655-661

Bevan, J. A., and Yung, B. 1974. Longitudinal propagation of the myogenic activity in rabbit arteries and in the rat portal vein. Acta Physiol Scand 90:703-714

Bohr, D. F. 1963. Vascular smooth muscle: dual effect of calcium. Science 139:597-599

Brodie, D. C., Bohr, D. F., and Smith, J. 1963. Dual contractile response of the aorta strip. Am J Physiol 197:241-246

Fleckenstein, A. 1977. Specific pharmacology of calcium in myocardium, cardiac pacemakers, and vascular smooth muscle. Ann Rev Pharmacol Toxicol 17:149-166

Ginsburg, R., Bristow, M. R., Stinson, E. B., and Harrison, D. C. 1980. Histamine receptors in the human heart. Life Sciences 26:2245-2249

Ginsburg, R., Schroeder, J. S. 1980. Coronary artery spasm: Approach to diagnosis and treatment. Pract Cardiol 6:62-82

Johansson, B., and Bohr, D. R. 1966. Rhythmic activity in smooth muscle from small subcutaneous arteries. Am J Physiol 210:801-806

Kalsner, S. 1975. Endogenous prostaglandin release contributes directly to coronary artery tone. Can J Physiol Pharmacol 53:560-565

Karaki, H., Kubota, H., and Urakowa, N. 1979. Mobilization of stored calcium for phasic contraction induced by norephinephrine in rabbit aorta. Eur J Pharm 56:237-245

Kulkarni, P. S., Roberts, R., Needleman, P. 1976. Paradoxical endogenous synthesis of a coronary dilating substance from arachidonate. Prostaglandins 12:337-353

McGrath, M. A., and Shepherd, J. T. 1976. Inhibition of adrenergic neurotransmission in canine vascular smooth muscle by histamine. Cir Res 39:566-573

McLaughlin, P. R., Doherty, P. W., Martin, R. P. Goris, M. L., and Harrison, D. C. 1977. Myocardial imaging in a patient with reproducible angina. Am J Cardiol 39:126-129

Mohrman, D. E., and Feigl, E. O. 1978. Competition between sympathetic vasoconstriction and metabolic vasodilation in the canine coronary circulation. Circ Res 42:70-86

Müller-Schweinitzer, E., and Stürmer, E. 1974. Investigations on the mode of action of ergotamine in the isolated femoral vein of the dog. Br J Pharmacol 51:441-446

Needleman, P., and Isakson, P. C. In *Handbook of Physiology*, Section 2: The Cardiovascular System. Bohr, D., Somlyo, A., and Sparks, H., eds. 1980. Bethesda: American Physiological Society, pp. 613-633

Orlick, A. E., Ricci, D. R., Cipriano, P. R., Guthaner, D. F., Alderman, E. L., and Harrison, D. C. 1978. The contributions of alpha-adrenergic tone to resting coronary vascular resistance in man. J Clin Invest 62:459-467

Ricci, D. R., Orlick, A. E., Cipriano, P. R., Guthaner, D. F., and Harrison, D. C. 1979. Altered adrenergic activity in coronary arterial spasm: insight into mechanism based on study of coronary hemodynamics and the electrocardiogram. Am J Cardiol 43:1073-1079

Ricci, D. R., Orlick, A. E., Doherty, P. W., Cipriano, P. R., and Harrison, D. C. 1978. Reduction of coronary blood flow during coronary artery spasm occurring spontaneously and after provocation by ergonovine maleate. Circulation 57:392-395

Rosenthal, R., Ginsburg, R., Baim, D., and Schroeder, J. S. 1980. Efficacy of diltiazem in variant angina. Am J Cardiol 46:1027-1032

Ross, G., Stinson, E. B., Schroeder, J. S., and Ginsburg, R. 1980. Spontaneous phasic activity of isolated human coronary arteries. Cardiovascular Research 14:613-618

Schroeder, J. S., Bolen, J. L., Quint, R. A., Clark, D. A., Hayden, W. G., Higgins, C. B., and Wexler, L. 1977. Provocation of coronary artery spasm with ergonovine maleate: New test with results in 57 patients undergoing coronary arteriography. Am J Cardiol 40:487-491

Sitrin, M. D., and Bohr, D. F. 1971. Ca and Na interaction in vascular smooth muscle contraction. Amer J Physiol 220:1124-1128

Steinsland,O. S., Furchgott, R. F., and Kirpekar, S. M. 1973. Biphasic vasoconstriction of the rabbit ear artery. Circ Res 32:49-58

Van Breemen, C., and Siegel, B. 1980. The mechanism of α-adrenergic activation of the dog coronary artery. Circ Res 46:426-429

Yasue, H., Touyama, M., Shimamoto, M., et al. 1974. Role of autonomic nervous system in the pathogenesis of Prinzmetal's variant form of angina. Circulation 50:534-539

Yokoyama, M., and Henry, P. D. 1979. Sensitization of isolated canine coronary arteries to calcium ions after exposure to cholesterol. Circ Res 45:479-489

Discussion

Dr. Kirk: I have a comment about ergononvine on large vessels. We found it very disturbing not to be able to get a constriction in dogs, since this is the way of provoking spasm in human catheter studies, and I think Dick Conti has shown some luminal changes in angiographic recordings even in patients who didn't show evidence of spastic disease. I was shown some data just very recently by Edward Hart that suggested that the response does occur in dogs if one instruments the animal and waits for a long period of recovery, as though something about the acute preparation in the animal diminishes the sensitivity. I am not sure that this is altogether correct, but the studies that Steve Vatner and colleagues are doing in instrumented animals may show a broader range of vessel reactivity, perhaps to the ergots as well.

Dr. Winbury: Well, I think we have to separate the two responses in terms of an increase in tone versus the actual production of something that resembles spasm. I do not know if one is an extension of the other. The point you bring out is well taken and I think we have to keep in mind that the two (vasoconstriction and spasm) may be different.

Dr. Kirk: True, but I still think that the large vessel constriction is a good beginning model to study spasm. That was the reason in fact in that the study that we, Dr. Foreman and I, did using ergots. We thought we were going to develop a model for testing drugs that might be antispastic but we just couldn't get the ergots to constrict. I think if one had a good response to ergonovine, one might be able then to work into testing for effective anticoronary spasm drugs.

Dr. Smith: A comment and a question for Dr. Aiken. First, when you are considering the local formation of PGI_2, I don't think you have to limit it to the local formation of prostacyclin because the amount of prostacyclin that you would have to form to get a hypertensive effect in your dogs is much more massive than I think you would see in your protocol here.

I think possibly also you should look at increases in cyclic AMP with PGI_2 as cyclic AMP levels might be falling by the time you assay your platelets for cyclic AMP. So you may be having a significant prostacyclin formation but not enough to see any physiological effects. The question I have is concerning your thromboxane synthetase inhibitor. I was wondering if you have looked at any other thromboxane synthetase inhibitors, for example, amysole, and if you get similar results with that.

Dr. Aiken: We have looked at a few related compounds that behave similarly in this model, but none of them were imidizole-like compounds, so I can't comment on that. Your initial comment is true. It is possible that there is a small increase in circulating PGI_2, perhaps released from lung, but the increase in circulating prostacyclin, if it occurred, could not account for the prevention of blockage of the coronary artery in our model. We know that even threshold doses of prostacyclin, infused at 15 ng/kg/min, which have only a marginal affect on the rate of aggregation in the coronary artery, will cause a detectable increase in cyclic AMP levels and about a 5-mm Hg drop in blood pressure. So, although what you say is true, it can't explain the action on the drug in our particular model. We feel it is local production that is important.

Dr. Winbury: These of course are very elegant experiments, but I am wondering how do they differ from some of the earlier and perhaps simpler studies using peripheral blood vessels or intact rats where occluders were put in or filters were put in. Is there anything particularly unique about the coronary bed in your type of preparation?

Dr. Aiken: No, this particular technique can be done on other blood vessels in which there is not a substantial amount of collateral flow. For example, you can measure an aggregating response in renal artery but it is very difficult to obtain in the femoral artery because you can't really get rid of reactive hypermia. I think the unique thing about this study is being able to distinguish quantitative differences in efficacy between cyclooxygenase inhibitors and prostacyclin or any other substance that elevates cyclic AMP in the platelets. The other techniques that, for example, have shunts with artificial surfaces do not allow you to do this sort of study where you can look at the importance of local production of prostacyclin. There are not many ways of monitoring platelet aggregation in vivo where the aggregation is occurring on the vessel wall as opposed to some other artificial surface. I think this is a particularly good method.

Dr. Maseri: I wish to compliment you on having been able to achieve such nice standardization of the model that allows you to test these interventions so carefully. I wondered if you don't flip the vessels, does the vessel remain occluded or does it spontaneously open up?

Dr. Aiken: No, it will usually not spontaneously open up. The heart usually fibrillates.

Dr. Maseri: It will close and the dog will fibrillate?

Dr. Aiken: Yes, but we usually don't wait that long. But it does happen occasionally. There are some animals in which the aggregates are always spontaneously shed, and we have wondered if perhaps that is due to local prostacyclin production. It is probably not; if we topically apply a prostacyclin synthetase inhibitor, we cannot convert spontaneously shed aggregates to ones having to be shaken loose. In those particular cases, and I emphasize that there are not many of them, if that is due to prostacyclin, it must be due to some other circulating prostacyclin, but it is not local production. It is for that reason that we think the blood vessel normally is not making enough prostacyclin to prevent the platelet from aggregating and blocking the vessel. Now, we acknowledge that this is a very severe model, we have set up so that it is a very severe stimulus for aggregation. But we feel that under normal conditions the blood vessel doesn't make enough prostacyclin to prevent it from being completely occluded.

Dr. Gould: The tracings you showed, showed a regular release every 4–5 min. Did you flick it then every 4 or 5 min?

Dr. Aiken: Yes. Every time there is an "SL" above the record, we shook the aggregate loose by sliding the obstructor up the artery and then placing it back.

Dr. Gould: Why is it that a beating heart, which is usually pretty violent, couldn't open the artery up? Is there something about your finger?

Dr. Aiken: No. We actually move the obstructor away from the place where the thrombus has formed and then move it back, and that allows the blood to sweep the thrombus away.

Dr. Gould: But the blood flow doesn't change because you haven't taken it off, right?

Dr. Aiken: Correct. But what we have done is to allow the vessel to expand by moving the obstructor away, and I think that dislodges the thrombus. The thrombus is small in relation to the normal lumen diameter of the vessel. When we slide the obstructor away, I think that is enough to dislodge it.

Dr. Gould: The Japanese group, as you and Folts know, thinks that effect is peripheral. Just for the purpose of discussion maybe you would like to get back to the basic model. With the concentrations that you used, you may be affecting distal vasculature even though locally applied, particularly with 5-min cycles. With that tight a stenosis, the instability of the peripheral vascular bed and critical closure, I am a little uncomfortable with the model. What are your comments?

Dr. Aiken: Let me elaborate just a little bit. We of course were very concerned with that when we first started, that either the response might be due to vascular effect or be influenced by vascular effects. The types of things that we have done to try and rule that out are the following. Regarding the downstream vascular bed, the vessel is obstructed to the point where there is no longer any reactive hyperemic response, so we are assuming that now the point of greatest resistance to flow is at the obstructor, and any further reduction in lumen size at that site would cause reduction in flow. Now, as I mentioned earlier, we can drip prostacyclin on the vessel upstream of the obstructor and prevent aggregation. If we drip prostacyclin just downstream from the obstructor, there is no effect at all in the cyclical flow pattern. Just as much prostacyclin would be absorbed through the blood vessel downstream from the obstructor as there would be upstream from the obstructor. Yet only upstream from the obstructor does it prevent the cyclical flow pattern. Well, then you might argue that the smooth muscle right under the obstructor can constrict or thin out. We took rings of circumflex coronary arteries and determined how much nitroglycerin it took to block contractions to angiotensin, norepinephrine or prostaglandin F2α, and then we used a great excess of nitroglycerin applied topically right on the vessel. That does not alter the cyclical decline of flow either. So, I don't think the blood vessels under our experimental conditions are in spasm and I don't think any further dilation is possible because of the restriction of the obstructor. The records I show are mean coronary flow so it isn't obvious how rapidly flow is restored when the aggregate comes loose. It is an almost instantaneous restoration of blood flow. I have never seen blood vessels dilate that way. The pattern of response and the effects of drugs on it are inconsistent with it being due to vasospasm or influenced by vascular effect drugs.

Dr. Berkowitz: Recently, from Olsson's laboratory, he published an abstract where, in patients with angina, he was able to block thromboxane synthetase completely using aspirin, yet angina was unaffected in the patients. Do you know that work, could you comment on it and what are your feelings on the importance of thromboxane in angina?

Dr. Aiken: Well, I am not exactly sure which abstract you are referring to. Angina is due to ischemia, but what is causing it could be multiple factors, and it may not be thromboxane dependent in all cases. Platelet aggregation can occur in blood vessels for a number of reasons. Platelets release not only thromboxane but serotonin and other substances that are going to affect the vasculature.

Dr. Wolf: If you poison the platelets before you create the constriction, in some manner, do you still get this phenomenon of repeated aggregation? In other words, if you pretreat with cyclooxygenase inhibitors or poison them in some other manner, by depleting the patient of platelets or just making them sick platelets, will you get the same phenomenon?

Dr. Aiken: It depends. I had a couple of dogs that were thrombocytopenic, and you can't get the cyclical declines in flow in those dogs. We have pretreated some animals with aspirin and with some difficulty you can get some response, but you have to really severely obstruct the vessel. Under the normal degree of obstruction, you would not get an effect.

Dr. Wolf: There has been a large debate in clinical medicine on whether you can help patients, if you will, by giving them aspirin long term. The model that you create would have hopefully suggested that if you had a tight stenosis and you gave such patients aspirin, that you could prevent a total occlusion. However, it is difficult to produce this aggregation over and over again. I am a little despondent in that this model may not depict the same kind of problem we see in patients.

Dr. Aiken: I think the results with aspirin for prevention of reinfarction are rather disappointing. I don't know the cause of that. Our model would suggest that aspirin treatment, with a relatively mild degree of obstruction, would suppress platelet aggregation and prevent blockage of the vessel. However, under more severe stenosis, it may not prevent platelets from occluding blood vessels. For example, we found that efficacy of cyclooxygenase inhibitors was dependent on degree of obstruction. This is somewhat consistent with the observation that aggregation induced by shear forces cannot be blocked with the cyclooxygenase inhibitors, even though the release reaction is blocked. So, one might hypothesize that the more severe the obstruction, the greater the shear effects on the platelet membranes. That type of stimulus for aggregation is not susceptible to inhibition by aspirin-like drugs.

Dr. Gould: When you look at the coronary arteries from humans externally and watch if they constrict or not, do you have any data on the geometric changes? Interestingly, you said that diseased coronary arteries in humans contract just as well as the normal arteries. Did you mean in terms of force development, or of circumferential shortening?

Dr. Ginsburg: In the muscle bath, I am measuring isometric tension generated by a ring segment, and not geometrical changes. The force generated by a ring segment decreases with the increase in amount of atherosclerosis. However, rhythmicity or spontaneous contraction and relaxation can be found in any ring segment regardless of the extent of atherosclerotic disease.

Dr. Gould: I don't quite understand that. We don't see rhythmic contraction of the vessel during arteriography. If you could extrapolate what that means, please?

Dr. Ginsburg: Rhythmicity will not be seen during arteriography for several reasons. First, the periods of rhythmicity are longer than the length of a coronary injection; second, renografin has potential dilating properties; and lastly, the changes may be too small to detect without the aid of computer imaging.

Dr. Gould: What is the time period in those fluctuations?

Dr. Ginsburg: Those are usually seen anywhere between 40 and 120 sec depending upon the physiological conditions.

Dr. Gould: If it is that periodic, one should see it during arteriography.

Dr. Ginsburg: Changes in coronary diameter can be seen during several repetitive coronary injections of the same vessel. This is best detected with the aid of computer-imaging techniques. I believe that if it is looked for, it can be found. However, the physiologic significance of this rhythmicity is unknown.

Dr. Beacon: You implied in the beginning of your talk that prostaglandins might be involved in some of your responses, but you didn't come back to that.

Dr. Ginsburg: It is possible and purely speculative that resting basal tone is mediated by prostaglandins. Receptor antagonists of histaminic, muscarinic or adrenergic receptors do not affect tone. However, the addition of ibuprofen or indomethacin causes contraction. It is possible that these cyclooxygenase inhibitors are decreasing PGI_2 production, resulting in increased tone.

Dr. Kent: These rhythmic contractions you are talking about can be obtained in vitro with almost any animal species. In fact, in 1969 Biamino and Thron (Pfluegers Arch 305:361) said that this was a natural property of rat aorta, hung under the same conditions that you hung the human coronaries. These days, many people can hang rings of rat aorta and not get these oscillations, so a lot of it is in the preparation of hanging vessels. I can get rhythmic contractions with dogs, rat and even rabbit vessels, stretched excessively.

Dr. Ginsburg: It is possible. We have seen it rarely in dog and frequently in bovine coronaries and rabbit iliac, femoral and distal abdominal aortic vessels.

Dr. Kent: I was more interested because you were looking at norepinephrine causing calcium uptake in human coronary. Are you implying that norepinephrine does not cause any cellular calcium uptake in human coronary arteries?

Dr. Ginsburg: Norepinephrine does cause an increase in $^{45}Ca^{2+}$ uptake into the smooth muscle cell. This occurs at a different rate than that of potassium and this unidirectional uptake is not altered in the presence of calcium entry blockers (i.e., D-600 or diltiazem).

Dr. Watkins: Could you tell us if you have had the opportunity to try thromboxane A_2 and angiotensin in this system and if so, could you tell us what calcium pools they mobilize?

Dr. Ginsburg: We do not have a system to generate thromboxane A_2 or its analog, carbocyclic thromboxane A_2, and therefore we have not performed any studies with it. I have used angiotensin on one occasion to demonstrate that it can contract the segments, but have not studied it further. I assume it triggers the same calcium pools as any other vasoactive agent.

Dr. Watkins: In responding to the previous question, you indicated that norepinephrine in the human coronary artery, unlike many other vascular smooth muscle preparations, was an incomplete agonist and caused a minimal amount of contraction. Could you rank the contractile response to the agonist? Ordinarily we think of norepinephrine and histamine as being full agonists in a rabbit or rat aorta followed by perhaps acetylcholine, and angiotensin comes in around two-thirds' worth.

Dr. Ginsburg: Norepinephrine and histamine are complete agonists operating through specific receptors. In the human coronary, histamine=carbachol>norepinephrine>serotonin>ergonovine.

Dr. Pepine: Have you had the opportunity to study the coronary arteries of anybody with angiographically documented spasms? If so, what are the changes in rhythmic contractions in the coronary areas where the spasm was observed angiographically?

Dr. Ginsburg: Fortunately or unfortunately, we have not studied anyone with documented coronary spasm in the in vitro setting.

Dr. Greenberg: I would like to answer some questions that people have been asking about the prostaglandin effect on coronaries; and maybe illustrate a difference between what people call spasm and what may be just a contraction. We have been looking at bovine coronary arteries and have found that PGH_2, a coronary analog thromboxane agonist, causes a very nice contraction followed by these rhythmic contractions that you have shown. The rhythmic contractions are definitely calcium dependent. The contraction of the vessel is not. So that if you cause a contraction with the thromboxane agonist, it is not calcium dependent; the rhythmic contractions and relaxation that follow the contraction are.

Dr. Ginsburg: PGH_2 or U-44069 is one of the most potent agents we have studied. More interesting is that the tension generated by PGH_2 is due to intracellular Ca^{2+} release. Rhythmicity is only seen if Ca^{2+} is present in the physiologic solution.

Dr. Texon: Earlier in your presentation, you showed four sections of coronary arteries progressively becoming worse. You said that the interval in time was about 10 years? The implication that I got was that the severity of atherosclerosis is age dependent. Is that what you meant to say?

Dr. Ginsburg: Atherosclerosis is not age dependent. It can occur at any age, and probably begins at the time of birth. What is important is realizing that, unlike animal models, there is no such thing as a normal human coronary artery. What we are dealing with is gradations from mild to moderate to severe atherosclerosis.

Dr. Greenberg: Dr. Perhach, I would like to comment on your interpretation of the inhibition of the bradykinin bronchoconstriction and also on the clinical findings of nifedipine and exercise-induced asthma. I think that there is no doubt that the bradykinin-induced bronchoconstriction in the guinea pig is thromboxane mediated, probably through the activation of a calcium phospholipase. It is possible that a calcium antagonist would prevent the activation of the phospholipase, however, you would also have to consider that calcium also is necessary for smooth muscle contraction. Therefore, you would have to show that histamine or acetylcholine release is blocked in exercise-induced asthma, I looked at the clinical study reported on nifedipine and came to the conclusion that it wasn't due to the fact that the mediator release was prevented, but it was the bronchodilation effect on the smooth muscle.

Dr. Perlach: Perhaps we have overgeneralized. I agree with your concerns and comments.

Dr. Lentini: Dr. Ginsburg, did you notice any change in the response to the sensitivity of the coronary receptors as a function of the postmortem interval? Now, I know sometimes it is rather difficult to go ahead and get specimens within 30 min from the pathologist, so could you please clarify that particular problem?

Dr. Ginsburg: The coronary arteries for my studies are obtained from recipient hearts of patients within 1–2 min of removal of the heart from the patient. Although coronary segments from postmortem hearts will respond to various agents, I do not know if these are different from our experimental work. I doubt that $^{45}Ca^{2+}$ tracer studies could be performed on postmortem vessels because of the loss of membrane integrity.

Dr. Watkins: There is a great deal of information that is beginning to come out now that is telling us that there is more to conducting an experiment with vascular smooth muscle, than just taking a strip, hanging it up and adding the drug. What I am referring to is some of the complex relationships that the endothelium seems to have in the response to the drug, and this refers to something of the work done by Dr. Kirschner and Dr. Van Hooten. I just wonder in your characterization of the response, the vascular smooth muscle of human origins, have you tried to assess that question by rubbing off the endothelium and that sort of thing?

Dr. Ginsburg: No, we have not studied the influence of the endothelium on the contractile responses of the human coronary.

Dr. Watkins: I realize that work is just beginning and you have a unique opportunity of studying this particular kind of muscle. Just curious though, can you get acetylcholine-induced relaxation?

Dr. Ginsburg: No, acetylcholine or carbachol always cause contraction in human coronary ring segments.

Dr. Walinsky: I have a question for Dr. Aiken. You mentioned two of the three possible therapeutic modalities related to the thromboxane and prostacyclin interaction. That is, prostacyclin and thromboxane synthetase inhibitor; I wondered if you have any experience with a thromboxane receptor-blockade compound.

Dr. Aiken: No, I haven't worked on them myself. There is one epoxyamino analog in PGH_2 that has been reported by Fitzpatrick to be a receptor antagonist of thromboxane on platelets. That compound, however, had no antagonistic properties on blood vessels. Our main interest was in blood vessels, and in that preparation it behaved like an agonist. That tells us something immediately. The receptors for thromboxane in platelets are different from the receptors for thromboxane in blood vessels. But it didn't help us in receptor analysis of thromboxane-like compounds on blood vessels. We don't have any other receptor level antagonists.

Dr. Wendling: One of the difficulties in working with prostacyclin and cyclooxygenase is that they are rapidly inactivated. Are there prostaglandin analogs that could be used that would be longer lasting such as longer lasting prostaglandin constrictors or relaxants? I guess another question is, could prostaglandin F2α or prostaglandin E_2 be used in lieu of thromboxane A_2 or prostacyclin?

Dr. Aiken: Several compounds that have been used are 9,11-substituted analogs of PGH_2. These are stable substances (unlike the PGH_2) analogs; pharmacologically they behave a lot more like thromboxane. I am not sure are true thromboxane analogs. One of the things that we have done with these compounds is to look at the effect of removing calcium from the Krebs solution on the ability of these substances to contract arteries and compared that to what happens with real thromboxane A_2. If you leave calcium out of the Krebs solution, PGH_2 analogs still give you a full maximum response, whereas you greatly attenuate the response to authentic thromboxane. So there is at least suggestive evidence that, although these compounds are very potent vasoconstrictors (in fact they are more potent than authentic thromboxane), the mechanism by which they contract vascular smooth muscle is different from the mechanism involved with thromboxane. The second part of the question, regarding whether $PGF_2\alpha$ would substitute for thromboxane, I don't think that is known yet. We don't have the antagonists needed to prove those points. Dr. Ginsburg referred to high doses of prostacyclin-contracting arteries. If you look at a vessel such as, for example, the rat aorta, every prostaglandin will contract the rat aorta at some concentration. I think that there is at least one contractile receptor that all the prostaglandins may interact with at some dose. So when you see contractions to PGE_2 and $PGF_2\alpha$ and prostacyclin, it is very likely that they each have a weak agonist effect on the thromboxane receptors. In the rat aorta, we calculated the ED_{50} for authentic thromboxane; it is around 3×10^{-9} M. Interestingly, the epoxymethano analog of PGH_2 is five to six times more potent than that.

Dr. Winbury: There is one question I want to pose regarding the calcium entry blockers in general. We are seeing more and more of them coming on the horizon. I am posing this question to anyone on the panel; are they going to all exhibit the same general profile or therapeutic modality? Or can the calcium entry blockers be directed to different areas or regions of the body?

Dr. Perhach: I will make one brief comment. I think the hope exists that there is some relative degree of selectivity for vascular smooth muscle. There are some indications that the chemistry can be rearranged to further direct its activity; this remains to be seen.

Dr. Ginsburg: There is not enough time for an in-depth discussion of calcium entry blockers, but several points should be emphasized. Although the soon-to-be released drugs verapamil, nifedipine and diltiazem belong to the pharmacologic class called calcium entry blockers, their mechanism of action as well as adverse side-effects are all very different. Unlike beta-adrenergic blockers, which differ very little from one another, each of the calcium entry blockers differs to the extent that each one will be used for specific indications. Thus calcium blockers will be for the 1980s what the beta-blockers were for the 1970s.

Section III

Etiology of Coronary Artery Disease

K. Lance Gould, *Chairperson*

The Hemodynamic Basis of Coronary Atherosclerosis

Meyer Texon

Introduction

Application of the laws of fluid mechanics to the natural conditions in the circulatory system reveals a rational and demonstrable basis for the localization, inception and progressive development of atherosclerosis. Atherosclerosis does not occur at random locations. It does occur uniformly at specific sites of predilection that can be precisely defined, predicted and produced by applying the principles of fluid mechanics. The areas of predilection for atherosclerosis are consistently found to be the segmental zones of diminished lateral pressure produced by the forces generated by the flowing blood. Such segmental zones of diminished wall pressure are characterized by tapering, curvature, branching, bifurcation or external fixation (Figs. 1–5). Although these anatomic configurations occur in many variations of geometry, their common feature is a pattern of flow conducive to the production of localized areas of diminished lateral pressure. This is the initial stimulus. Atherosclerosis may therefore be considered the reactive biological response to the effect of the laws of fluid mechanics, namely, the forces (diminished lateral pressure) generated by the flowing blood at sites of predilection determined by local hydraulic specifications in the circulatory system.

Reports from this laboratory beginning in 1957 (Texon, 1957; 1960; 1963; 1967; 1971; 1972; 1973; 1974; 1976a,b; 1980) have described the prerequisite hydraulic conditions and basic laws of fluid mechanics that are relevant to the development of atherosclerosis in the circulation. Character-

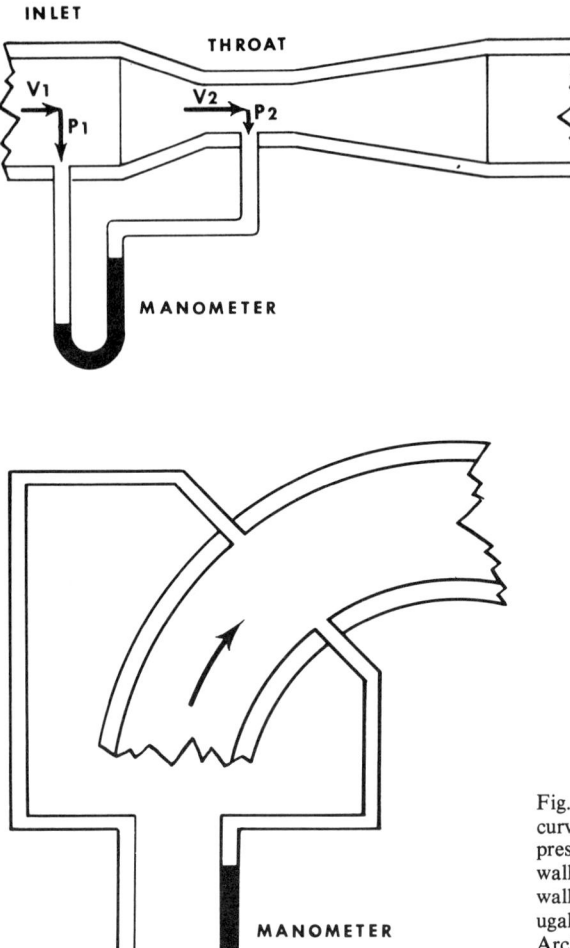

Fig. 1. Venturi meter. Flow in a tube with converging boundaries causes the lateral pressure to be reduced at the narrow portion where the velocity is increased. Bernoulli's theorem states that the sum of the pressure and the square of the velocity times $\rho/2$ is constant if fluid flows from Point 1 to Point 2 on the same streamline. (From Texon, M. 1957. Arch Intern Med 99:418–427, copyright 1957, American Medical Association; reproduced with permission.)

Fig. 2. Elbow flow meter. In curvilinear motion, the lateral pressure is increased along the outer wall and decreased along the inner wall, owing to the effective centrifugal force. (From Texon, M. 1957. Arch Intern Med 99:418–427, copyright 1957 American Medical Association; reproduced with permission.)

istics of blood flow in arteries, flow patterns and certain theoretical calculations have been identified (Texon et al., 1960; 1962; 1965). In addition, hemodynamically induced atherosclerotic lesions in dogs have been produced by the surgical alteration of vascular configurations under controlled conditions (Texon et al., 1962). The naturally and experimentally produced lesions in dogs and the naturally occurring lesions in humans have been illustrated and analyzed both pathologically and mathematically. The localization and atherosclerotic changes are demonstrated to be due consistently to the same

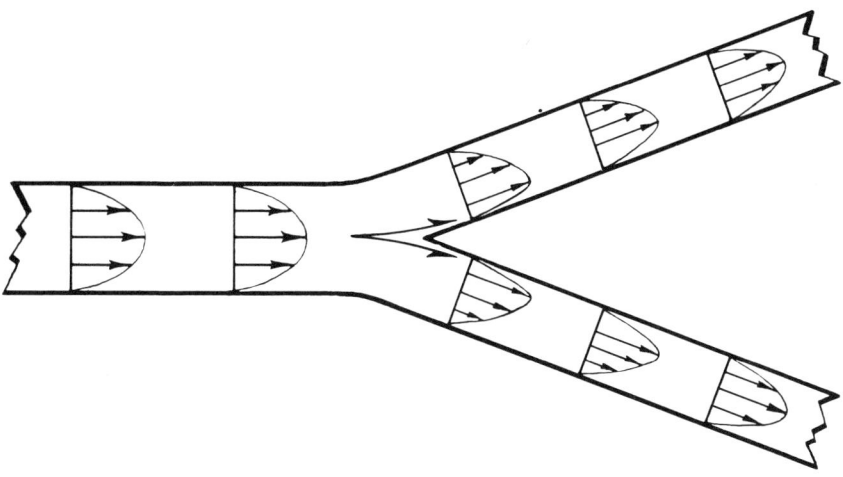

Fig. 3. Velocity distribution for streamline flow along a tube and bifurcation. The velocity of flow at a cross-section of a tube increases from the wall toward the center. Division of the axial stream results in a relative increase in velocity and a decrease in lateral pressure at the medial walls, due to the local curvatures required of the streamlines. (From Texon, M. et al., 1960. Arch Surg 80:47–53, copyright 1960, American Medical Association; reproduced with permission.)

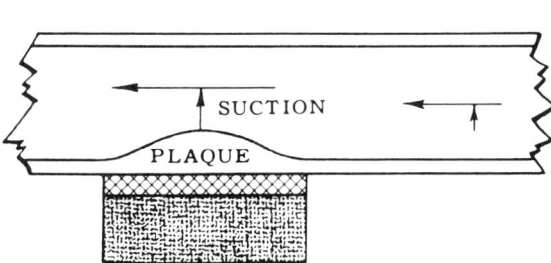

Fig. 4. Effect of diminished lateral pressure at zone of external attachment. The fixation resists the tendency of the flowing blood to move the wall of the vessel inward toward the axial stream. (From Texon, M. 1963. In *Atherosclerosis and Its Origin,* eds. M. Sandler and G. H. Bourne, pp. 167–195, New York: Academic Press, with permission.)

specific stimulus—the diminished lateral pressure—as determined by the characteristics of flowing blood and the local hydraulic conditions.

The localized decrease in static pressure at zones of predilection produces, in effect, a local suction action upon the intima at some phase of pulsatile flow in the cardiac cycle. The intima is subjected to the lifting or pulling effect of the flowing blood upon the endothelium and subjacent cells. The response is the logical biologic change, a reparative or reactive thickening, resulting from the proliferation of endothelial cells, fibroblasts and smooth muscle cells. With continuing blood flow, progressive changes occur in situ. These may include elastic tissue changes, cellular infiltration, collagen deposition, lipid changes, calcification and vascularization. The pathologic processes inherent in atherosclerosis may be stationary for long periods of time or slowly progressive. Relatively quick or sudden changes may also occur. Ulceration of an atherosclerotic plaque may result from lifting off or shearing off of the superficial layers. Blood elements may form a thrombus at the raw or ulcerated surface. The thrombus may enlarge to a partially occlusive or totally occlusive degree by the accretion of additional blood elements. The progressive pathologic process, by encroaching on the lumen, produces occlusive changes of all degrees that are the result of the biologic or cellular response to the continuing mechanical stresses at segmental zones of the intima, determined by the flowing blood and local hydraulic specifications.

Variations as well as similarities in the severity of atherosclerosis in different individuals and in different locations in the circulatory system of the same individual are principally due to differences as well as similarities in local hydraulic specifications (Fig. 6). These include the velocity of blood flow, the pattern of blood flow, the caliber of the lumen and the anatomical pattern or geometry. A biological factor must also be considered, namely, the local

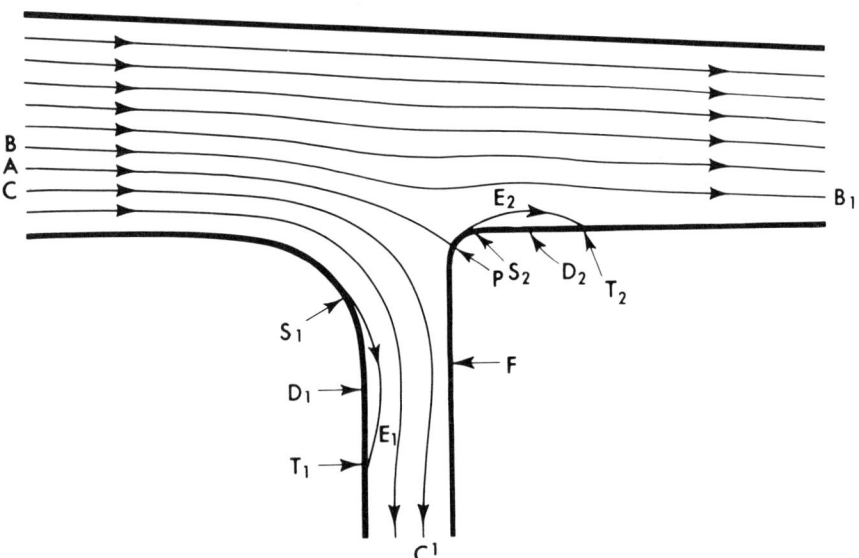

Fig. 5. Flow pattern at site of branching in a two-dimensional flow showing zones of low pressure and sites of atherosclerotic changes. Precise localization of the atherosclerotic plaque is determined by local hydraulic specifications, which include velocity of flow, angle of branching, ratio of diameter of main stem to diameter of branch and shape of ostial orifice. (From Texon, M. 1972. Bull NY Acad Med 48:733–740, with permission.)

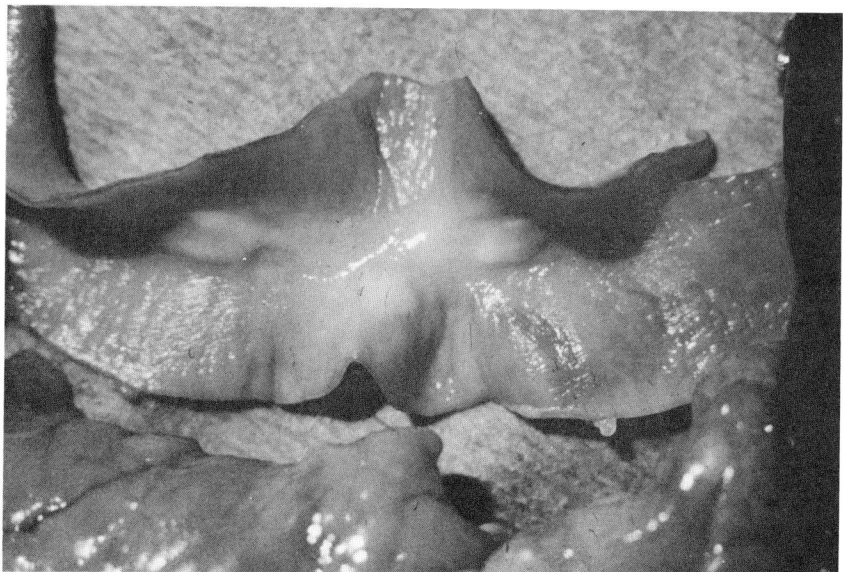

Fig. 6. Splenic artery—curvature lesions. Note the atherosclerotic plaque on each of three similar curvatures. (From Texon, M. 1963. In *Atherosclerosis and Its Origin,* eds. M. Sandler and G. H. Bourne, pp. 167–195. New York: Academic Press, with permission.)

reparative reaction or pathophysiological response of the intima to the diminshed lateral pressure generated by the flowing blood. It is here that the nature and degree of atherosclerotic change may be modified or influenced by differences in tissue structure and differences in tissue or cellular response arising from genetic and species characteristics.

In summary, all the data from human specimens, model hydraulic systems, the laws of fluid mechanics and experimental production of hemodynamically induced arterial lesions in dogs support the hemodynamic basis of atherosclerosis and compel the conclusion that the effect of the laws of fluid mechanics, vascular dynamics, is a major causative factor in the localization, inception and progressive development of atherosclerosis.

The Coronary Circulation

The precise correlation of atherosclerotic lesions with their localization at sites of predilection, namely, regions of diminished lateral pressure, in accordance with the laws of fluid mechanics, is demonstrated in the coronary circulation.

The coronary circulation is unique with respect to its hydraulic characteristics. The flow of blood is intermittent as a result of systolic contraction of the heart. The blood stream is subject to abrupt, rapid and wide fluctuations in velocity, with increased velocity and volumetric flow occurring during diastole, and reduced velocity and volumetric flow occurring during systole. Retrograde or reversal of flow under certain conditions also occurs. The coronary arteries are unique in the body with respect to such wide phasic variations in blood flow. It is notable that the caliber of the extramural coronary arteries tapers rapidly. The anatomic curvatures inherent in the coronary circulation are also notable. The composite effects of these hydraulic factors (namely, the rapid changes in velocity of flow, the nozzle effect of tapering and the inherent anatomical curves) are significant factors in the predisposition of the coronary arteries toward atherosclerotic changes.

Pathological examination of coronary arteries reveals uniformly that the atherosclerotic process develops at sites of predilection that are determined by local hydraulic conditions. A free and straight vessel presents correspondingly more concentric atherosclerotic change (Fig. 7). The forces generated by the flowing blood in a zone of curvature determine a greater degree of involvement of the inner (convex) wall compared to the outer (concave) wall (Fig. 8). The free epicardial aspect of a coronary artery may be less affected by atherosclerotic change than the tethered or attached surface. The reduced lumen at the site of atherosclerosis due to curvature or attachment is, of necessity, eccentrically placed. A frequent finding is a segmental lesion or atherosclerotic plaque involving the left coronary artery beginning approximately 1 cm from its origin at a zone where it curves and forms the left anterior descending branch. This is aptly described as a "waterfall" lesion.

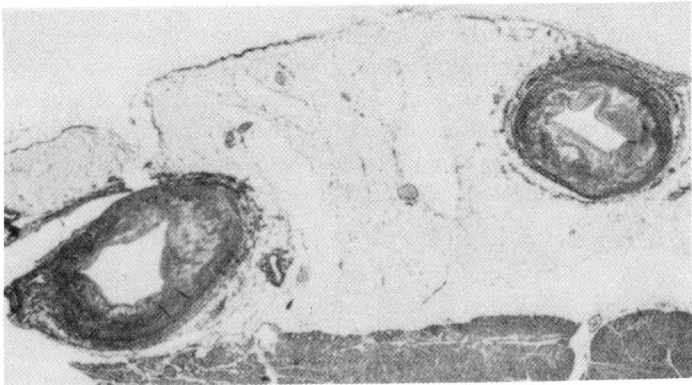

Fig. 7. Coronary atherosclerosis showing concentric occlusive disease in relatively free and straight portions of left anterior descending branches. (From Texon, M. 1957. Arch Intern Med 99:418–427, copyright 1957, American Medical Association, reproduced with permission.)

Implications

Atherosclerosis, beginning with the intimal proliferation, is an ongoing process that appears in utero as soon as blood begins to flow in definitive channels. The continuous operation of local hydraulic forces throughout life makes progressive pathological changes inherently possible. Atherosclerotic lesions are consistently found at sites of predilection at all ages, and the severity of the process does not bear a linear relation to age but rather to time in relation to local hydraulic specifications (Fig. 8).

Atherosclerosis, as a progressive arterial disease, and its pathological complications are a major cause of human illness, disability and death. Apart from localized dilating procedures, bypass operations and the replacement of surgically accessible diseased vessels, atherosclerosis, which affects all individuals in varying degrees, cannot be cured in the sense of curing or eliminating an infectious disease. However, I would suggest that we can minimize or retard the development of atherosclerosis by controlling the relevant hydraulic specifications that determine the development of atherosclerosis. It may be noted that not all the hydraulic factors that contribute to the development of atherosclerosis are of equal importance, nor are they all amenable to change, manipulation or control. Thus, the anatomic patterns, such as angles of branching, radii of curvature, attachments and calibers of lumens, are largely determined by hereditary and development. Similarly, the biological response of the intima to the stimulus of the hyraulic forces is probably determined by heredity as a racial, species or cellular characteristic.

In contrast to steady flow, which characteristically produces either a relatively constant compressional or tensile stress at a given site in a blood vessel, pulsatile flow is characterized by alternating compressional and tensile stresses. In a pulsatile flow, a high mean velocity, a high peak velocity, and a high rate of change of velocity may be more prone to promote the development of intimal proliferation and atherosclerotic change than a lower rate of flow, a lower peak velocity and a lower rate of change of velocity. In this sense, a pulsatile flow that can be made to approach the characteristics of steady flow may be less prone to produce atherosclerosis.

Modifications of the features of pulsatile flow that may be expected to retard the development of atherosclerosis are: 1) a slower pulse rate, 2) a slower rate of change of velocity from minimum to maximum, 3) a decreased peak velocity, 4) a decreased mean velocity and 5) a smaller range of blood velocity.

It may be noted that the velocity of blood flow is largely determined by the contractility or ejection force of the myocardium (vis a tergo) and the peripheral resistance. It should also be noted that velocity of flow is determined by the gradient—the difference in pressure between two points in a continuous system—not the absolute pressure. If there is no difference in

136 Section III Etiology of Coronary Artery Disease

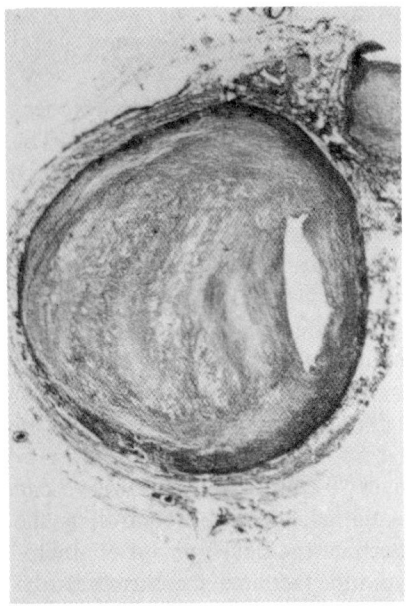

Fig. 8a. White female, aged 29 years.

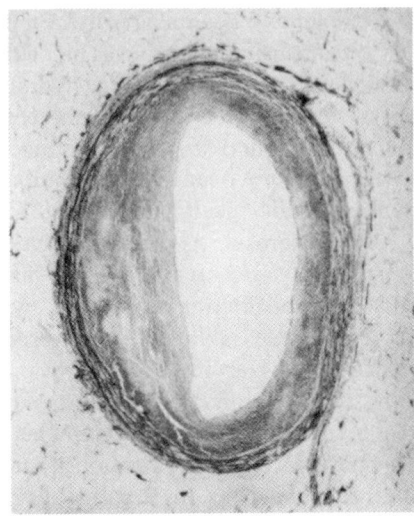

Fig. 8b. White male, aged 56 years.

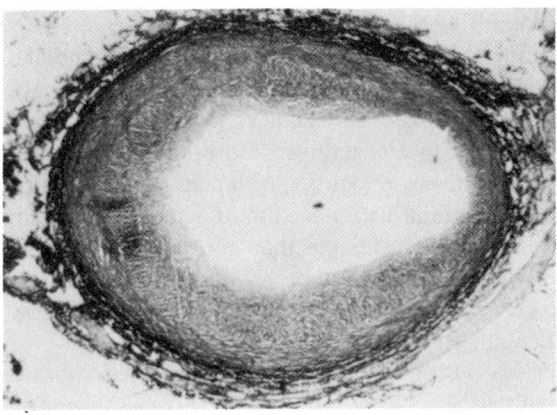

Fig. 8c. Black male, aged 5 months.

Fig. 8. Coronary arteries (L.A.D.) showing eccentric atherosclerotic disease in "curvature" lesions. Note that reduction in lumen by atherosclerosis does not bear a linear relation to chronologic age (see text).

pressure between two points, there is no flow, regardless of the absolute pressure present.

A promising area of specific research lies in the study of the velocity of blood flow. An increase in blood velocity, if other factors remain unchanged, must produce more severe atherosclerosis (McAllister et al., 1960). A decrease in blood velocity, if achieved without impairing the metabolic requirements of vital centers or organs, may be expected to minimize or retard the development of atherosclerosis and its progressive pathological complications. A pharmacological or a physiological method may be found or developed to achieve this goal and consequently extend the human life span.

Acknowledgments

This project was supported in part by the Fan Fox and Leslie R. Samuels Foundation, the Swift Newton Research Fund, the Doctor and Mrs. Henry Raphael Gold Research Fund, the Therma and Alan Jones Research Fund, the Metzger-Price Research Fund, New York, NY, and National Institutes of Health Research Grant H-3590.

References

Imparato, A. M., Lord, J. W., Texon, M. and Helpern, M. 1961. Experimental atherosclerosis produced by alteration of blood vessel configuration. Surg Forum 12: 245–247

McAllister, F. F., Bertsch, R., Jacobson, J. and D'Allesio, G. 1960. The accelerating effect of muscular exercise on experimental atherosclerosis. Arch Surg 80:54–60

Texon, M. 1957. A hemodynamic concept of atherosclerosis with particular reference to coronary occlusion. Arch Intern Med 99:418–427

Texon, M. 1960. The hemodynamic concept of atherosclerosis. Bull NY Acad Med 36:263–274

Texon, M. 1963. The role of vascular hemodynamics in the development of atherosclerosis. In *Atherosclerosis and Its Origin*, eds. Maurice Sandler and Geoffrey H. Bourne, pp. 167–195. New York: Academic Press

Texon, M. 1967. Mechanical factors involved in atherosclerosis. In *Atheroslerotic Vascular Disease*, eds. Albert N. Brest and John H. Moyer, pp. 23–42. New York: Appleton-Century-Crofts

Texon, M. 1971. The role of vascular dynamics (mechanical factors) in the development of atherosclerosis. In *Coronary Heart Disease*, eds. Henry I. Russek and Burton L. Zohman, pp. 121–136. Philadelphia: Lippincott Co

Texon, M. 1972. The hemodynamic basis of atherosclerosis. Further observations: The ostial lesion. Bull NY Acad Med 48: 733–740

Texon, M. 1973. Vascular dynamics and the prevention of coronary heart disease. In *The Paul D. White Symposium: Major Advances in Cardiovascular Therapy*, ed. Henry I. Russek, pp. 116–119. Baltimore: The Williams and Wilkins Co.

Texon, M. 1974. Atherosclerosis—its hemodynamic basis and implications. In *Med Clin North Am—Symposium on Atherosclerosis*, ed. Mark D. Altschule, 58:257–269. Philadelphia: Saunders

Texon, M. 1976a. The hemodynamic basis of atherosclerosis. Further observations: The bifurcation lesion. Bull NY Acad Med 52:187–200

Texon, M. 1976b. The hemodynamic basis of atherosclerosis with special reference to physical exercise. In *Advances in Cardiology*, vol. 18, eds. Vesa Manninen and Pentti I. Hallonen, pp. 122–135. Basel: Karger

Texon, M. 1980. *Hemodynamic Basis of Atherosclerosis*. New York: Hemisphere, McGraw-Hill

Texon, M., Imparato, A. M. and Lord, J. W. 1960. Hemodynamic concept of atherosclerosis: Experimental production of hemodynamic arterial disease. Arch Surg 80:47–53

Texon, M., Imparato, A. M., and Lord, J. W. and Helpern, M. 1962. The experimental production of arterial lesions furthering the hemodynamic concept of atherosclerosis. Arch Int Med 110:50–52

Texon, M., Imparato, A. M. and Helpern, M. 1965. The role of vascular dynamics in the development of atherosclerosis. JAMA 194:1226–1230

The Pathogenesis of Atherosclerosis

Russell Ross

Introduction

Although coronary artery disease has been known and described for centuries, the pathogenesis of this disease process has been poorly understood. Consequently, the lesions such as those found in the coronary arteries have largely been regarded to represent a degenerative process. During the past decade, a different point of view has become accepted—namely, that the lesions of atherosclerosis begin as an intimal smooth muscle cell proliferative response that appears to go through several stages of evolution that culminate in the classic lesion of atherosclerosis, the fibrous plaque (Anonymous, 1971). These lesions go on to occlude the affected arteries, often with accompanying thrombosis. The recognition that the lesions are essentially proliferative rather than degenerative has stimulated the development of several new hypotheses of atherogenesis. Recently, many investigators have begun to study this problem by utilizing the concept that understanding the biology of the cells of the artery wall, coupled with factors associated with the initiation and promotion of cell proliferation, could lead to better understanding of the process of atherogenesis, and ultimately to its control and prevention.

With this in mind, at least three important hypotheses have been formulated concerning the etiology and pathogenesis of atherosclerosis. These are discussed briefly together with new data concerning the biology of the four cells that principally interact in this process: endothelium, smooth muscle, platelets and the blood monocyte. With this data a clearer picture is developing of how this disease process comes about, and possible steps have been accepted that may lead to its prevention. The three hypotheses that are considered in this review are the lipid infiltration hypothesis, the response-to-injury hypothesis, and the monoclonal hypothesis. Each of these hypotheses is in some way interrelated with the others, and each has stimulated development of new information concerning the role of the different cells in the pathogenesis of atherosclerosis.

The Lipid Infiltration Hypothesis

This hypothesis is perhaps one of the oldest concerning the etiology and pathogenesis of atherosclerosis and was developed during the period when atherosclerosis was thought to be primarily related to the degree of hypercholesterolemia in individuals. From the outset, it has been associated with the capacity of investigators to induce atherogenesis by feeding animals high-fat, high cholesterol diets (Armstrong et al., 1966; Armstrong et al., 1974; Mahley et al., 1975; Manning and Clarkson, 1972; Scott et al., 1967; Vesselinovitch et al., 1971).

Simply stated, the hypothesis that suggests lipids somehow filter through the endothelium and accumulate in the intima. These lipids are thought to be associated with the subsequent cellular changes that are found in the disease. A modern version of this hypothesis has been developed as a result of the recognition that many of the lipoprotein subfractions present in plasma do not contain cholesterol, nor are they equally atherogenic. In addition, some hyperlipoproteinemias can result in experimental animals from diets that are not necessarily rich in cholesterol. The low density class of lipoproteins (LDL) has been shown to be most closely associated with atherogenesis in man as well as in experimental animals, although there is data to support the role of the triglyceride-rich lipoproteins: chylomicrons and very low density lipoproteins (VLDL) in atherogenesis as well. In contrast, the high density lipoproteins (HDL) somehow appear to be antiatherogenic or protective against atherosclerosis. The reasons for this protective effect, which has been observed in epidemiologic studies, are not well understood.

Most studies suggest that the clinical complications of atherosclerosis are related to the concentrations of LDL-cholesterol in given individuals. In persons who have a single gene defect that results in large increases in LDL in the plasma, the development of atherosclerotic lesions and their complications are greatly accelerated (Goldstein and Brown, 1977). This observation, coupled with the fact that atherosclerotic lesions can be experimentally produced in a number of different experimental animals by dietary increases in plasma LDL, provide a definite role for this lipoprotein in atherogenesis. The accumulation of lipids in atherosclerosis has been known for many years; however, the mechanism by which the lipoproteins induce atherosclerosis is not well understood. The observation that chronic hypercholesterolemia is somehow injurious to endothelial cells has provided a link between the lipid-infiltration hypothesis and the second hypothesis considered in this review, the response-to-injury hypothesis of atherosclerosis (Ross and Harker, 1976).

The Reponse-to-Injury Hypothesis

The response-to-injury hypothesis (Ross and Glomset, 1973; 1976) proposes that some form of "injury" to the lining endothelial cells results in a sequence of events that include intimal smooth muscle cell proliferation, new connective

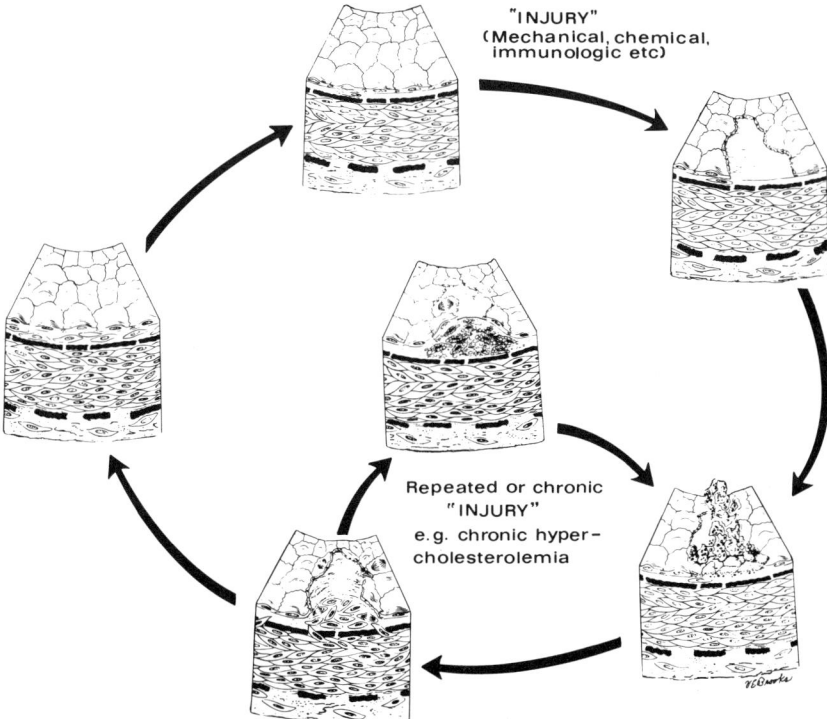

Fig. 1. In the response-to-injury hypothesis, two different cyclic events may occur. The outer, or regression cycle, may represent common single occurrences in all individuals in which endothelial injury leads to desquamation, platelet adherence, aggregation and release, followed by intimal smooth muscle proliferation and connective tissue formation. If the injury is a single event, the lesions may go on to heal and regression occur. The inner or progession cycle demonstrates the possible consequences of repeated or chronic endothelial injury, as may occur in chronic hyperlipidemia. In this instance, lipid deposition as well as continued smooth muscle proliferation may occur after recurrent sequences of proliferation and regression, and these may lead to complicated lesions that calcify. Such lesions could go on to produce clinical sequelae such as thrombosis and infarction.

tissue formation and accumulation of both intracellular and extracellular lipid that leads to the different forms of the lesions of atherosclerosis.

One of the most difficult aspects of this hypothesis has been to define the nature of the endothelial cell injury and to understand how this injury leads to the intimal smooth muscle proliferative lesions of atherosclerosis. (See Chapter 9 for further discussion of endothelial injury.)

Endothelial cells serve several functions in the artery wall. They act as a blood container, as a thromboresistant surface, as a permeability barrier and they form specific types of connective tissue, as well as several vasoactive substances. Injury to these cells may include alteration in their morphologic integrity as well as in their functional capacities, including their ability to provide a thromboresistant surface.

The hypothesis suggests that when endothelial structure or function are altered, interactions occur between elements from the blood, specifically platelets or monocyte/macrophages and the plasma, including lipoproteins, at sites of injury. These interactions lead to the migration of smooth muscle cells from the media of the artery into the intima, and to the subsequent proliferation of these migratory smooth muscle cells. During the process of smooth muscle proliferation, these cells form new connective tissue constituents and accumulate variable amounts of lipid in the cells as well as the connective tissue they have formed. The hypothesis as shown in Figure 1 states that if the injury is continuous or chronic, the lesions become progressive and ultimately enlarge to a point where they may lead to clinical sequelae. If the injury is delimited and healing occurs, the lesions may regress and remain clinically silent. A great deal of evidence has accumulated in relationship to this hypothesis and is briefly described below.

The Monoclonal Hypothesis

The third hypothesis of atherogenesis considered in this review is the monoclonal hypothesis of atherosclerosis. This hypothesis also assumes that the lesions of atherosclerosis are proliferative. Its unique aspect suggests that all of the proliferated smooth muscle cells in the lesions are derived from a single progenitor cell (Benditt and Benditt, 1973). If this is the case, the hypothesis goes on to suggest that the lesions are benign neoplasms with all of the implications that neoplasia might have upon the pathogenesis of the process, as well as its clinical outcome.

The data from which this hypothesis evolved was derived from observations of a series of atherosclerotic lesions taken from black females, at autopsy, who where heterozygous for the enzyme glucose-6-phosphate dehydrogenase (G-6-PD). In these studies the majority of the lesions of atherosclerosis appeared to contain one or the other of the isozymes of G-6-PD, whereas the normal artery wall was observed to be a mixture of the two isozymes. This approach is based upon an analysis of the monoclonality of neoplastic lesions such as leiomyomas of the uterus (Lindner and Gartler, 1965). All lesions that contain a single isozyme are not necessarily monoclonal (Fialkow, 1971). There are two mechanisms by which lesions could contain a single isozyme. The first of these could be due to the fact all of the cells in the lesion are derived from a single cell and are truly monoclonal; the second possibility is that the majority of the cells in the lesion contain the same isozyme as a result of a process of selection that had occurred over a period of many years involving lesion progression and regression resulting in a population of cells that were genetically identical, but which were derived from a population of identical cells and not from a single cell. Such a lesion would be monotypic. The potential relationship between these observations and those that led to the response-to-injury hypothesis are that many of the lesions of atherosclerosis could be of a single isozyme type based upon selection, whereas others may be truly monoclonal. Research concerning these hypotheses continues in terms of determining the relative importance of each hypothesis in the pathogenesis of atherosclerosis.

The Role of the Cells of the Artery Wall and the Blood in Atherosclerosis

The Endothelium

Each of the hypotheses of atherosclerosis has stimulated new research into the biology of the cells of the artery wall: endothelium and smooth muscle, and of two cells from the blood: the platelet and the monocyte.

Endothelial cells have been studied extensively during the past several years. It is now possible to grow arterial endothelium derived from cow, swine, human umbilical vein and nonhuman primate arteries in culture. The cells retain their capacity to grow in a single layer in culture, and to form prostacyclin (PGI_2), Factor VIII antigen and specific types of collagen (Jaffe et al., 1973; Gimbrone et al., 1974). Studies are underway to determine what happens to endothelial cells after they have been injured mechanically and to elucidate the factors that control the growth of these cells in culture, as well as in vivo. Recently, it was discovered that arterial endothelial cells produce a growth factor in culture that is a mitogen for smooth muscle cells and fibroblasts, and that may potentially play a role in the process of atherogenesis (Gajdusek et al., 1980). Further understanding of the nature of endothelium, the basis for its thromboresistant characteristics and the means by which it controls arterial permeability, all of which can be studied in culture, should provide an opportunity to better understand how injury to endothelium and alterations in its functions may be associated with atherosclerosis.

Smooth Muscle

Arterial smooth muscle cells are the cells that proliferate within the intima of affected arteries. Like endothelium, these cells can be grown in culture, remain differentiated as smooth muscle and retain a number of functional characteristics associated with smooth muscle cells in vivo (Ross, 1971; Chamley-Campbell et al., 1980). They synthesize specific types of collagen in culture, and remain contractile under particular circumstances. If the cells are obtained for culture by a process of collagenase and elastase digestion of the media of the artery they are contractile, contain relatively large amounts of myosin and are nonresponsive to growth factors such as the platelet-derived growth factor (Chamley-Campbell et al., 1981). If they are then placed sparsely in culture, the cells lose their contractility and their myosin over a period of 7–9 days. After this period they become susceptible to mitogens such as the platelet-derived growth factor, and undergo extensive proliferation if they are exposed to this factor. It has been suggested that the cells in the media of an intact artery are in a density-inhibited, contractile, refractory state; whereas after smooth muscle cells migrate into the intima of the artery in response to exposure to the platelet-derived growth factor, they modulate, lose their contractility and become susceptible to the mitogen. Understanding the nature of the smooth muscle cell and its response to different environmental factors should help us to comprehend the role of this cell in the process of atherogenesis.

The Platelet

The platelet may play an important role in the initiation and possibly in the progression of the lesions of atherosclerosis. Platelets have been observed adherent at sites of endothelial injury where the subendothelial connective tissue becomes exposed after a prolonged period of chronic hypercholesterolemia. After mechanical injury to the endothelium, platelets adhere and degranulate, releasing a number of substances including a potent mitogen, the platelet-derived growth factor (PDGF) (Ross et al., 1974). PDGF is extraordinarily potent. It has been purified to homogeneity. Five nanograms of pure PDGF will initiate a number of phenomena in susceptible smooth muscle cells, including DNA synthesis, increased cholesterol synthesis and LDL binding (Chait et al., 1980), increased pinocytosis (Davies and Ross, 1978) and increased connective tissue synthesis. After exposure to PDGF, smooth muscle cells under go multiple rounds of division. Of particular interest is a recent observation that this mitogen is specifically chemotactic for smooth muscle cells (Grotendorst et al., 1981). When platelets adhere at sites of endothelial injury, the chemotactic property of the released PDGF could attract smooth muscle cells to migrate in a gradient of increasing concentrations of PDGF. Thus, platelets, which are known to contain a number of substances including lysosmal enzymes, ADP and ATP, as well as anti-heparin activity, contain a mitogen that could play a critical role in the genesis of atherosclerosis.

The Monocyte/Macrophage

The other blood cell that has been implicated in atherogenesis is the monocyte/macrophage. Studies of human atherosclerosis have shown that monocytes are present in most lesions. In fibrous plaques these cells range in amount from 5–50% of the cells of the lesions. Together with the smooth muscle cells, they represent an important source of foam cells. The macrophage, which is derived from the peripheral blood monocyte, is capable of forming a large number of biological substances. The monocyte/macrophage can form a growth factor that is as potent as the mitogen derived from the platelets. It has been termed the monocyte/macrophage-derived growth factor (Leibovich and Ross, 1976). The role of this growth factor in atherogenesis, particularly in the progression of the lesions of atherosclerosis, remains to be established.

Summary

Thus, all three of the hypotheses of atherogenesis, the lipid infiltration hypothesis, the response-to-injury hypothesis and the monoclonal hypothesis, are each concerned with the intimal proliferation of smooth muscle cells, lipid accumulation within and around these cells and new formation of connective tissue by them. Each hypothesis attempts to explain the pathogenesis of atherosclerosis on a somewhat different basis. Each has provided an opportunity to enhance our understanding of the biology of the cells of the artery wall, as they interact with elements in the blood, in the etiology and pathogenesis of atherosclerosis.

Acknowledgment

The research presented in this review was supported in part by grants from the United States Public Health Service, AM 13970 and HL 18645.

References

Anonymous. 1971. Atherosclerosis: A Report by the National Heart and Lung Institute Task Force on Arteriosclerosis. (DHEW Publication No. [NIH] 72–219). Vol. 2. Washington, D.C: Government Printing Office

Armstrong, M. L., Lee, K. T., Pastori, S. et al. 1966. Atherosclerosis in rabbits: Architectural and subcellular alterations of smooth muscle cells in aortas in response to hyperlipemia. Exp Mol Pathol 5:273–310

Armstrong, M. L., Megan, M. B. and Warner, E. D. 1974. Intimal thickening in normocholesterolemic rhemus monkeys fed low supplements of dietary cholesterol. Circ Res 34:447–454

Benditt, E. P. and Benditt, J. M. 1973. Evidence for a monoclonal origin of human atherosclerotic plaques. Proc Natl Acad Sci USA 70:1753–1756

Chait, A., Ross, R., Albers, J. and Bierman, E. 1980. Platelet derived growth factor stimulates low density lipoprotein receptor activity. Proc Natl Acad Sci USA 77:4084–4088

Chamley-Campbell, J., Cambell, G. R. and Ross, R. 1981. Penotype-dependent response of cultured aortic smooth muscle to serum mitogens. J Cell Biol in press

Davies, P. F. and Ross, R. 1978. Mediation of pinocytosis in cultured arterial smooth muscle and endothelial cells by platelet-derived growth factor. J Cell Biol 79:663

Fialkow, P. J. 1971. The origin and development of human tumors studied with cell markers. N Engl J Med 291:26–35

Gajdusek, C., DiCorleto, P., Ross, R. and Schwartz, S. 1980. An endothelial cell derived growth factor. J Cell Biol 85:467–472

Gimbrone, M. A., Jr., Cotran, R. S. and Folkman, J. 1974. Human vascular endothelial cells in culture: growth and DNA synthesis. J Cell Biol 60: 673–684

Goldstein, J. L. and Brown, M. S. 1977. The low-density lipoprotein pathway and its relation to atherosclerosis. Ann Rev Biochem 46:879

Grotendorst, G. R., Seppä, H., Kleinman, H. K. and Martin, G. R. 1981. Attachment of smooth muscle cells to collagen and their migration toward platelet-derived growth factor. Proc Nat Acad Sci USA 78:3669–3672

Jaffe, E. A., Nachman, R. L., Becker, C. G. et al. 1973. Culture of human endothelial cells derived from umbilical veins: Identification by morphological and immunologic criteria. J Clin Invest 52:2745–2756

Leibovich, S. J. and Ross, R. 1976. A macrophage-dependent factor that stimulates the proliferation of fibroblasts in vitro. Am J Pathol 84:501–513

Linder, D. and Gartler, S. M. 1965. Glucose-6-phosphate dehydrogenase mosaicism: Utilization as a cell marker in the study of leiomyomas. Science 150:67–69

Mahley, R. W., Weisgraber, K. H., Innerarity, T. et al. 1975. Swine lipoproteins and atherosclerosis: Changes in the plasma lipoproteins and apoproteins induced by cholesterol feeding. Biochemistry 14:2817–2823

Manning, P. J. and Clarkson, T. B. 1972. Development, distribution, and lipid content of diet-induced atherosclerotic lesions of rhesus monkeys. Exp Mol Pathol 17:38–54

Ross, R. 1971. The smooth muscle cell. II. Growth of smooth muscle in culture and formation of elastic fibers. J Cell Biol 50:172–186

Ross, R. and Glomset, J. A. 1973. Atherosclerosis and the arterial smooth muscle cell. Science 180:1332–1339

Ross, R. and Glomset, J. A. 1976. The pathogenesis of atherosclerosis. N Engl J Med 295:369–377 & 420–425

Ross, R., Glomset, J., Kariya, B. et al. 1974. A platelet-dependent serum factor that stimulates the proliferation of arterial smooth muscle cells in vitro. Proc Natl Acad Sci USA 71:1207–1210

Ross, R. and Harker, L. 1976. Hyperlipidemia and atherosclerosis. Science 193:1094–1100

Scott, R. F., Jones, R., Daoud, A. S. et al. 1967. Experimental atherosclerosis in rhesus monkeys. II. Cellular elements of prolifrative lesions and possible role of cytoplasmic degeneration in pathogenesis as studied by electron microscopy. Exp Mol Pathol 7:34–57

Vesselinovitch, D., Getz, G. S., Hughes, R. H. et al. 1971. Atherosclerosis in the rhesus monkey fed three food fats. Atherosclerosis 20:303–321

Discussion

Dr. Wolf: We note clinically two groups of patients. One group appeared to have stable angina for many years with multiple coronary lesions that didn't seem to progress immediately. The other group has a terrible course that goes very briskly, and yet on catheterization appears to have one lesion. Do you think the pathogenesis of these two types of coronary disease is the same? Secondly, the lesion you described appears to follow a predictable kind of course that should be going at a certain speed; and yet we note patients change their course quickly. Could you comment?

Dr. Ross: Obviously, my answer is going to have to be speculative. I think the factors that lead to lesion formation (and I am speaking in relation to the response-to-injury hypothesis) progress at a reasonably constant rate over a period of time, because of the flow characteristics and the shear stresses that Fry and his collaborators have described. Only in high shear areas does one get platelet adherence. Baumgartner has very beautifully shown that platelet adherence to the artery wall is directly related to the shear stress at that site, and the higher the shear the greater the tendency for adherence. The rheology is a complicated problem. Nevertheless, as lesions progress, the shear stress will change. There probably is a critical point (I think Dr. Brown has some data on this) where, as the lesions get larger, the shear stress changes. Then one could get to the point where platelet adherence and release and possibly monocytic attractions will become more pronounced conceivably, to a point where proliferative response would accelerate at a more rapid pace than previously. There are many factors, however, that could modify this. We know virtually nothing about the genetic susceptibility of the patient. Some patients are obviously more susceptible than others. What is the genetic basis of this? There are other factors that complicate this problem as well, because the rheology of the situation itself, things such as senescence in the proliferating cells. There are a lot of data that suggest the smooth muscle cells can only go through a limited number of doublings. The number of cells available to participate in this proliferative response is going to be critical. If the cells have not gone through too many doublings, the response can go on at a rapid pace. If the cells have undergone too many doublings, it is conceivable that the response may not be able to go much further.

Dr. Nanarday: You mentioned injury, but now we are seeing more and more angioplasty has been done. Yesterday, I was in the lecture where Dr. Grunzig showed that immediately after the dilation there is improvement in coronary circulation; and after 2 or 3 years, there is a much better looking coronary angiogram. Now we are producing injury by dilating the coronary. Is it possible that we are transferring the smooth muscle from intima back into the media, and is this why you see the rapid regression?

Dr. Ross: No, I think it would be very difficult to transfer the cells from the intima back into the media. I am not sure that after angioplasty one is seeing regression, but rather lack of further proliferation. Why one has lack of further proliferation is a very important question that has to be answered.

Dr. Bergey: Do calcium blockers have any effect on either proliferation or chemotactic response?

Dr. Ross: Calcium blockers in vitro certainly have an effect on proliferation. Calcium is a requirement of cell proliferation, calcium ions. Whether these agents would have such an effect in vivo remains to be seen. I don't think there are any data.

Dr. Bergey: But verapamil and nifedipine would block the proliferative response.

Dr. Ross: If they prevent calcium uptake by the cells, yes.

Dr. Simpson: There is a thrombocytopenic rabbit model with antibodies directed toward platelets that clearly implicates the platelet in the fairly complex atherogenesis beyond such a lesion that you describe here. Have you tested your antibodies to platelet-derived growth factor; and does it have a similar effect, a predictable effect on atherogenesis such as we see in the thrombocytopenic rabbit?

Dr. Ross: Well, of course, there are four models that have shown the platelets in vivo. Actually three. The thrombocytopenic rabbit that you already have implied was studied both at Moore's lab, McMaster and Spaet's Lab at Monteer. There are the studies that we have done with Harker with homocytopenia where one could pharmacologically inhibit platelet interaction and prevent the proliferation response. And then there is the group at Mayo who have shown in the Von Willebrand's swine that if platelet adherence is inhibited, one doesn't get a proliferate response and atherosclerosis; whereas normal animals develop atherosclerosis. In terms of the platelet-derived growth factor, the antibodies in cell culture completely prevent cell proliferation. Now, this is going to be a difficult experiment to do in vivo, because there are mouse antibodies. Monoclonal antibodies were made from mouse cells; and to inject into nonhuman primates or humans, the mouse antibody poses, as you immediately see, a number of problems. We have some hope to be able to test this, however, because it is now possible to make human-human hybridomas. These human-human hybridomas are in a very early stage of development in other laboratories. It is human platelet-derived growth factors

that we are attempting to make monoclonal antibodies against. But we can't use this mouse antibody in primates, and we do not have human-human hybridomas in the laboratory. We would like to be able to develop human-human hybridomas because we think it may be important. There are other ways of getting around this problem; but they are complicated, because they involve sandwich reactions and indirect means of studying the tissue. What one might do is use a radioimmunoassay to detect levels of PDGF in the circulation of the plasma of individuals, and this is something we do want to look at. My guess is PDGF won't be seen as elevated even after platelet release, because it is so sticky that it probably binds very rapidly to sites where it is released, which would make it a very effective means of function, but would not permit levels that one could detect that could be seen in circulation.
Dr. Aiken: Will cell proliferation be suppressed by prostacyclin? You implied that was true with any agent that had elevated platelet cyclic AMP. The second part of the question is: do you have any evidence or any approach to the problem of demonstrating that in vivo prostacyclin might suppress proliferation at these intramural sights?
Dr. Ross: We went through the data fairly rapidly, so let me go back and explain. It depends upon the state of modulation of the smooth muscle cells, as to whether they are affected by prostacyclin. If they are contractile cells, such as the cells in the media are, or if they are in high density in an early state of culture (I didn't go through all the details of how we get them in these two states of culture) then prostacyclin, because it is an adenylcyclase activator, maintains cyclic AMP high enough. If prostacyclin levels are high enough or cyclic AMP levels are high enough, the cells will remain in a contractile state and will be refractile to PDGF. On the other hand, if the cells are sparse and go through this modulation process, so they lose their contractility, then presumably (and this is now speculation) the sparse cells cannot generate sufficient PGI_2 to keep cyclic AMP levels high enough to maintain them in a contractile, refractile state; and therefore, they become susceptible. So it is clearly dependent upon the state of the cells. Once the cells get into a synthetic noncontractile state and go through multiple doublings, they become refractile to this; and then they remain continually susceptible to PDGF, and prostacyclin then does not appear to have an effect on this situation.
Dr. Aiken: That implies to me that in vivo there might be some reciprocal relationship between the vascular prostacyclin production and the platelets. Have you any evidence to suggest that would be true?
Dr. Ross: The notion that we are entertaining for the moment is that cells in the lesion are now quite different from the cells in the media. The cells in the lesion, depending upon the density and how many cell proliferations they have undergone, may be in a different state of susceptibility to PGI_2 and cyclic AMP and thus to PDGF compared to cells in the media, which would be refractile to PDGF and quite susceptible to prostacyclin. This idea is based

on observations of immunoflourescence and myosin content in lesion cells versus medical cells. Those are very preliminary observations, and we have a lot of work to do to determine whether, in fact, that is correct.

Dr. Gould: Dr. Ross, Malinow made the point that the atheromas often are uniformly covered with endothelial cells and that the ongoing injury in the development of the atheroma is opened to question, as a mechanism towards its progression. Could you respond to that?

Dr. Ross: Yes, some lesions are covered with endothelium; and I don't know how to respond to that statement that all lesions are uniformly covered with endothelium because in our hyperlipemic monkeys, after 2 years of hyperlipemia, many of the lesions still do not have endothelial coverage. We don't know if this is true earlier in lesion development. We obviously have no way of knowing in man whether the lesions are covered with endothelium because one can't perfuse and fix man; and the only way one can be absolutely certain about endothelial stability is if you have appropriate endothelial fixation under appropriate pressure conditions. That is not possible in man, so we may never have an accurate answer to this. In primates, there are lesions, however, that do have endothelium cover. Whether this relates to different phases of lesions, I don't know. But at the same time, I certainly don't want to leave you with an impression that all lesions depend on platelet interactions. I think there are many different factors and now we know that endothelial cells, particularly regenerating endothelial cells, also make a growth factor. The process of endothelial regeneration and its relationship to lesion progression has to be examined. That, certainly, is another area related to lesion formation.

Dr. Simpson: Question for Dr. Ross. Would you comment on the evidence that dipyridamole is useful in the homocysteine-induced lesion as an agent to reduce atherogenesis; and are there patient data that pharmacologic antiplatelet intervention is useful in terms of atherogenesis?

Dr. Ross: Well, unfortunately, the dipyridamole levels that we are using in homocysteinemic baboons are higher than one can use pharmacologically in patients. There were very high levels, and they were effective in our homocysteinemic baboons, probably because of the very high levels. Greg Brown and others have data to demonstrate that dipyridamole at the levels commonly used in man are not terribly effective, at least in preventing recurrence of a previous infarct. I don't think we have any data at all about the prevention of early infarcts, prevention of atherosclerosis per se. What one would hope for is that there are several levels of potential intervention, if one assumes that the hypothesis I presented to you has some merit; and I repeat, it is a hypothesis and not a fact. One presumes that one can intervene by protecting the endothelium; therefore, agents or means of protecting endothelium at the rheologic level or cellular level would be one mode of intervention. Agents that potentially would prevent platelet-blood vessel wall interactions at a second level—I think we don't yet have available an agent that

The Pathogenesis of Atherosclerosis   153

is terribly effective in that mode. Agents that will potentially inhibit the growth factor are still another area that might work. We now know that PDGF, and I didn't show you the data, is bound to a high affinity receptor on the surface of smooth muscle cells; therefore, a factor that would block the receptor binding is another potential area of intervention. At yet another level, one could somehow block the intracellular signals that relate to mitogens, once mitogenesis has been induced. So I think there are multiple levels of intervention that one needs to look for. Particularly, to answer your question directly, I don't think we have an effective antiplatelet pharmacologic agent.

Dr. Kiely: Dr. Ross, could you tell us anything more about the biochemical mechanisms of the platelet-derived growth factor in terms of the receptors, internalizations and any enzyme systems that turn it on; and is it feasible to interfere with these pharmacologically to inhibit the action of the growth factor?

Dr. Ross: Yes, we have a great deal of very preliminary data, which is in the process of being studied. I can tell you that the platelet-derived growth factor binds to a high affinity receptor on the surface of cells. This binding triggers a signal that does many things that I showed you this morning. In addition, a postdoctoral fellow, Linda Pike, working in Krebs' lab in collaboration with us, has already shown that within 60 sec after binding to the cell surface, a cyclic AMP-dependent protein kinase is activated that ends up in phosphorylation of tyrosine molecules in the membrane, which leads to a cyclic AMP-level alterations in the cell that lead to cell proliferation via DNA synthesis. But there are a number of very early events at the molecular level that we are only just beginning to understand. We have only been able to do these studies, and what I am telling you is only 6 weeks old, because we just obtained large levels of completely pure iodination platelet-derived growth factor. It took us 8 years to purify the protein, 2 years to make antibodies to it and about a year to to get pure material sufficiently well ionated so that we could begin studying with confidence the molecule at the cellular and molecular level. The next several years are going to be very exciting because we can now do all these studies; we have been literally working for 8 years to get to this point. Hopefully, over the next 2 years, studies at the cellular and molecular level will unfold; and then we can begin to ask questions to lead us to experiments that will ask how can we really attack this at cellular and molecular levels.

Section IV

Hemodynamic Consequences of Coronary Artery Disease

K. Lance Gould, *Chairperson*

Alterations in the Severity of Coronary Stenosis: Effects of Intraluminal Pressure and Proximal Coronary Artery Vasoconstriction

William P. Santamore and Alfred A. Bove

Introduction

With the advent of coronary angiography, some coronary artery stenoses were shown to rapidly alter their shape in response to vasoconstriction stimuli (Weiner et al., 1976; Schroeder et al., 1977; Curry et al., 1977). From postmortem examination, Maseri (Maseri et al., 1978) showed that part of the arterial wall in coronary stenosis could be normal and apparently able to contract. Conversely, if a coronary artery stenosis contains a normal segment, then that wall segment should also respond to changes in intraluminal pressure: as the pressure increases the radius would increase, and as the pressure decreased the radius would decrease. With a fixed underlying stenosis occluding part of the arterial lumen, these changes in vessel radius would greatly modulate the luminal area and thereby influence coronary blood flow. We examined the active (proximal coronary artery vasoconstriction) characteristics and passive (intraluminal pressure) characteristics of arterial stenosis using mathematical models, in vitro preparations and a closed chest animal model.

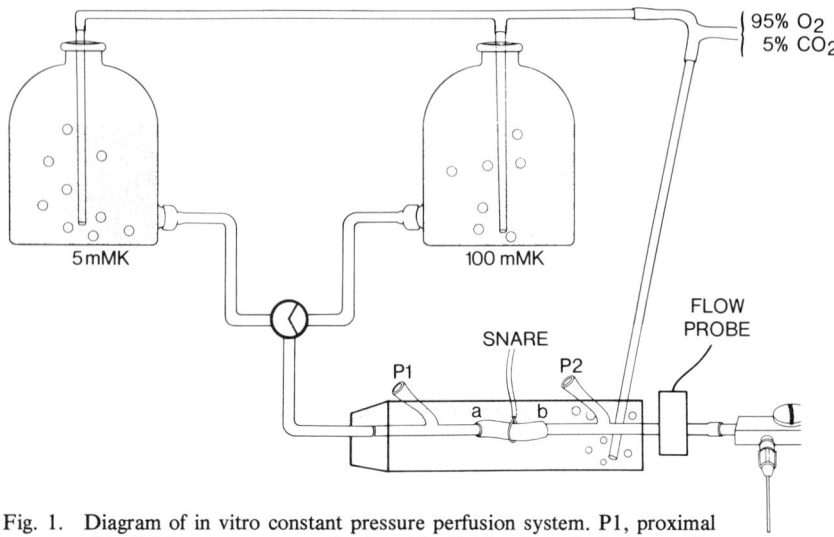

Fig. 1. Diagram of in vitro constant pressure perfusion system. P1, proximal pressure; P2, distal pressure; a, proximal and b, distal points of attachment for artery; and R1, 20-gauge Longdwel needle. (From Am Heart J 100:851–856, with permission)

Active Characteristics

The effects of proximal coronary artery vasoconstriction on stenotic hemodynamics were examined in an in vitro coronary artery preparation (Santamore et al., 1980). The proximal circumflex coronary arteries obtained from mongrel dogs were attached to the perfusion apparatus (Fig. 1). Figure 2 shows the effects of coronary artery vasoconstriction on pressure and flow in the artery. An initial stenosis was created with an external circumferential snare. With a 1.5 mM K physiologic salt solution perfusing the artery, the initial stenosis was established and allowed to stabilize. The perfusate was switched to a 100 mM K salt solution, indicated by the arrow in Figure 2. The 100 mM K solution was used to induce arterial vasoconstriction (Nakayama et al., 1978). As can be seen in Figure 2, maximum arterial vasoconstriction caused no observable effects on the flow through or the pressure across the stenosis produced by an external, circumferential snare.

For the same artery, Figure 3 shows the effects of coronary artery vasoconstriction on pressure and flow in a stenosis that was created with an intraluminal Grundzig balloon catheter. With a 1.5 mM K physiologic salt solution perfusing the artery, the initial stenosis was established and allowed to

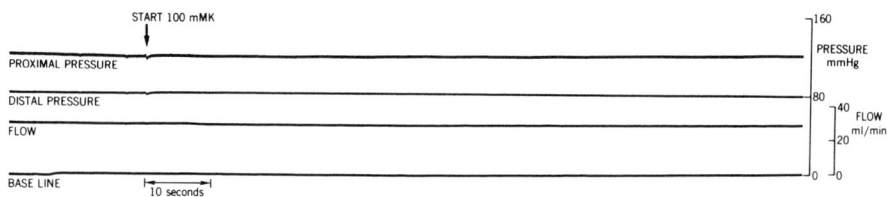

Fig. 2. Typical stenotic hemodynamic response to coronary artery vasoconstriction with an external circumferential snare.

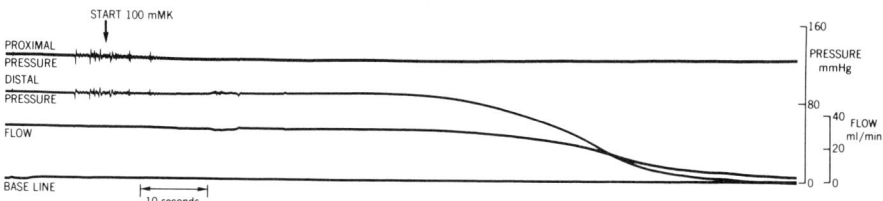

Fig. 3. Typical stenotic hemodynamic response to coronary artery vasoconstriction with an intraluminal obstruction.

stabilize. The perfusate was then switched to a 100 mM K salt solution. As can be seen in Figure 3, arterial vasoconstriction severely reduced the flow through and increased the pressure across the stenosis. Thus, stenosis created by internal obstruction was extremely sensitive to arterial vasoconstriction.

Table 1 summarizes the results from the eight coronary arteries studied. Table 1 is based upon 8 observations with no constriction, 16 observations with external constriction and 24 observations with internal obstruction. The diameter data are from two experiments. Before the creation of an arterial stenosis, vasoconstriction had no significant effect on the measured and calculated variables. Similarly, with arterial stenosis produced by an external circumferential snare, arterial vasoconstriction had no significant effect on the measured and calculated variables. In striking contrast, with the stenosis produced by an intraluminal balloon catheter, arterial vasoconstriction caused significant hemodynamic changes. Distal pressure, flow and distal diameter decreased and the stenoic resistance increased markedly. Thus, internal obstruction potentiated the effects of arterial vasoconstriction causing significant hemodynamic changes.

Table 1. Hemodynamic Effects of Coronary Artery Vasoconstriction.

Solution	Proximal Pressure (mm Hg)	Distal Pressure (mm Hg)	Flow (ml/min)
No Constriction			
1.5 mMK	94.7 ± 1.2	91.1 ± 1.3	31.1 ± 1.0
100 mMK	94.5 ± 1.6	90.5 ± 1.8	30.1 ± 1.4
External Constriction			
1.5 mMK	93.0 ± 1.8	68.4 ± 4.9	25.9 ± 2.0
100 mMK	93.5 ± 2.0	68.0 ± 5.3	25.5 ± 2.0
Internal Constriction			
1.5 mMK	94.9 ± 0.9	69.3 ± 4.9	27.1 ± 1.7
100 mMK	94.9 ± 1.0	18.2 ± 1.0	11.8* ± 2.0

All data values are mean ± standard error of mean.
*$P \pi 0.01$ compared to 1.5 mMK response by Student's t test.
From Am Heart J 100: 851–856, with permission

Passive Characteristics—Effects of Intraluminal Pressure

Mathematical Model

The coronary circulation was modeled as two resistors in series. R_d represents the resistance to flow offered by the coronary artery distal to the stenosis, while R_s represents the flow resistance of the stenosis. The pressure gradient ($\triangle P$) across the stenosis would be:

$$\triangle P = \frac{0.55 \times L_s \times Q}{A_s^2} + 3.76[\frac{1}{A_s} - \frac{1}{A_n}]^2 Q^2 \quad (1)$$

where Q is the flow; L_s is the length of the stenosis; A_n is the normal, unstenosed cross-sectional area; and A_s is the remaining luminal area by the stenosis (May et al., 1963; Young et al., 1975; Gould, 1978). A_s would be equal to:

$$A_s = \pi r_s^2 - \text{plaque area} \quad (2)$$

where r_s is the vessel radius by the stenosis. In turn, the vessel radius, r_s, was related to the pressure by the stenosis, P_s. For a rigid or noncompliant vessel (r_s independent of P_s):

$$r_s = d$$

Alterations in the Severity of Coronary Stenosis 161

Stenotic Resistance (mm Hg/ml • min⁻¹)	Distal Resistance (mm Hg/ml • min⁻¹)	Proximal Diameter (cm)	Distal Diameter (cm)
	2.94 ± 0.08	3.1 ± 0.3	
	3.00 ± 0.13	3.0 ± 0.3	
1.07 ± 0.25	2.66 ± 0.07	3.1 ± 0.1	2.9 ± 0.1
1.13 ± 0.28	2.68 ± 0.09	3.1 ± 0.1	2.9 ± 0.1
1.12 ± 0.29	2.52 ± 0.07	3.2 ± 0.1	2.9 ± 0.1
10.62* ± 2.86	1.76 ± 0.2	3.1 ± 0.1	2.0* ± 0.2

For a compliant vessel:

$$r_s = a(1 - e^{-cP_s}) + b$$

This is the approximate relation for normal vessels described by Cox (1976). According to the Bernouilli equation, P_s, the pressure by the stenosis, would be equal to or less than:

$$P_s < Q \times R_d \quad (3)$$

The total pressure-flow relationship would be:

$$P = \frac{0.55 \times L_s}{A_s^2} \times Q + 3.76 \left[\frac{1}{A_s} - \frac{1}{A_n}\right]^2 Q^2 + R_d Q \quad (4)$$

Using a digital computer, Equations 1, 2, 3 and 4 were used to calculate the flow through the vessel as the plaque within the vessel was gradually increased. For demonstration purposes, $a = 1.14$, $b = 1.0$, $c = 0.02$, $d = 2.0$ and $L_s = 1$ mm. So that at $P_s = 100$ mm Hg, $r_s = 2$ mm for both noncompliant and compliant vessels, at $P_s = 0$ mm Hg, $r_s = 2$ mm for rigid, noncompliant vessels and $r_s = 1$ mm for compliant vessels; and at $P_s = 200$ mm Hg, $r_s = 2$ mm for rigid vessels and $r_s = 2.12$ mm for compliant vessels.

Figure 4a shows the effects of plaque area on flow through the rigid vessel at two levels of distal resistance. With a high distal resistance, flow is not affected until approximately 92% stenosis, and flow falls rapidly with further stenosis. With a low distal resistance, the maximum flow is limited at much lower levels of stenosis. For a rigid vessel, decreasing distal resistance always increases flow, even at high levels of stenosis. In contrast, Figure 4b shows the effects of distal resistance on flow through a compliant vessel (r_s dependent upon P_s). With a high distal resistance, flow is not affected until approximately 78%

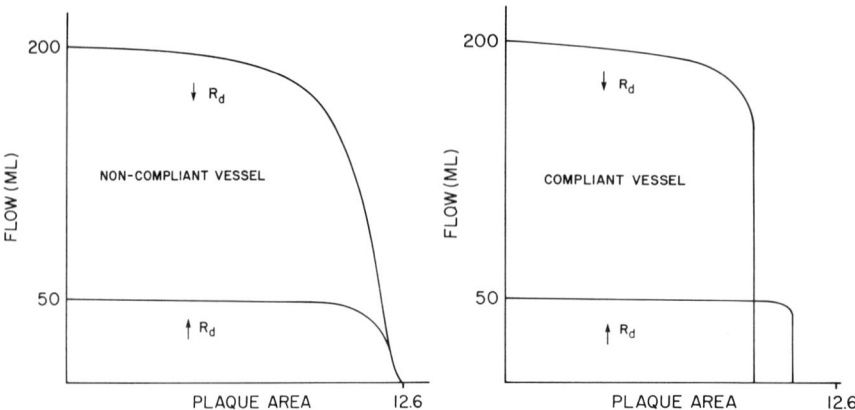

Fig. 4 a and b. Theoretical influence of distal resistance on flow through a stenotic vessel. ↑R_d, increased or high distal resistance; ↓R_d, decreased or low distal resistance.

stenosis. The flow then falls very rapidly with further increases in the underlying plaque. With a low distal resistance, flow is affected at a lower percent stenosis. Interestingly, with a low distal resistance flow goes to 0 with a smaller underlying plaque, as compared to a high distal resistance. In other words, theoretically with a compliant stenosis, flow can conceivably decrease in response to a reduction in distal resistance. This paradoxical response would only occur in a compliant vessel with a severe underlying stenosis.

Figure 5 shows the effects of perfusion pressure on flow. Three levels of perfusion pressure were examined: 50, 100 and 200 with a high distal resistance. The initial flow rates were normalized. As can be seen in Figure 5, in a rigid vessel, perfusion pressure had no effect on normalized flow: changing perfusion pressure has very little effect on the flow versus stenosis curve. In contrast, perfusion pressure has a profound influence of flow through a compliant vessel. Increasing perfusion pressure can re-establish flow, even with a larger underlying stenosis. Conversely, decreasing perfusion pressure caused the flow to decrease even with a smaller initial stenosis.

In Vitro Preparation

An in vitro preparation was used to verify the theoretical effects of distal resistance on flow through a compliant arterial stenosis. The in vitro preparation excluded alpha- and beta-adrenergic stimulation, reflexes, systemic blood pressure changes, pulsatile blood flow and pressure, collateral

Table 2. Constant Pressure-external Constrictor.

Distal Resistance (mm Hg/ml•min^{-1})	Distal Pressure (mm Hg)	Flow (ml/min)	Stenotic Resistance (mm Hg/ml•min^{-1})
Group A: Flow Increase			
5.03 ± 0.11	94.0 ± 2.7	18.7 ± 0.5	1.08 ± 0.17
2.47 ± 0.07*	74.1 ± 3.5*	30.1 ± 1.5*	1.37 ± 0.20
1.27 ± 0.04*†	49.4 ± 4.2*†	38.7 ± 2.9*†	1.78 ± 0.26*
0.70 ± 0.03*†	30.4 ± 3.7*†	43.1 ± 4.4*	2.12 ± 0.28*
Group B: Initial Flow Increase			
4.99 ± 0.05	77.3 ± 2.1	15.5 ± 0.4	2.40 ± 0.19
2.45 ± 0.03*	50.1 ± 2.2*	20.4 ± 0.8*	3.24 ± 0.24*
1.22 ± 0.02*†	25.1 ± 1.5*†	20.8 ± 1.4*	4.74 ± 0.43*†
0.73 ± 0.02*†	12.2 ± 0.9*†	17.0 ± 1.6	7.15 ± 0.95*†

All data values are mean ± standard error of mean.
*Change from control value significant at $P \leq 0.05$ by Wilcoxon test.
† Change from preceding value significant at $P \leq 0.05$ by Wilcoxson test.
From Am J Cardiol 45: 276–285, with permission

vessels and platelet plugging as potential causes of the stenotic resistance changes. In each study, after removal from anesthetized dogs, the carotid arteries were frozen, thawed, suspended in air and kept moist by externally applied saline solution. By design, therefore, only the passive characteristics of arterial stenosis were studied with the preparation. The carotid arteries were attached to a constant pressure perfusion apparatus (Santamore and Walinsky, 1980) and stretched to their original in vivo length. Table 2 summarizes the results of these experiments. Table 2 is based on 31 observations in five

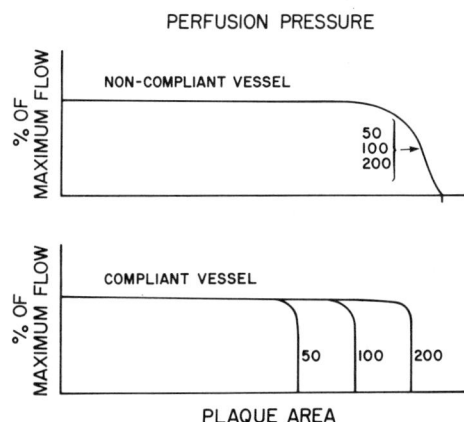

Fig. 5. Theoretical effects of perfusion pressure on flow through a stenotic vessel.

arteries. The mean perfusion pressure was 112.4 ± 0.2 mm Hg. On the basis of the flow response, the data were divided into two groups. In Group A, the flow always increased as the distal resistance decreased. In Group B, the flow initially increased as the distal resistance was decreased. With subsequent lowering of the distal resistance, flow decreased. The decrease in flow was due to the large increase in stenotic resistance. The initial stenotic resistance was significantly higher ($P \leq 0.05$) and the distal pressure significantly lower ($P \leq 0.05$) in Group B than in Group A. Thus, the data indicate that a severe stenosis (Group B) was required for flow to decrease as the distal resistance was decreased.

In Vivo Preparation

Lastly, the consequences of distal coronary arteriolar resistance on flow were studied in an intact, open chest anesthetized animal preparation. Catheters were placed in the aorta and the anterior marginal branch of the circumflex coronary artery. Additionally, a flow probe and snare occluder were placed on the circumflex coronary artery. Isoproterenol was used to induce distal coronary artery vasodilation, while methoxamine was used to induce distal coronary artery vasoconstriction (Santamore and Walinksy, 1980).

Isoproterenol

The typical response to intracoronary isoproterenol (1 μg) given before tightening the snare occluder is shown in Figure 6 (top). After the isoproterenol injection, there was a large increase in coronary flow subsequent to the decrease in distal coronary resistance. Heart rate also increased. After partial coronary arterial constriction, there was a strikingly different response to isoproterenol (Fig. 6, bottom). Coronary flow and coronary pressure now decreased and stenotic resistance and heart rate increased. The decrease in coronary flow was associated with a large increase in stenotic resistance.

Methoxamine

Figure 7 (top) shows the typical response to intracoronary methoxamine (500 μg) before tightening the snare occluder. After administration of methoxamine, coronary flow decreased, whereas distal coronary resistance increased. Figure 7 (bottom) shows for the same experiment the response to methoxamine after partial coronary occlusion. Methoxamine then caused a slight increase in coronary flow, an increase in coronary pressure, an initial increase in distal coronary resistance and a decrease in stenotic resistance.

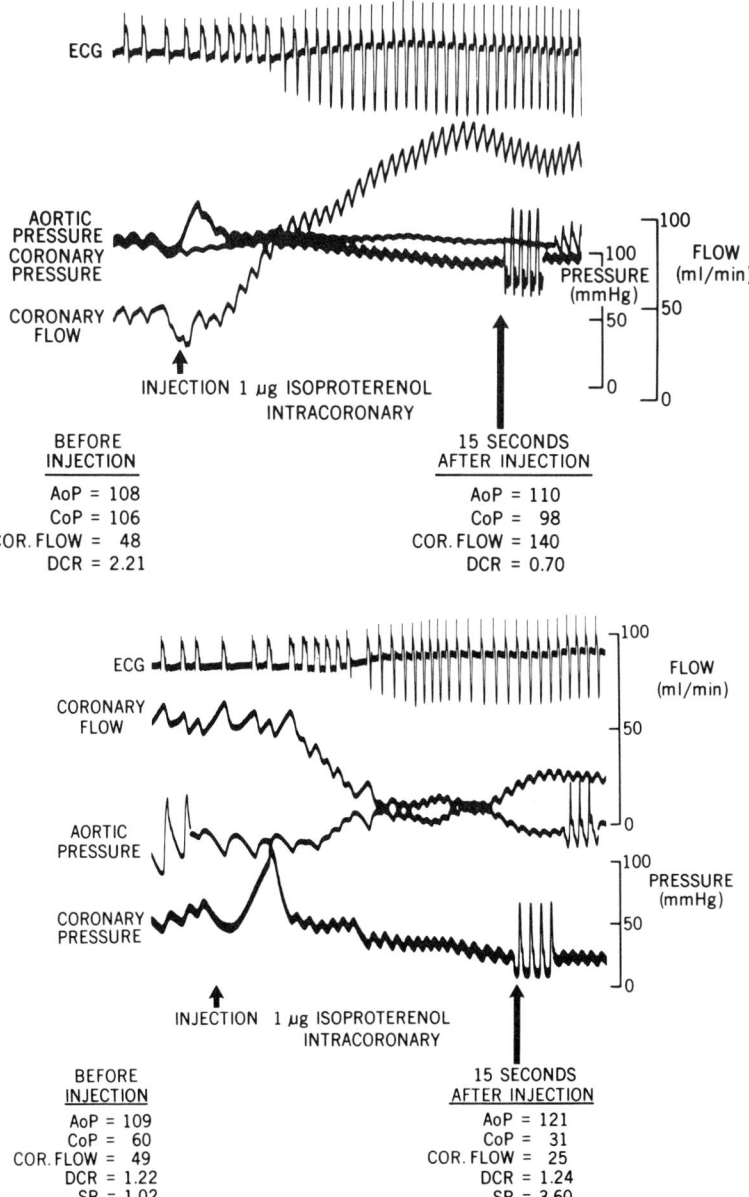

Fig. 6. The response of one experiment to intracoronary administration of isoproterenol (1 µg) before (top) and after (bottom) partial coronary artery occlusion. AoP, mean aortic pressure; CoP, mean coronary pressure; Cor. Flow, mean coronary blood flow; DCR, distal coronary resistance: ECG, electrocardiogram; and SR, stenotic resistance. (From Am J Cardiol 45:276–285, with permission).

Discussion

Traditionally, coronary artery stenoses were assumed to be fixed, rigid lesions that could not respond to changes in intraluminal pressure or proximal coronary artery vasoconstriction. However, with the advent of coronary angiography, the concept of all coronary artery stenoses being hard, fixed structures was no longer tenable. In this review, the influences of proximal coronary artery vasoconstriction and intraluminal pressure on stenotic hemodynamics were examined theoretically, and in in vivo and in vitro preparations. While obviously the mathematical model was too simplified to give quantitative results, the qualitative predictions were enlightening. The model predicted that, for rigid vessels, stenotic hemodynamic severity would not be influenced by perfusion pressure or distal resistance, while, in compliant vessels, stenotic hemodynamics would be greatly affected by perfusion pressure or distal resistance. The in vitro preparation confirmed the model prediction. In a carotid artery, distal resistance greatly modulated stenotic hemodynamic severity. Decreasing distal resistance increased stenotic resistance. In some experiments, flow paradoxically decreased after a decreased distal resistance due to the large stenotic resistance increase.

The theoretical predictions and in vitro observations were also confirmed in the in vivo preparations. Isoproterenol was used to selectively dilate the distal coronary arteriolar bed. Without an underlying stenosis, isoproterenol caused a large flow increase. In the presence of a severe, underlying stenosis, isoproterenol caused a paradoxical flow decrease. This flow decrease was associated with a large stenotic resistance increase. Conversely, methoxamine selectively constricted the distal coronary arteriolar bed (Santamore and Walinsky, 1980). Without stenosis, methoxamine decreased flow. In the presence of a severe, underlying stenosis, methoxamine caused a stenotic resistance decrease. In some experiments, this stenotic resistance decrease caused a flow increase. Thus, from a theoretical basis and from in vitro and in vivo preparations, intraluminal pressure was shown to affect stenotic severity. This effect was present in compliant, but not rigid vessels.

This study also demonstrated the striking hemodynamic effect of proximal artery vasoconstriction when a partial luminal obstruction is present. Neither the arterial vasoconstriction alone in the normal vessel, nor the stenosis alone caused a significant flow change; but when present together, they acted synergistically to produce a marked reduction in arterial lumen, a large pressure gradient and a significant reduction of flow (see Fig. 8).

This study would suggest clinically that in the presence of a severe underlying stenosis, with part of the arterial wall normal and able to contract, a vasoconstriction stimulus could cause a reduction in flow and myocardial ischemia.

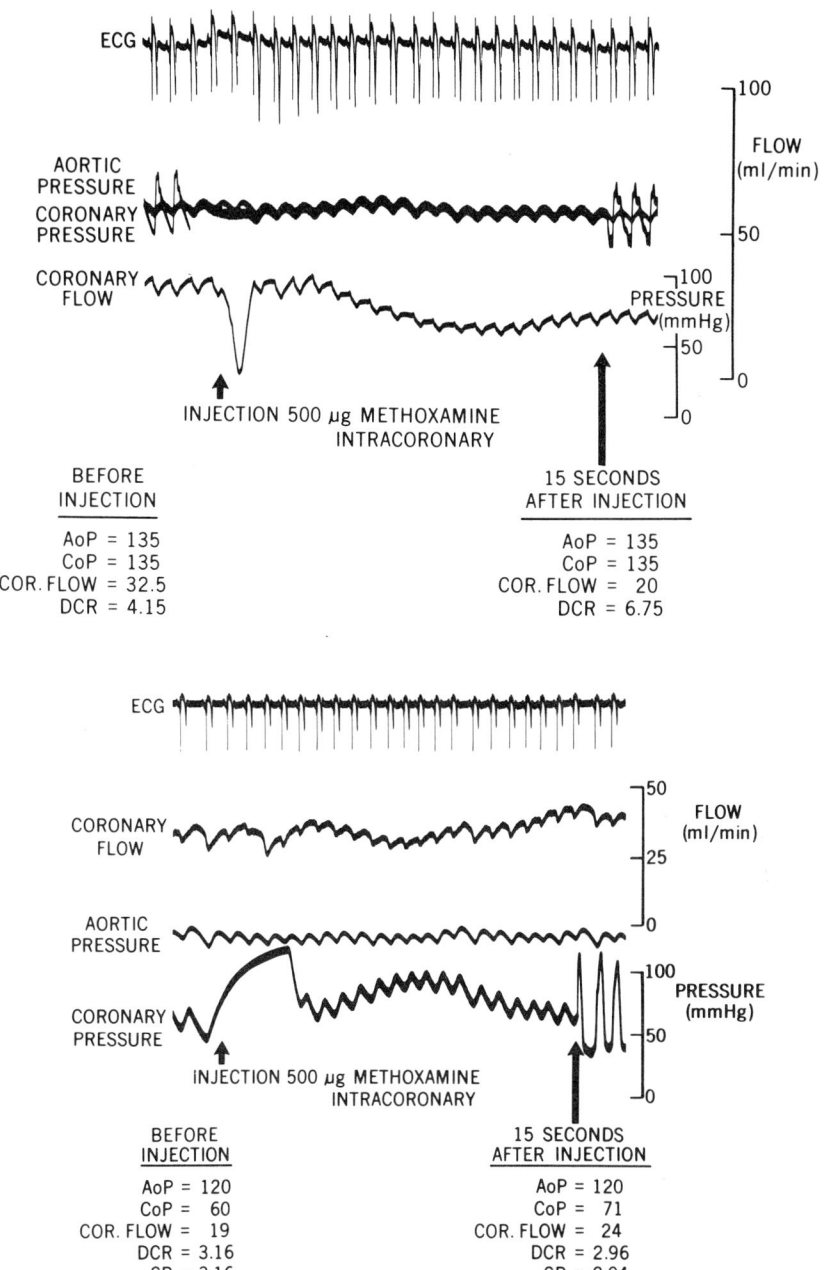

Fig. 7. The response in one experiment to intracoronary administration of methoxamine (500 μg) before (top) and after (bottom) partial coronary arterial constriction. Abbreviations as in figure 6. (From Am J Cardiol 45:276–285, with permission)

POTENTIATING EFFECTS OF STENOSIS PLUS VASOCONSTRICTION ON REDUCING FLOW

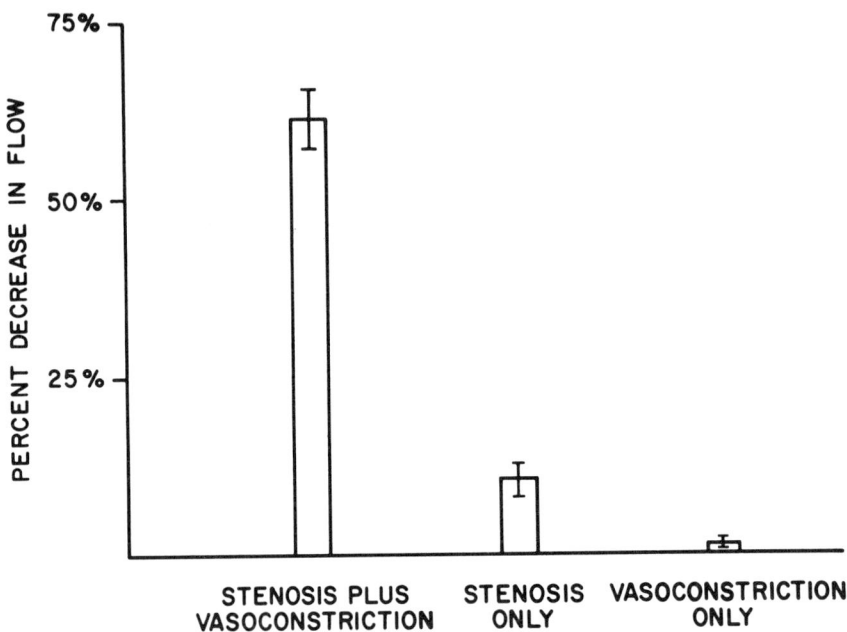

Fig. 8. Diagram showing synergistic effects of stenosis and proximal coronary arterial vasoconstriction on reducing flow. (From Am Heart J 100: 851–856, with permission)

Conversely, with partial stenosis created by a circumferential snare, subsequent arterial vasoconstriction had little effect on stenotic hemodynamics. One possible explanation for this lack of effect may be that the external snare had created a circumferential vessel fiber shortening to a maximal degree so that further shortening was impossible by vasoconstriction. This observation may be relevant to the clinical situation where, although two patients may have a similar degree of stenosis, only one patient will exhibit coronary artery spasm.

Theoretically, the dynamic changes in stenotic severity were caused by changes in geometry of the stenosis. As Gould (1980) points out, this view is supported by the observed stenotic resistance increase with a flow decrease in both the in vitro and in vivo preparations. Normal coronary arteries are known to change their geometry when intraluminal pressure changes or proximal coronary artery vasoconstriction occurs (Cox, 1976). In the presence of stenosis, distal coronary arteriolar vasodilation reduces the intraluminal pressure and thereby decreases the vessel diameter. Proximal coronary artery vasoconstriction also decreases the vessel diameter. In the presence of an underlying stenosis or plaque, the vessel diameter reduction could decrease the luminal area by the stenosis and thereby increase the hemodynamic severity of the stenosis. With an underlying stenosis of 80 or 90%, a 10% decrease in luminal area would greatly alter flow through the vessel.

In a previous study, an in vitro arterial preparation was used to analyze the stenotic geometry changes that occurred after distal dilation (Santamore and Walinksy, 1980). Microangiographic techniques were employed to measure the vessel diameter at the stenosis. Distal dilation increased stenotic resistance and decreased flow through the stenosed vessel. The distal dilation, by reducing intraluminal pressure, caused a decrease in stenoic luminal area. The change in stenotic geometry partially explained the increase in stenotic resistance (Santamore and Walinsky, 1980). We would speculate that the observed stenotic resistance increases after isoproterenol or proximal coronary artery vasoconstriction were also partially caused by a decrease in stenosis area.

Several experimental studies have demonstrated changes in stenotic resistance induced by intraluminal pressure reduction or distal coronary vasodilation. These studies reported either no increase or a decrease in blood flow through the stenosed vessel caused by vasodilation distal to the stenosis. This paradoxical flow response was associated with a large increase in stenotic resistance. Because the flow decreased, the stenotic resistance increases were postulated to be caused by changes in geometry of the stenosis.

Kreuzer and Schenk (1973) demonstrated an increase in stenotic resistance in the iliac artery caused by distal vasodilation. They believed that vasodilation altered the degree of stenosis by increasing the unstenosed cross-sectional luminal area. Previously, we demonstrated an increase in stenotic resistance caused by momentary coronary arterial occlusion (Walinsky et al., 1979) or drug-induced distal coronary arteriolar vasodilation (Santamore and Walinsky, 1980; Walinsky et al., 1980). Conversely, increasing distal coronary arteriolar resistance caused a stenotic resistance decrease. The stenotic resistance changes could be related to the distal coronary pressure and were caused, in part, by changes in stenotic geometry. Schwartz et al. (1979) observed similar changes in stenotic resistance after momentary coronary artery occlusion, and postulated that the increase in stenotic resistance was due to a passive decrease in the stenotic area secondary to the reduction of intraluminal pressure. In another study, Schwartz et al. (1980) further demonstrated the pressure dependency of coronary artery lesions. The aortic pressure was elevated by inflating a balloon in the ascending aorta. The rise in aortic pressure resulted in an increase in coronary blood flow through the stenosed coronary artery and a decrease in stenotic resistance. Conversely, lowering aortic pressure by bleeding the animal resulted in an increased resistance. These experimental observations could only be explained by a dynamic change in stenotic geometry, secondary to the changes in intraluminal pressure.

In human coronary arteries with eccentric lesions (a plaque on one side not completely surrounding the lumen), Logan (1975) also found that the resistance to flow was dependent upon the perfusion pressure. At lower perfusion pressures, the resistance increased, whereas at higher perfusion pressures, the resistance decreased. In unsedated dogs in which instruments were chronically in place, Gould (1978) observed dynamic increases in the hemodynamic severity of coronary arterial stenosis after coronary vasodilation. The increase in stenotic resistance after coronary vasodilation was believed to be due to the dilation of the epicardial artery adjacent to the stenosis, which caused more severe related percent narrowing and a larger divergence angle of the stenosis. However, Libscomb and Hooten (1978), using stenotic models, found that the pressure gradient across the coronary stenosis was not affected by varying the exit angle of the stenosis from 10°–90°. Dr. Brown, in Chapter 12, describes changes in luminal area by stenoses in patients after proximal coronary artery vasoconstriction (hand-grip) or distal coronary arteriolar vasodilation (dipyridamole). More studies appear to be necessary to determine the exact mechanism or mechanisms involved in the increase in stenotic resistance after a reduction in the distal pressure and the clinical significance of these passive changes.

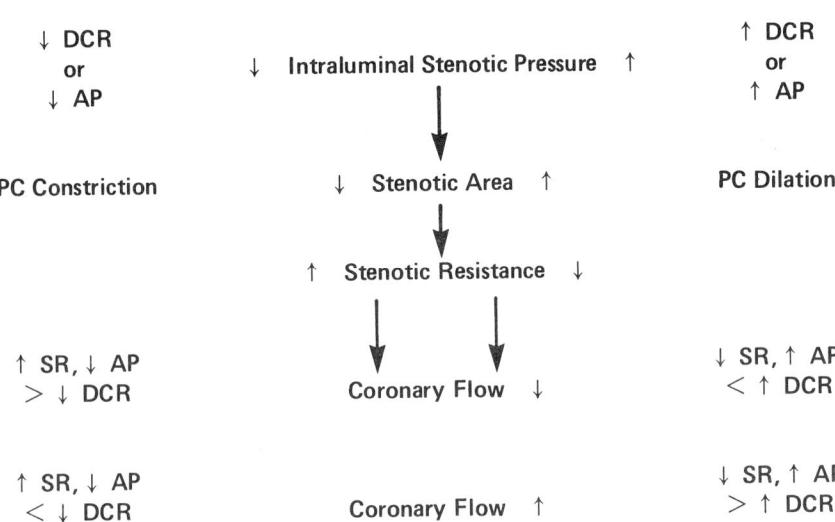

Fig. 9. Postulated mechanism for effects of distal coronary resistance (DCR), aortic pressure (AP) or proximal coronary artery (PC) vasomotor tone on coronary blood flow.

Figure 9 summarizes how distal resistance, aortic pressure and proximal coronary artery vasoconstriction may affect coronary blood flow. Decreasing distal coronary arteriolar resistance or aortic pressure decreases the intraluminal pressure; and in turn, causes a decrease in stenotic area. Proximal coronary artery vasoconstriction would directly reduce the stenotic area. This change in stenotic area would only occur in a compliant stenosis. The stenotic area decrease would increase the severity of the stenosis. Coronary blood flow would decrease if effects of reduced pressure or stenotic resistance increases were greater than any compensatory distal coronary arteriolar resistance changes. If the distal resistance were able to provide compensatory changes, the flow increase would be attenuated. Conversely, stenotic resistance would decrease with a distal coronary resistance increase, aortic pressure increase or proximal coronary artery vasodilation. Coronary blood flow would increase or decrease depending upon the interactions between the distal resistance, stenotic resistance and aortic pressure.

In summary, clinical and experimental studies have indicated that coronary arterial stenosis may be dynamic. If so, the coronary lesions could be influenced by aortic pressure, distal coronary arteriolar resistance and proximal coronary artery vasoconstriction. The interaction of these variables ultimately determines myocardial blood flow.

Acknowledgment

This work was supported in part by National Institutes of Health Grants HL 19425 and HL 26592.

References

Cox, R. H. 1976. Mechanics of canine iliac artery smooth muscle in vitro. Am J Physiol 230:462–470

Curry, R. C., Pepine, C. J., Sabom, M. B., Feldman, R. L., Christie, L. G. and Conti, C. R. 1977. Effects of ergonovine in patients with and without coronary artery disease. Circulation 56:803–809 56:803–809

Gould, K. L. 1978. Pressure-flow characteristics of coronary stenoses in unsedated dogs at rest and during coronary vasodilation. Circ Res 43:242–253

Gould, K. L. 1980. Dynamic coronary stenosis. Am J Cardiol 45:236–292

Kreuzer, W. and Schenk, W., Jr. 1973. Effects of local vasodilation on blood flow through arterial stenosis. Eur J Surg Res 5:233–242

Libscomb, K. and Hooten, S. 1978. Effect of stenotic dimensions and blood flow on the hemodynamic significance of model coronary arterial stenoses. Am J Cardiol 42:781–792

Logan, S. E. 1975. On the fluid mechanics of human coronary artery stenosis. IEEE Trans Biomed Eng 22:327–334

Maseri, A., L'Abbate, A., Baroldi G., Chierchia, S., Marzilli, M., Ballestra, A. M., Severi, S., Parodi, O., Biagini, A. Distante, A. and Pesola, A. 1978. Coronary vasospasm as a possible cause of myocardial infarction. A conclusion derived from the study of "perinfarction" angina. N Engl J Med 299:1271–1277

May, A. G., Van den Berg, L., DeWeese, J. A. and Rob, C. G. 1963. Critical arterial stenosis. Surgery 54:250–259

Nakayama, K., Fleckenstein, A., Byon, Y. K. and Fleckenstein-Gron, G. 1978. Fundamental physiology of coronary smooth musculature from extramural stem arteries of pigs and rabbits (electric excitability, tension development, influence of Ca, Mg, H and K ions). Eur J Cardiol 8:319–323

Santamore, W. P., Walinsky, P., Bove, A. A., Cox, R. H., Carey, R. A. and Spann, J. F. 1980. The effects of vasoconstriction on experimental coronary artery stenosis. Am Heart J 100:851–856

Santamore, W. P. and Walinsky, P. 1980. Altered coronary flow responses to vasoactive drug in the presence of coronary artery stenosis in the dog. Am J Cardiol 45:276–285

Schroeder, J. S., Bolen, J. L., Quint, R. A., Clark, D. A., Hayden, W. G., Higgins, C. B. and Wexler, L. 1977. Provocation of coronary spasm with ergonovine maleate. New test with results in 57 patients undergoing coronary arteriography. Am J Cardiol 40:487–497

Schwartz, J. S., Carlyle, P. F. and Cohn, J. N. 1979. Effect of dilation of the distal coronary arteries in the dog. Am J Cardiol 43:219–224

Schwartz, J. S., Carlyle, P. F. and Cohn, J. N. 1980. Effect of coronary arterial pressure on coronary artery stenosis. Circulation 61:70–76

Walinsky, P., Santamore, W. P., Wiener, L. and Brest, A. N. 1979. Dynamic changes in the hemodynamic severity of coronary artery stenosis in a canine model. Cardiovasc Res 13:113–118

Walinsky, P., Santamore, W. P., Wiener, L. Cho, S. Y. and Brest, A. N. 1980. Effect of epinephrine on coronary hemodynamics in coronary stenotic canine model. Am Heart J 99:494–502

Weiner, L., Kasparian, H., Duca, P. R., Walinsky, P., Gottlieb, R. S., Hanckel, F. and Brest, A. N. 1976. Spectrum of coronary arterial spasm. Clinical, angiographic, and myocardial metabolic experience in 29 cases. Am J Cardiol 38:945–955

Young, D. F., Cholvin, N. R. and Roth, A. C. 1975. Pressure drop across artifically induced stenoses in the femoral arteries of dogs. Circ Res 36:735–743

Hemodynamics of Coronary Stenoses

K. Lance Gould and Katharine O. Kelley

Introduction

A satisfactory hemodynamic analysis of coronary artery stenosis has been restricted by a number of conceptual and experimental problems. Visual interpretation of coronary arteriography is so variable that its usefulness is limited as an objective standard for measuring severity of coronary stenosis. Although quantitative coronary arteriography has been described (Brown, 1977), the validity of this technique has not been proven by comparison of x-ray predicted pressure flow characteristics to directly measured pressure flow characteristics of stenoses. Dynamic changes in coronary constrictions have also been reported (Kreuzer and Schenk, 1973; Gould, 1978, 1980; Logan, 1975; Swartz et al., 1979; Santamore and Walinsky, 1980; Walinsky et al., 1979; 1980) but the quantitative magnitude and importance of these changes have not been documented. Finally, in evaluating stenosis severity the relative usefulness of measuring coronary volume blood flow in cubic centimeters per minute versus coronary flow velocity in centimers per second, as in classical fluid dynamics, have not been established.

The purpose of this review is to summarize current solutions to these problems and our state-of-the-art understanding of the hemodynamics of coronary stenosis.

Methods

Basic Fluid Dynamics

The fluid dynamic equations for relating $\triangle P$ to coronary flow velocity or volume flow are:

$$\triangle P = \frac{8\pi\mu L}{A_s} \frac{A_n}{A_s} V + \frac{\rho k}{2}\left(\frac{A_n}{A_s} - 1\right)^2 V^2 \quad \text{or} \quad \triangle P = FV + SV^2 \quad (1)$$

$$\triangle P = \frac{8\pi\mu L}{A_s} \frac{1}{A_s} Q + \frac{\rho k}{2}\left(\frac{1}{A_s} - \frac{1}{A_n}\right)^2 Q^2 \quad \text{or} \quad \triangle P = fQ + sQ^2 \quad (2)$$

where P is pressure loss across the stenosis, μ is absolute blood viscosity, L is stenosis length, A_n is the cross-sectional area of the normal artery, A_s is the cross-sectional area of the stenotic segment, V is flow velocity, ρ is blood density, k is a constant related to the exit or divergence angle, here equal to 1, Q is volume flow, F and S are the coefficients of pressure loss due to viscous friction and exit separation in the velocity equation (Equation 1) and f and s are corresponding coefficients in the flow equation (Equation 2). The total pressure drop across a stenosis may be predicted by multiplying these coefficients as determined from x-ray geometry times a selected value of flow or flow velocity according to the equations on the right hand side above (Equations 1 and 2).

In the flow equation (Equation 2), $1/A_n$ is much smaller that $1/A_s$ for stenoses of modest to severe degree. Therefore, A_n, or the normal size of the artery, has little influence on severity of stenosis in the flow equation and therefore changes in the normal arterial diameter due to vasomotion have small effects on resulting pressure gradient. The effects of stenosis in the flow equation are dependent primarily on the absolute diameter of the stenotic segment, not on relative percent stenosis or diameter of the normal adjacent artery. However, severity of stenosis in the velocity equation (Equation 1) is highly dependent on relative stenosis as well as on absolute stenosis diameter, and the pressure gradient would therefore increase with vasodilation of the normal part of the artery in the presence of a fixed stenotic segment. In addition, both equations show that the pressure gradient across a stenosis increases sharply and in a progressive curvilinear fashion with increases in coronary flow. Therefore, the effects of a stenosis will be least at resting coronary flow and greatest at high flows.

Surgical Preparation

For the data presented subsequently, male field hounds weighing 22–28 kg were anesthetized with intravenous thiopental sodium and a mixture of nitrous oxide and methoxyflourane. The left circumflex coronary artery was dissected free from a sterile, left thoracotomy. A small tapered tygon catheter was implanted at the origin of the left circumflex artery for injection of contrast media in order to obtain coronary arteriograms and for measurement of proximal coronary perfusion pressure. A Doppler flow velocity transducer was placed around the left circumflex coronary artery distal to the proximal coronary catheter tip.

Distal to the Doppler transducer a saline-filled circumferential balloon constrictor was placed and a second tygon catheter was inserted in the distal main circumflex artery before major branches for measurement of coronary pressure distal to the constrictor. Dogs were treated with 100 mg of dipyridamole and 600 mg of aspirin for 2 days preoperatively and for 10 days after surgery to prevent formation of platelet clots on the catheters in the postoperative period. Catheters were flushed daily and filled with herapin.

The coronary catheter construction and implantation technique used in this laboratory have been described in detail previously (Gould, 1978; Gould et al., 1978).

Instrumentation

Instantaneous mean cross-sectional flow velocity in the circumflex artery was measured with a continuous wave directional Doppler (L and M Electronics) operating at 8–9MHz. The construction and calibration of the Doppler transducer has also been described previously (Gould,1978, Gould et al., 1978). These tranducers had a linear response from zero velocity up to 156 cm/sec (600 ml/min through a 3-mm I.D. tube) with maximum Doppler shifts of up to 12 kc and signal-to-noise ratios of 50:1–100:1.

Proximal and distal coronary pressures on either side of the constrictor were measured with Bio-Tec BT-70 pressure transducers and differential pressures were recorded simultaneously using a differential pressure gauge (National Semiconductor Corp., part no. Lx1701D) mounted in a plastic manifold to which the BT-70 transducers were also attached. Needle obturators, stopcocks and plastic parts were filled by immersion under sterile saline in a vacuum chamber to remove microscopic air bubbles and maximize frequency response. The response of the Bio Tec catheter manometer system was flat ($\pm 5\%$) to 15 Hz with debubbled saline, and that of the differential gauge with two simultaneous pressures applied to catheters used for implantation was flat to 30 Hz. For each experiment, pressure calibrations were recorded with 100-

mm Hg pressure applied by mercury column to the coronary and differential transducers at the beginning and end of each study.

ECG standard lead II, mean and phasic flow, proximal and distal coronary pressure and differential coronary pressure were recorded on an Electronics for Medicine DR 12 with a direct writer and on a Honeywell 7600 tape recorder for analog to digital computer conversion and subsequent analysis.

Coronary arteriograms were obtained by injecting radiopaque contrast media (Renografin-76) into the proximal coronary catheter while triggering exposure of a single spot film from the electrocardiogram in late diastole. The injection/x-ray sequence was automated and precisely controlled using a timing circuit triggered by the R wave from the ECG. The contrast medium was injected using a Thermodilution Injector 3700 (OMP Lab Inc.) modified with an energized solenoid connected to the output of the ECG channel. The injector was powered with compressed air regulated to inject the contrast medium through the catheter at a flow rate not exceeding the dog's coronary arterial flow. With this system, less than 2 cc of contrast medium produced adequate filling for visualization of the stenotic, the proximal and distal normal sections of the circumflex artery. X-rays were taken with a general Electric Maxiray 100 tube with a 0.3-mm focal spot, a 6.5° target angle and a 26-inch tube-to-film distance. Exposures were at 1/60 or 1/30 sec, 200 mA, at 90–116 kV using Ultra Detail, Cronex 4, Dupont 3 x-ray film and either Ultra Detail phosphor Radelain cassettes or Kodak X-Omatic cassettes with Regular intensifying screens. The entire system had a resolution of 11 lines pairs/mm or 215 line pairs/inch.

Protocol

The dogs were positioned on their right side for biplane x-rays. Some animals were lightly sedated with xylazine (1 mg/kg i.m.) to facilitate a stable position during filming. During a 5-min rest period initial flow and pressure calibrations were made and the flow response to a 10-sec total occlusion was recorded. The coronary constrictor was then expanded with saline under pressures up to 1000 mm Hg (20 psi) depending on the severity of stenosis desired. The expansion pressure was held constant at the chosen level by a water-sealed ball valve in line with an automatic pressure regulator attached to a compressed air source.

The stenosis was allowed to stabilize for 20 min. Four sets of data were then obtained to characterize the pressure/flow relationships resulting from this stenosis.

1. X-rays at rest: Orthognal x-rays were taken during baseline flow conditions in the left anterior oblique and left posterior oblique view. The

two x-rays were taken sequentially separated by at least 3 min, such that flow and heart rate had returned to baseline values before the second x-ray was taken. In preliminary studies repeated x-rays in the same plane demonstrated return of all dimensions to control baseline at 3 min.
2. Measured pressure-flow data at rest: The pressure and flow velocity transducers were recalibrated and baseline control recordings were made of the electrocardiogram, coronary flow velocity and proximal, distal and differential coronary pressures.
3. Measured pressure-flow data at vasodilation: A dose of 0.4–0.8 ml of papaverine in a concentration of 2.0 mg/ml was injected as a bolus through the distal coronary catheter to produce a transient increase in flow while phasic pressures and flow velocity were recorded. Transducer calibrations were verified at the end of data collection.
4. X-rays at vasodilation: The same dose of papaverine was injected again and then x-rays were taken at 10 sec and 60 sec after the injection. The dog was repositioned for the opposing biplane view and the same hypermia x-ray sequence was repeated. X-rays were developed with the stenosis still in place and were repeated if films were of poor quality. The entire experiment lasted 1 hour. Data were obtained over a wide range of coronary constrictions for each dog during repeated studies over a period of 4–6 weeks.

Data Analysis

Measured Pressure-flow Data

For each stenosis the relation of differential pressure to flow velocity was determined for each of four to six heart cycles for flow levels ranging from resting control to peak flow during pharmacological vasodilation. Analog voltage recordings of phasic flow velocity and phasic differential pressure (stenosis pressure gradient) from the diastolic portion of the selected cardiac cycles were converted to digital signals at 100 samples/sec with a PDP-8e computer. Data were processed by a digital filter equivalent to a low pass filter flat to 15 Hz and having linear roll off from 15–30 Hz (-40 db down at 30 Hz with no phase shift). During each cardiac cycle, the pressure gradient and flow velocity were correlated by a quadratic equation having the general form $\triangle P = FV + SV^2$, where $\triangle P$ is the pressure loss in millimeters of mercury, V is coronary flow velocity in centimeters per second, F is the coefficent of pressure loss due to viscous friction, and S is the coefficient of pressure due to flow separation or localized turbulence downstream from the stenosis. For single heart cycles, we determined the constants F and S, which best fit this general equation to the experimental data by computer, using a general purpose curve-fitting algorithm. The computer output consisted of the coefficients F and S, the mean velocity, the average velocity, and the mean differential pressure for each heart cycle as well as a plot of the differential pressure versus flow velocity and the calculated best fit curve for each heart cycle.

For each stenosis the quadratic relation between $\triangle P$ and V for several cardiac cycles at different flows was used to establish a composite relation for $\triangle P$ and V over the entire range of flows for that stenosis. Five individual beats were selected, one at rest and four over a range of increased flow during vasodilation. Every flow velocity data point in centimeters per second was then converted by computer to volume flow in cubic centimeters per minute by multiplying velocity times the cross-sectional area of the vessel at the site of the Doppler flow probe determined from orthogonal arteriograms taken in each experiment. The cross-sectional area of the artery at the site of the velocity transducer from the rest x-ray was used with the hydraulic data for the rest beat, and the cross-sectional area of the artery at the velocity transducer from the vasodilated x-ray was used with the hydraulic data for the high flow beats following vasodilators. We demonstrated by sequential arteriograms that this arterial cross-sectional area was relatively constant after injection of the vasodilator for the 60-sec period of data collection. For each stenosis the pressure gradient and volume flow in cubic centimeters per minute (Q) from the five beats was combined into a single composite $\triangle P$-Q relation. The combined data was curvilinear and did not fit a simple quadratic relationship due to changing stenosis geometry during vasodilation. Therefore, a general purpose curve-fitting algorithm was used to derive a cubic equation that best fit the composite experimentally recorded data in the form $y = ax + bx^2 + cx^3$. This cubic equation was used to determine a single pressure gradient at any particular flow rate for that stenosis. The pressure gradient for different stenoses in different experiments could then be compared at identical flow rates. The cubic equation has no physiologic significance but was simply used to determine a single pressure gradient falling within the range of pressure gradients measured experimentally at any given flow.

X-ray Analysis

X-ray films were printed directly in reverse image with a 4 × 5 enlarger at 3× magnification using Kodac polycontrast, lightweight paper, contrast grade 2. Exposure times were individually adjusted to maximize contrast at the vessel border. Vessel borders on the prints were outlined lightly in pencil independently by the authors and then jointly re-evaluated for a final "concensus" tracing. One copy of each x-ray was always left unmarked for visual reference. The penciled vessel outlines were traced into a PDP 11/45 computer using an x-y cursor system on a back lighted drafting board with resolution of 250 lines/inch. The outline of a 3.18-mm stainless steel ball surgically implanted next to the stenosis was also traced into the computer as a size reference.

Tracings of paired orthogonal arteriograms and the steel ball as a size reference were processed by a previously described computer program (Brown et al., 1977). The program corrected for pincushion distortion and absolute size to produce a true scale, three-dimensional reconstruction of the vessel and stenotic segment. In this computer program, cross-sectional area of the coronary artery at any given location was calculated as an ellipse using the diameter of the vessel from two orthogonal x-rays as the two axes. Arterial diameters in each orthogonal view were matched spatially at 0.25-mm increments along the long axis of the artery starting from a reference point chosen as the site of greatest narrowing in the stenosis. The starting and ending points of the stenosis on the photographic prints were carefully defined manually as points where the vessel appeared to be normal size and was not changing dimensions. The percent area stenosis was calculated as $(A_n - A_s)/A_n \times 100$, where A_n = area of distal normal vessel and A_s equals the minimum stenosis area, and refers to the percent reduction in normal vessel area. The percent diameter stenosis reported here was calculated as the average of the percent diameter reduction in each of the two orthogonal views where percent diameter reduction equals $D_n - D_s/D_n \times 100$; D_n = diameter of distal vessel and D_s = diameter of the stenosis. The divergence angle is the angle between the longitudinal axis and arterial wall at the distal, exit end of the stenosis as it broadens and flares away from the straight line continuation of the stenotic segment. The full divergence angle was the sum of the two angles formed by the two sides of the vessel.

A hard copy printout included stenosis dimensions, the cross-sectional area of the vessel at the Doppler flow probe and the computer reconstruction of the digitized vessels in each view. Each x-ray print was traced three times. Data from the most disparate trace were discarded. Data from the remaining two traces were averaged together and stored in the Data Base of a PDP 10 computer.

We then could compare the measured pressure-flow data and the x-ray data for a given stenosis at a given flow. For each stenosis the experimental pressure gradient was determined at the selected flow level using the cubic equation coefficients from the hydraulic analysis. Pressure gradient was then also determined at the same flow using the resistance equation from the x-ray analysis.

Reproducibility of tracing and digitizing the x-rays was evaluated in two ways. In the first, the difference between the stenosis dimensions in the two traces used was divided by 2, averaged for all stenoses and then compared to the mean resting value. Reproducibility of the stenosis x-ray system and digitizing was also assessed by taking five paris of biplane x-rays of the same stenosis, sequentially, moving and repositioning the dog between each set of

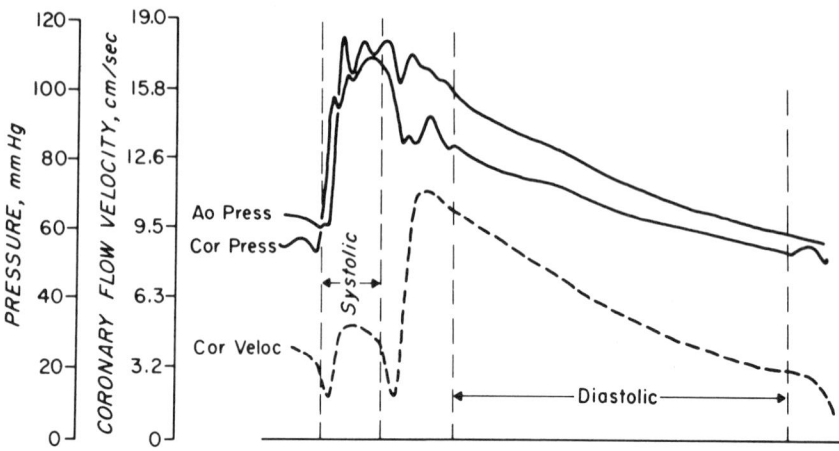

Fig. 1. Coronary flow velocity, aortic pressure and coronary pressure distal to a coronary stenosis at resting baseline conditions. Periods of deceleration and acceleration of coronary flow are indicated by light vertical dashed lines.

x-rays. Then the vessel border was outlined eight separate times, four each by two observers, for a total of 40 observations on a fixed stenosis. The mean and standard deviation of the 40 determinations of the percent stenosis were then determined. Intrinsic variability was defined as the standard deviation divided by the mean.

Results

Characteristics of Pulsatile Pressure Gradient and Flow

Figures 1 and 2 show examples of the pressure and velocity recordings in the presence of a mild coronary stenosis under control baseline conditions and during the increased flow produced by selective coronary vasodilation. Under control resting conditions, the pressure gradient was small and the velocity recording showed the characteristic phasic pattern of coronary flow. During coronary vasodilation after intracoronary injection of papaverine, the gradient became more severe as the flow increased. Systolic flow increased proportionately more than diastolic flow until there was little phasic variation. Thus, the phasic pattern of coronary flow in the presence of a "fixed," constant stenosis became damped during peak flow after a vasodilatory stimulus.

Coronary flow velocity and aorta-to-coronary differential pressure showed characteristic phasic patterns. In early systole, distal left circumflex coronary pressure rose slightly before aortic root pressure, thereby producing a sudden momentary pressure reversal, with coronary pressure being higher than aortic pressure. Immediately thereafter, coronary flow velocity fell with the typical early systolic phasic pattern due to systolic myocardial compression of the coronary capillary bed. In the presence of a stenosis, the momentary, early systolic drop or reversal of aortic-coronary pressure gradient always preceded systolic deceleration of coronary flow. In late systole and very early diastole, as myocardial compression ended, coronary flow increased rapidly during a phase of flow acceleration. In midsystole and throughout diastole, these sudden decelerative and accelerative changes in flow were absent.

During progressive coronary constriction under resting conditions, diastolic flow decreased and systolic flow increased until the characteristic phasic pattern of coronary flow was damped out with little fall in mean flow. Further constriction caused a fall in mean flow. When mean flow was reduced to half or less of control values, the phasic pattern of coronary flow resembled that of aortic pressure with systolic flow being higher than diastolic flow.

Figure 3a shows the primary recordings and Figure 3b shows a typical example of the relationship between coronary flow velocity and the pressure gradient due to a stenosis under resting conditions. Throughout diastole, the relation followed a curve of the general form $\triangle P = FV + SV^2$. During systolic deceleration, the pressure gradient was proportionately lower than flow

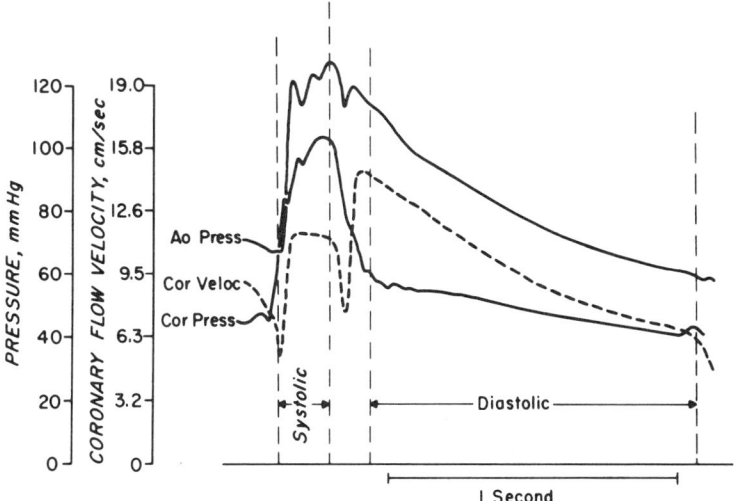

Fig. 2. Coronary flow velocity, aortic pressure and coronary pressure distal to a stenosis at higher blood flow after coronary vasodilation.

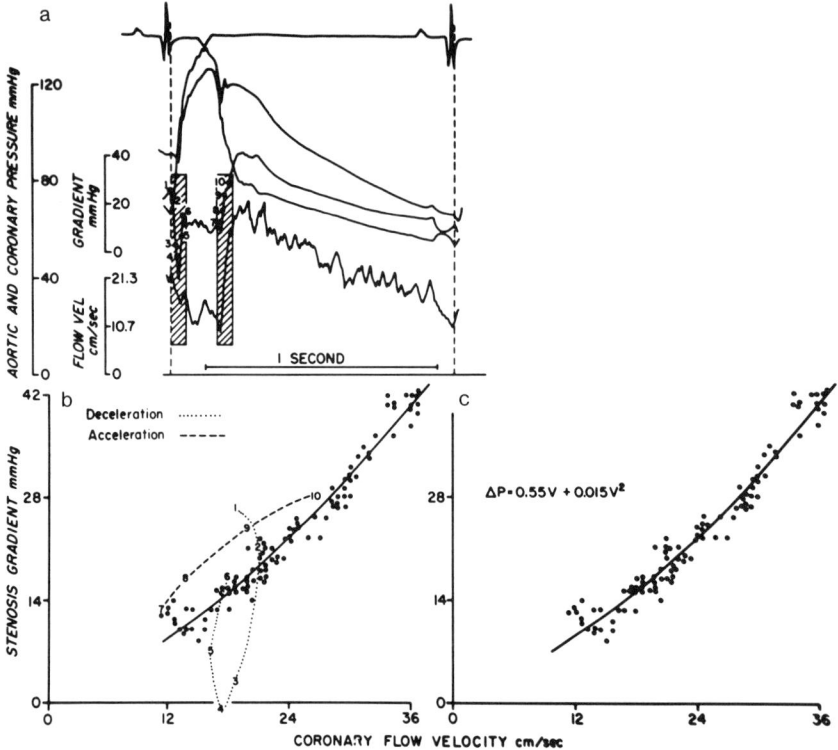

Fig. 3 Relation between coronary flow velocity and pressure gradient due to a stenosis under resting control conditions. Panel a shows the original pressure and velocity recordings. Panel b shows the relationship between the pressure gradient, ΔP, on the vertical axis and flow velocity, V, on the horizontal axis. The numbered points on the gradient-velocity relationship correspond to the numbered points on the original recordings and illustrate the effects of early systolic deceleration and late systolic acceleration of flow (shaded areas). Panel c shows the gradient-velocity relationship after the effects of deceleration and acceleration, unrelated to the severity of the stenosis, had been discarded. The diastolic relation is characterized by a quadratic equation. The first or linear term gives the pressure loss due to viscous friction and the second or nonlinear term gives the pressure loss due to flow separation. In the example shown, the coefficient of friction loss, F, is 0.55 and the coefficient of separation loss, S, is 0.015, both characteristic of moderate stenoses.

compared to the rest of the cardiac cycle. An early systolic decrease in the pressure gradient preceded the systolic fall in flow, and the gradient even became negative or reversed momentarily (coronary pressure greater than aortic root pressure), thereby producing a downward directed "tail" (dotted lines) at the lower, left end of the plotted curve. During diastolic acceleration, the pressure gradient increased before flow increased and was therefore proportionately larger than flow, compared to the rest of the cardiac cycle.

This increase in the pressure gradient in late systole and early diastole preceded the increase in flow until reaching peak values of flow at the upper, right end of the plotted curve. Consequently, the acceleration phase appeared as an open "loop" (dashed lines) extending from late systole at the lower left to early diastole at the upper right of the plotted gradient-velocity relation.

The deceleration tail and acceleration loop were due to the inertia of coronary blood flow and were therefore more dependent on strength of contraction, heart rate and epicardial artery compliance than on severity of stenosis. The purely fluid dynamic character of the stenosis, i.e., the pressure gradient-velocity ($\triangle$P-V) relation of the stenosis without the extraneous effects of deceleration and acceleration, is shown in Figure 3c, in which the data points during decelerative and accelerative phases of the cardiac cycle were edited out and discarded. The distortion of the gradient-velocity relationship by these inertial factors was marked for short cardiac cycles (tachycardia) having a narrow range of pressure and velocity data.

Figure 4 shows the pressure gradient-velocity relation of each of a series of cardiac cycles ranging from resting coronary flow up to maximum flow for one stenosis in one dog. During vasodilation and the transient increase in flow after intracoronary papaverine, this relationship became steeper than at rest due to a larger coefficient of separation, S. In other words, the apparently fixed stenosis

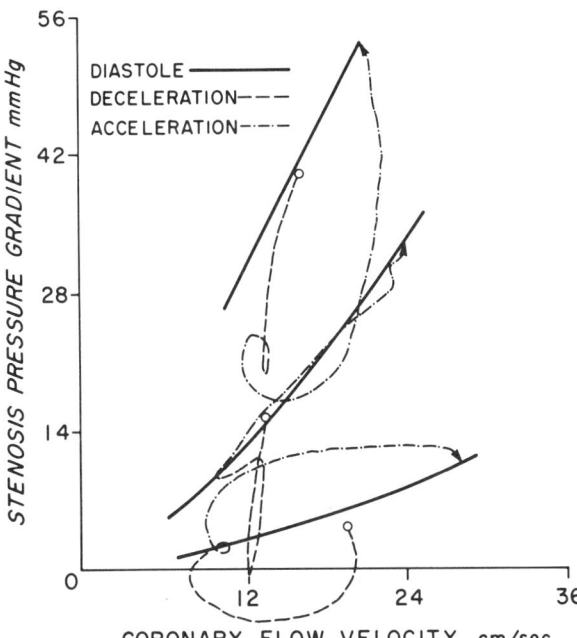

Fig. 4. Pressure gradient-velocity relation of three cardiac cycles, one at resting baseline coronary flow, one at maximum coronary flow and one at an intermediate range of coronary flow after vasodilators. The altered pressure gradient-velocity relation during systolic deceleration and early diastolic acceleration of coronary blood flow are also indicated by the broken lines.

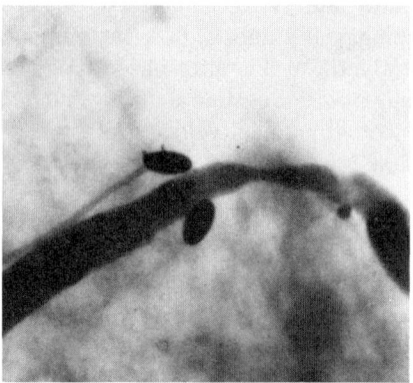 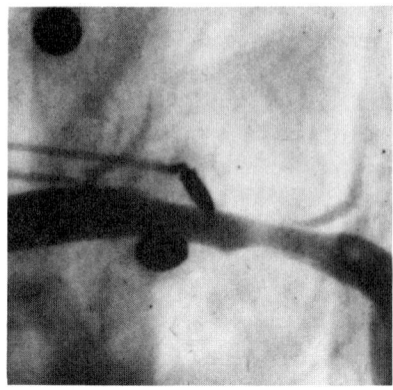

Fig. 5. Orthogonal coronary arteriograms taken in late diastole by triggering automated injection system and x-ray exposure from the electrocardiogram.

became hydraulically more severe during vasodilation with markedly greater pressure loss at any given velocity than would be predicted by the resting equation. Figure 4 also shows the changes in deceleration and acceleration that occurred with increasing steepness of the pressure gradient-flow velocity relation for each beat. The relative proportion or contribution of deceleration and acceleration effects on the $\triangle$ P-V relation are very different at high flows as compared to low flows. Therefore, if these phases of early systole and early diastole were not excluded the passive or diastolic pressure flow characteristics would be distorted to different degrees at low coronary flows as compared to high coronary flows. Therefore, the true hemodynamic characteristics of the coronary stenosis could not be evaluated unless these periods during the cardiac cycle were excluded. All subsequent data presented here consist of passive pressure gradient-velocity relations.

Validation of Quantitative Coronary Arteriography

Figure 5 illustrates orthogonal x-rays of a stenosis. The average diameter stenosis determined from biplane x-rays ranged from 45–78% diameter narrowing, mean 68%. The reduction in cross-sectional area of the artery at the stenosis ranged from 78–95%, mean 91%. The severity of the stenosis in the two orthogonal biplane views was quite asymmetric. The mean ratio of minimum stenosis diameter in one view to the stenosis diameter at the same point in the other orthogonal view was 0.64 ± 0.21 (standard deviation for all data).

Hemodynamics of Coronary Stenosis 185

After intracoronary injection of papaverine, coronary blood flow rose to peak values within 10 sec and gradually returned to resting values after 90 sec. The maximum flow following papaverine in each animal was dependent upon the severity of the stenosis and varied from 45–90 cc/min. The pressure gradient across the stenosis became more severe at the higher flows ranging up to 70 mm Hg for the most severe stenosis.

The pressure gradient-flow relation, $\triangle$P-Q, measured during a single diastole, was curvilinear and fit a quadratic relation, $\triangle P = fQ + sQ^2$, where $\triangle P$ is pressure gradient in millimeters of mercury, Q is flow in cubic centimeters per minute, f is the coefficient of viscous friction loss and s is the coefficient of separation loss. For a given stenosis the quadratic relation changed modestly as flow increased during vasodilation. The coefficient s for the quadratic relation became 22% greater at higher flow levels by indicating an increase in the resistance due to the disturbed flow caused by stenosis. Thus, for each stenosis there was a family of curves describing the $\triangle$P-Q relation over a range of flow from rest to vasodilation. This combined data for beats at several flow rates for a given stenosis did not fit a simple composite quadratic relationship due to changing stenosis geometry at high flows.

The $\triangle$P-Q relation and total pressure gradient at a given flow for each stenosis were also predicted from angiographic determinations of vessel geometry and dimensions of the stenosis at rest and after vasodilation. Because vasodilation caused a change in stenosis dimensions, a second $\triangle$P relationship for each stenosis was obtained from biplane x-rays taken during vasodilation. The composite pressure gradient-flow relation from the measured pressure-flow data and from the x-ray analysis at rest and at vasodilation were plotted together. Figures 6, 7 and 8 show the primary pressure gradient-flow data measured experimentally over a wide range of flows plotted by computer. The large heavy solid circles are the x-ray-predicted pressure gradient-flow points based quantitative analysis of coronary arteriograms by computer using the equations previously described. The lower solid circle is at rest and the upper is after coronary vasodilation. Figures 6, 7 and 8 are for 60%, 69% and 78% diameter narrowing, respectively. The $\triangle$P-Q curves ranges from hydraulically mild in Figure 6 to moderate in Figure 7 to severe in Figure 8. In Figures 9, 10 and 11 the solid lines are the composite $\triangle$P-Q relations fit to the raw data

Fig. 6 (*see page 186*). Primary pressure gradient-flow data measured experimentally over a range of coronary blood flow from resting control up to maximum flow after vasodilators, plotted by computer. Pressure gradient in millimeters of mercury is plotted on the vertical axis and coronary blood flow in cubic centimeters per minute is plotted on the horizontal axis. The numbers 02 or 03 following values on either axis indicate that the decimal point should be moved two or three places to the right. Thus, the range of values on the vertical axis is 0–70 mm Hg and the range of values on the horizontal axis is 0–100 cc/min. The large heavy solid circles indicate the x-ray-predicted pressure gradient-flow points based on quantitative coronary arteriography. The lower solid circle is for the x-ray-predicted pressure gradient-flow relation at rest and upper solid circle is after coronary vasodilators. The stenosis in this case averaged 60% diameter narrowing.

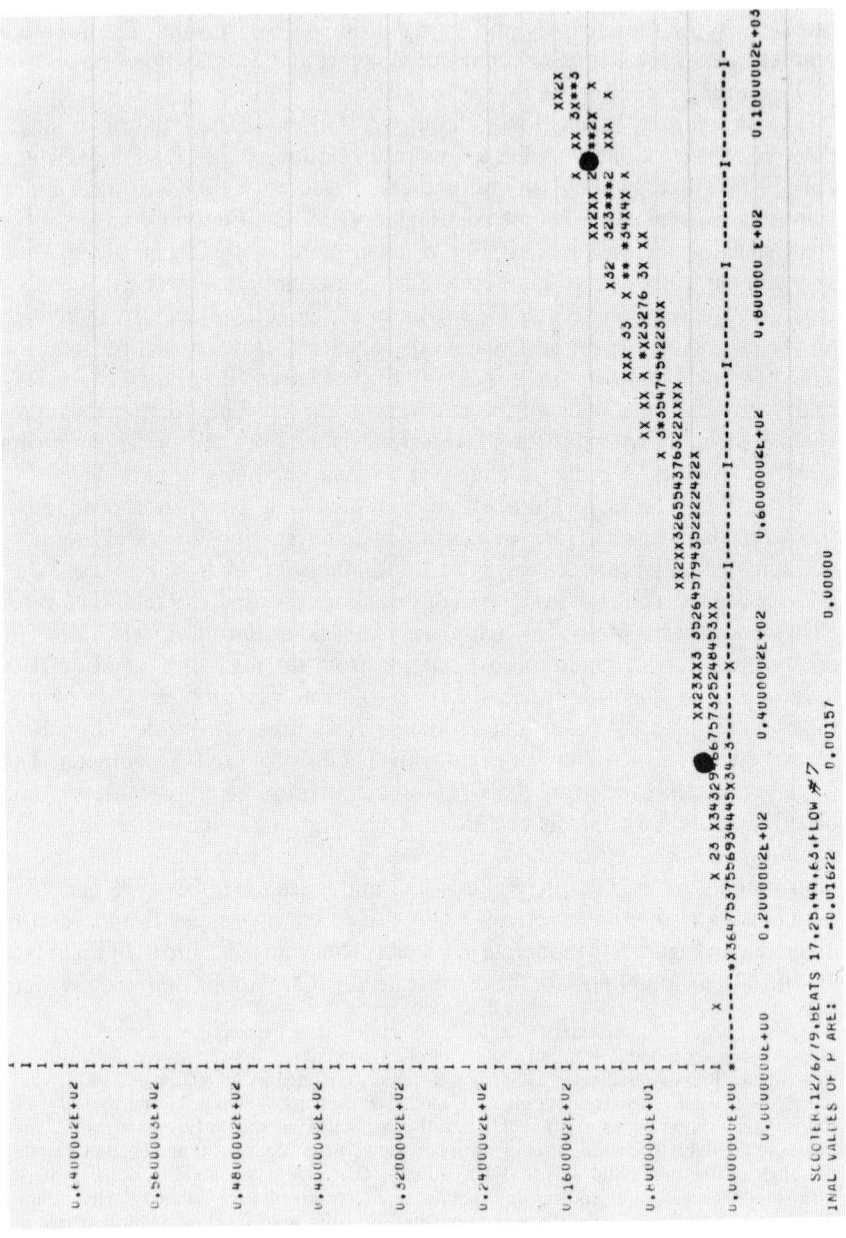

Fig. 6. legend see page 185.

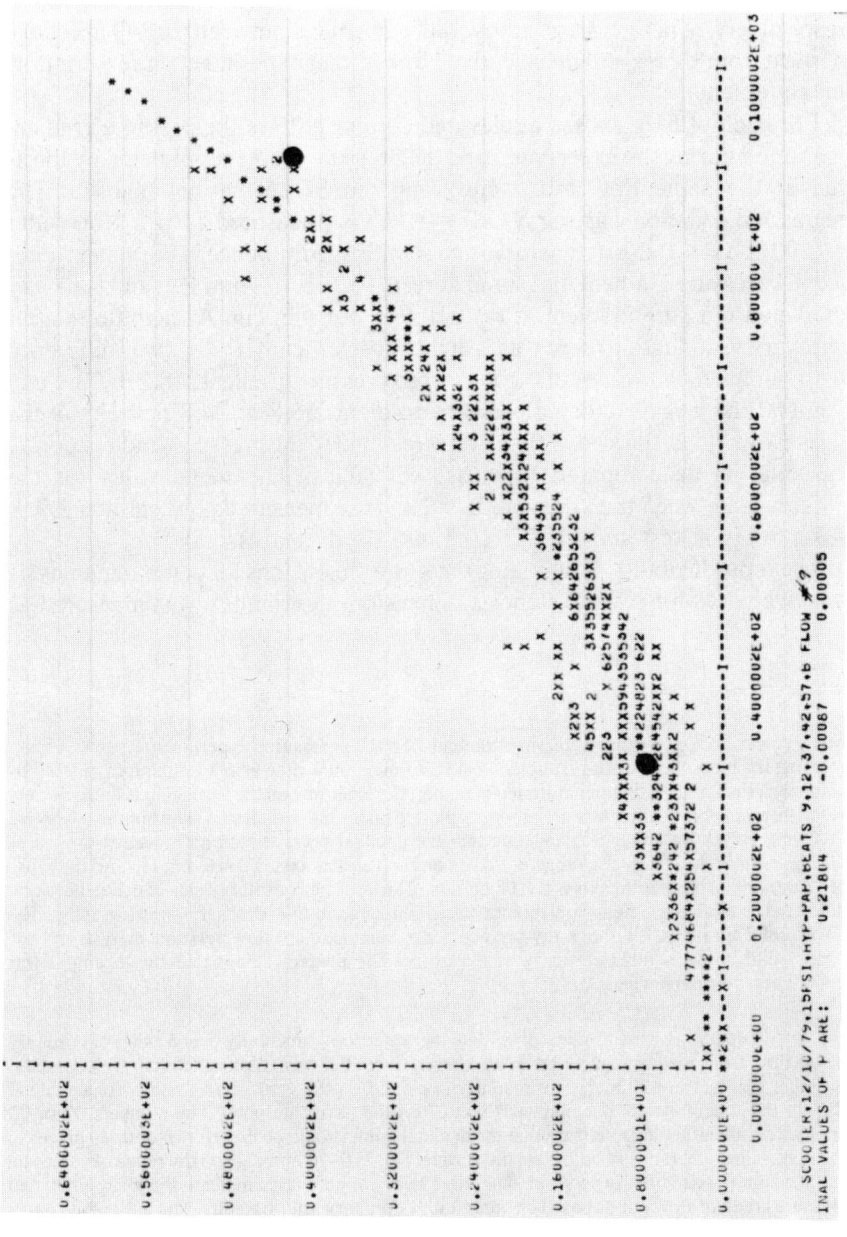

Fig. 7. legend see page 188.

points measured for each experiment shown above. The broken lines are the $\triangle$P-Q relations predicted from x-ray dimensions at rest and at vasodilation. Figures 9, 10 and 11 are computer-fit curves for data in Figures 6, 7 and 8, respectively. There was good overall agreement between $\triangle$P-Q relations derived from x-rays and those derived from direct experimental pressure-flow measurements.

For each of 51 stenoses at elevated coronary flows the pressure gradient measured during the experiment and the pressure gradient predicted by the x-ray at the same flow rate were compared by regression analysis. The regression equation was: x-ray $\triangle$P = 1.112 × (measured $\triangle$P) + 1.60 with r = 0.90 and $P < 0.0001$. There was no significant difference in the mean values for the pressure gradient measured at rest, 10.1 ± 7.7 mm Hg, and the x-ray predicted pressure gradient at rest, 10.9 ± 5.6 mm Hg. At high flows after coronary vasodilation there was a slight but significant ($P < 0.001$) difference between the mean values of the measured pressure gradient, 48.2 ± 23.1 mm Hg, and the x-ray-predicted pressure gradient, 55.8 ± 28.8 mm Hg, at the same flow. Thus, the x-rays slightly overestimated the pressure gradient during vasodilation as compared to measured values. The mean value for the difference between the x-ray-predicted and the measured gradient was 3.9 ± 4.3 mm Hg at rest and 11.9 ± 10.5 mm Hg during vasodilation.

The reproducibility of digitizing the x-ray dimensions for computer analysis was evaluated for several stenosis dimensions. Variability was measured as

Fig. 7 (see p. 187). Primary pressure gradient-flow data measured experimentally over a range of coronary blood flow from resting control up to maximum flow after vasodilators, plotted by computer. Pressure gradient in millimeters of mercury is plotted on the vertical axis and coronary blood flow in cubic centimeters per minute is plotted on the horizontal axis. The numbers 02 or 03 following values on either axis indicate that the decimal point should be moved two or three places to the right. Thus, the range of values on the vertical axis is 0–70 mm Hg and the range of values on the horizontal axis is 0–100 cc/min. The large heavy solid circles indicate the x-ray-predicted pressure gradient-flow points based on quantitative coronary arteriography. The lower solid circle is for the x-ray-predicted pressure gradient-flow relation at rest and the upper solid circle is after coronary vasodilators. The percent stenosis in this example was 69% diamenter narrowing.

Fig. 8. Primary pressure gradient-flow data measured experimentally over a range of coronary ▶ blood flow from resting control up to maximum flow after vasodilators, plotted by computer. Pressure gradient in millimeters of mercury is plotted on the vertical axis and coronary blood flow in cubic centimeters per minute is plotted on the horizontal axis. The numbers 02 or 03 after values on either axis indicate that the decimal point should be moved two or three places to the right. Thus, the range of values on the vertical axis is 0–70 mm Hg and the range of values on the horizontal axis is 0–100 cc/min. The large heavy solid circles indicate the x-ray-predicted pressure gradient-flow points based on quantitative coronary arteriography. The lower solid circle is for the x-ray-predicted pressure gradient-flow relation at rest and the upper solid circle is after coronary vasodilators. The percent coronary stenosis in this example was 78% diameter narrowing.

Hemodynamics of Coronary Stenosis

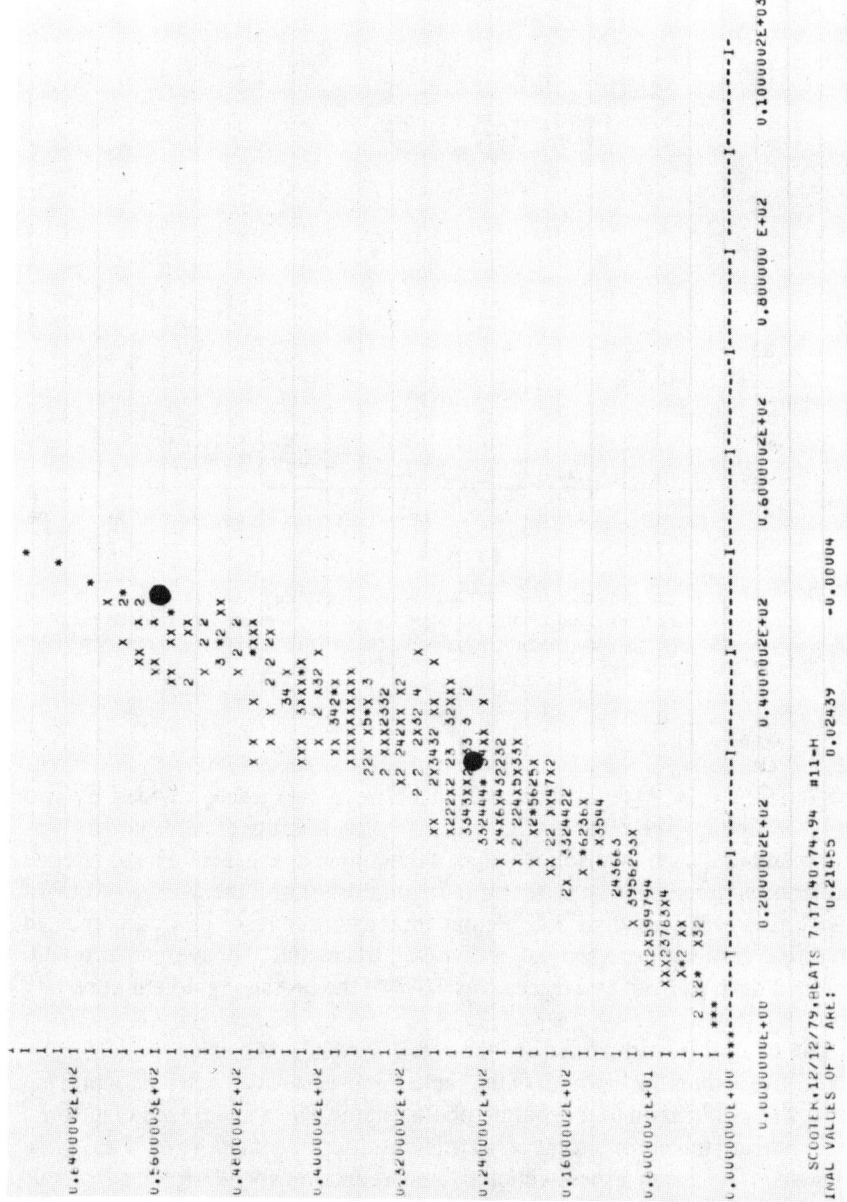

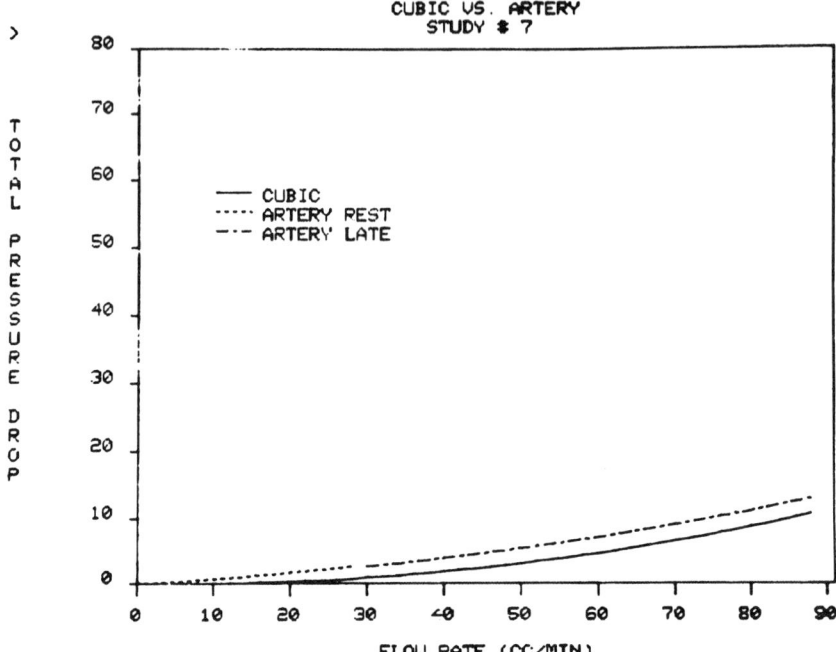

Fig. 9. Composite pressure gradient-flow relation over a wide range of coronary flow. The solid line is for directly measured experimental data and the broken lines are for angiographic data. These composite curves are based on raw, primary data shown in Figure 6 for a coronary stenosis of 60% diameter narrowing.

the difference in a stenosis dimension between two traces divided by two ($(T_1 - T_2)/2$). The mean of this measure of variability for all stenoses was compared to the mean absolute value of that dimension at rest. The difference in stenosis dimensions between an individual trace and the average value of two traces was less than 5% of that dimension at rest. The difference in pressure gradient between an individual trace and the average pressure gradient derived from two traces was 10% of the pressure gradient at resting coronary flow.

The overall reproducibility of the x-ray system was further evaluated by taking five sequential biplanes of the same stenosis at rest. Each pair of biplane films was outlined on four separate photographic prints and traced twice onto the digitizing tablet for a total of 40 tracings of orthogonal x-rays of the same stenosis. The mean cross-sectional area reduction for 40 tracings of this stenosis was 88.4 ± 1.8%. For this data the standard deviation of 1.8 is only 1.8/88.4 or 2% of the area reduction, indicating great reproducibility on

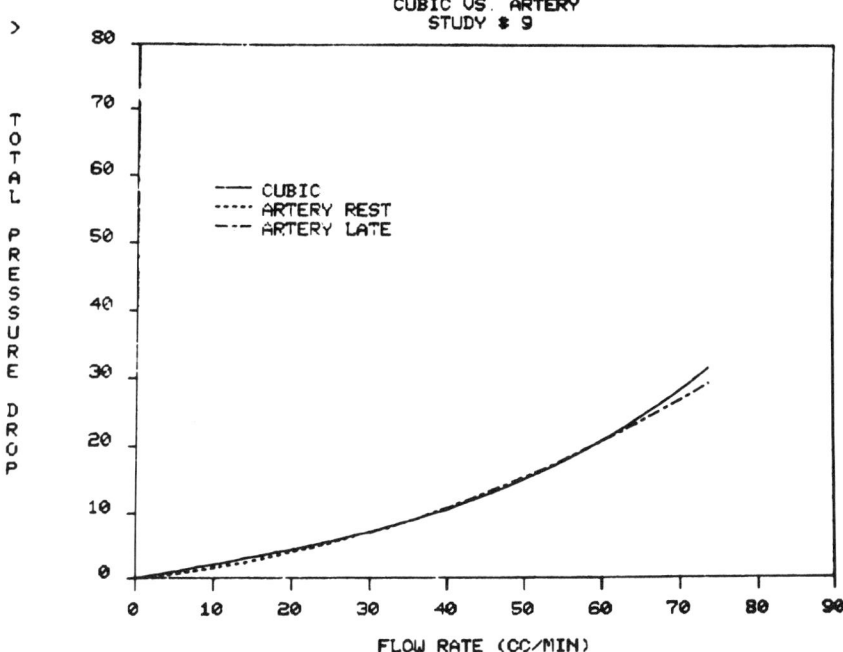

Fig. 10. Composite pressure gradient-flow relation over a wide range of coronary flow. The solid line is for directly measured experimental data and the broken lines are for angiographic data. These composite curves are based on the raw, primary data shown in Figure 7 for a coronary stenosis of 69% diameter narrowing.

sequential x-rays and tracings. The same analysis was performed for 40 traces on a second stenosis of 89.5 ± 1.9% area reduction with an identical 2% variability.

Dynamic Changes in Coronary Stenoses

Several previous reports on experimental coronary arterial stenoses described increased severity or greater stenosis resistance during elevated coronary blood flow (Shipley and Gregg, 1944; Kreuzer and Schenk, 1973; Gould et al., 1975; Logan, 1975; Swartz et al., 1979; Santamore and Walinsky et al., 1979; 1980). In these previous studies stenosis resistance was calculated as the pressure gradient across an arterial constriction divided by blood flow through the artery. Such calculated resistance is misleading because it is dependent on flow and increases as flow increases despite fixed stenosis geometry (Gould et al., 1975). However, more comprehensive analysis of the instantaneous pressure flow characteristics of arterial stenoses also indicate disproportionately increased severity at high blood flows (Gould, 1978). Mechanisms proposed for this apparent worsening of the stenosis at high blood flow have included a hypothesized vasodilation of the distal and proximal normal segments of the artery with more severe relative percent stenosis (Kreuzer and Schenk, 1973; Gould, 1978) or passive narrowing of the constricted segment of the artery due to a fall in intraluminal pressure at high coronary blood flow (Logan, 1975; Swartz et al., 1979; Walinsky et al., 1979; 1980; Santamore and Walinsky, 1980). In contrast to these experimental findings, quantitative coronary arteriography in man has indicated that the geometry of a coronary stenosis becomes less severe after coronary vasodilators (Doerner et al., 1979). Therefore, we analyzed orthogonal quantitative coronary arteriograms of these 51 coronary stenoses in order to define the geometric changes in the stenosis after coronary vasodilators.

For all 51 stenoses there was no significant change in the minimal cross-sectional area at the site of the constriction, the mean value at rest being 0.40 ± 0.16 mm^2 and at vasodilation $= 0.40 \pm 0.20$ mm^2, although early in the course of vasodilation there was a transient very small decrease in this dimension, which has no hemodynamic consequence as discussed subsequently. The divergence angle at the distal end of the stenosis did not change significantly: 31° versus 33°. However, there were significant changes in size of the normal vessel on either side of the stenosis. During vasodilation the cross-sectional area of the proximal portion of the vessel increased from 4.98 ± 2.09–5.87 ± 2.67 mm^2 and distal vessel cross-sectional area increased from 4.44 ± 107–4.97 ± 1.27 mm^2. These changes in the area of the normal vessel resulted in an increase in the percent diameter stenosis from 68 ± 7–$71 \pm 5\%$ and percent area stenosis from 90.7 ± 4.0–$92.1 \pm 3.1\%$. All these changes were significant ($P < 0.001$). The large standard deviations in all means in this study are due to averaging data from mild, moderate and severe stenoses together. These geometric changes during coronary vasodilation caused a 22% increase in the coefficient of pressure loss due to separation or disturbed flow but no change in the viscous coefficient.

As coronary flow increased the pressure gradient also increased as expected from the quadratic relation of pressure gradient to volume flow. The relative proportion of pressure losses due to viscous friction and separation also changed as coronary flow increased. Using the resting x-ray geometry and a resting coronary flow of 0.25 cc/sec (15 cc/min) the x-ray-predicted viscous losses accounted for 67% and the separation losses accounted for 33% of the total pressure gradient across the stenosis. Using x-ray geometry after coronary vasodilators at higher coronary flows of 1 cc/sec (60 cc/min) the x-ray-predicted viscous losses accounted for 32% and the separation losses accounted for 68% of the total pressure gradient across the stenosis. These

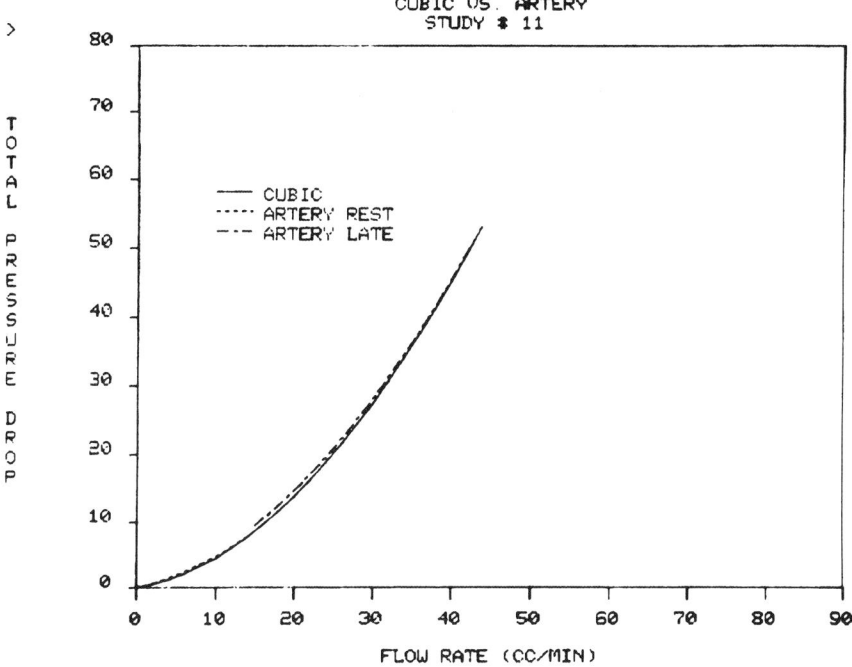

Fig. 11. Composite pressure gradient-flow relation over a wide range of coronary flow. The solid line is for directly measured experimental data and the broken lines are for angiographic data. These composite curves are based on the raw, primary data shown in Figure 8 above for a coronary stenosis of 78% diameter narrowing.

x-ray-predicted proportions are the same as those proportions of viscous and turbulent losses previously determined from pressure flow measurements alone without x-ray geometry (Gould, 1978).

The pressure gradient across the stenosis increased at elevated coronary blood flow for two reasons. The first is the expected increase in pressure gradient due to the quadratic $\triangle$P-Q relation and the second is that the separation coefficient of this equation became larger at higher blood flows as compared to rest. Therefore, in order to analyze any additional pressure losses due to altered geometry alone after vasodilators, it is necessary to calculate the pressure gradient from x-ray geometry at rest and from x-ray geometry after vasodilators but using the same coronary blood flow. At 1 cc/sec the pressure gradient predicted from resting x-ray geometry was 47 ± 41 mm Hg whereas the pressure gradient predicted from x-ray geometry at vasodilation, also at 1 cc/sec, was 58 ± 61 mm Hg, or a $16 \pm 39\%$ difference ($P < 0.002$). Thus, with coronary vasodilation and worsening stenosis severity the x-ray-predicted pressure gradient was 16% higher than it would have been had there been no geometric changes of the stenosis during coronary vasodilation.

In order to study the effects of geometric changes early in the course of coronary vasodilation a subset of 28 stenoses were studied by biplane arteriograms taken within 10 sec after injection of papaverine in addition to x-rays taken at the standard time of 60 sec for all 51 stenoses. During maximum coronary flow 10 sec after intracoronary papavarine there was a significant but very small reduction in minimum stenosis area from 0.39 ± 0.15 mm^2 at rest to 0.36 ± 0.16 mm^2 at peak flow ($P = 0.002$). Normal segments of the vessel on either side of the constricted segment increased somewhat in size during early vasodilation and increased still further at late vasodilation. The small decrease in the minimum stenosis area during early vasodilation was not associated with a significant change in the coefficients of viscous or separation losses as compared to the resting coefficients. Thus, although there was a very small passive collapse in the stenotic segment early in the course of vasodilation, this change did not persist into that period of time when the most marked changes in stenosis geometry were observed later in the course of coronary vasodilation.

In this experimental preparation with stenoses produced by external constriction of normal coronary arteries, the relative percent narrowing became more severe after coronary vasodilators due to vasodilation of the normal artery proximal and distal to the narrowed segment as previously hypothesized (Kreuzer and Schenk, 1973; Gould, 1978). This change in percent narrowing was quite modest, however, and the pressure gradient calculated from the vasodilated stenosis geometry was only 16% higher than the gradient calculated from resting stenosis geometry at the same coronary flow.

With severe stenoses some investigators have reported a decrease in coronary blood flow after distal vasodilation. They attributed this fall in flow to a passive collapse of the stenotic segment (Swartz et al., 1979; Santamore and Walinsky, 1980), as described in Chapter 11. Another explanation for their results is as follows: The maximal potential energy of aortic pressure is converted entirely to kinetic energy in the stenotic segment of severe "critical" stenoses. Distal pressure is then at a minimum and the pressure gradient at a fixed maximum (Berguer and Hwang, 1974). With epicardial arterial vasodilation and even slightly worse percent narrowing superimposed on a stenosis of this severity, there is insufficient total potential energy in aortic pressure to maintain or "carry" flow through the stenosis. Coronary blood flow therefore ceases. It is not even theoretically necessary that the stenotic segment completely collapse in order for blood flow to cease. We would conjecture that in this situation, if aortic pressure were then raised by pharmacologic agents or by diastolic counter pulsation, coronary blood flow would be re-established because additional potential energy is put into the system, which is then available for conversion to kinetic energy for "carrying" coronary blood flow through the stenotic segment. This mechanism may be the reason for relief of severe unstable angina pectoris by aortic balloon counterpulsation.

Relative Usefulness of △P-Q versus Relations for Defining Stenosis Severity

The results of our study experimentally confirm the theoretically predicted differences between pressure gradient flow velocity (△P-V) and pressure gradient-volume flow (△P-Q) relations as measures of hemodynamic severity (Gould, 1980). According to classical fluid dynamics the energy or pressure loss due to constriction of a tube is caused primarily by viscous friction between layers of fluid in the stenotic segment according to the Hagen-Poiseuille Law and by flow separation or disturbed flow at the downstream end of the stenosis (Binder, 1973; Young et al.; 1975). The pressure loss, △P, is related to flow velocity, V, through a stenotic tube according to a general equation that may be written in simplified form as $\triangle P = V + SV^2$ where F is the coefficient of pressure loss due to viscous friction and is dependent on relative percent narrowing, absolute diameter, and length of the stenosis; S is the coefficient of pressure loss due to flow separation and is dependent on relative percent stenosis; V is the first power of instantaneous, mean cross-sectional flow velocity and V^2 is the second power of velocity. The corresponding equation using a volume flow is $\triangle P = fQ + sQ^2$ where Q is volume flow in cubic centimeters per minute, f is the coefficient of pressure loss due to viscous friction and s is the coefficient of pressure loss due to flow separation. The values of f and s are several orders of magnitude larger than the values of F and S previously reported because of the differences in units of volume flow in cubic centimeters per second and flow velocity in centimeters per second.

A stenosis is most completely described by determining f and s or F and S, either by x-ray geometery or by direct pressure flow measurements experimentally (Gould, 1980). A graphic plot of △P versus V or Q is a visual presentation of these equations for a given stenosis. A leftward and upward shift in this graphic plot indicates a worsening of stenosis. We have previously reported that the pressure gradient observed at high coronary flow velocity was 36% higher than the pressure loss expected by extrapolation of the pressure gradient-velocity relationship observed at resting coronary flow (Gould, 1978). The comparable figure for the pressure gradient-flow relation is only 16%. Thus, the △P-V relations were steeper with a sharper upward break than the △P-Q relation, a difference that can now be explained as follows. The diameter of the coronary artery within the Doppler velocity transducer determined on orthogonal coronary arteriograms increased 32% after coronary vasodilators. Consequently, the flow velocity measured within the

Doppler transducer did not increase in proportion to flow because as flow increased, the diameter of the artery within the flow probe increased as well. Thus, the sharper break and steeper P-V curves of our previous report were due not only to worsening stenosis geometry but also due to dilation of the artery within the Doppler transducer, resulting in increased pressure gradient without corresponding increase in flow velocity. The differences in the results of these two studies are not experimental artifacts but are expected differences depending on whether coronary flow velocity in centimeters per second or quantitative coronary blood flow in cubic centimeters per minute were recorded. These conceptual or theoretical differences between $\triangle$P-V and $\triangle$P-Q relations have been extensively discussed previously (Gould, 1980) and are now confirmed by experimental results.

The characteristics of using either $\triangle$P-V or $\triangle$P-Q relations for describing stenosis severity can be summarized as follows.

Pressure Gradient-velocity Relation

1) The $\triangle$P-V relation is conceptually consistent with traditional assessment of stenosis severity in terms of relative percent stenosis because it is this dimension that is the dominant geometric influence on the $\triangle$ P-V relation. 2) The $\triangle$P-V curve, however, will break more sharply and become steeper when the artery on either side of the stenotic segment vasodilates because percent stenosis then increases and because flow velocity does not increase proportionately with $\triangle$ P due to increased cross-sectional area of the normal artery adjacent to the stenosis. 3) The velocity equation is broadly applicable to arteries of all sizes categorically and provides a uniform criterion for assessment of stenoses severity in terms of percent narrowing in both large or small vessels. Stenosis with similar $\triangle$ P-V relations have unequal resting and peak gradients with different flow reserve.

Pressure Gradient-volume Flow Relation

1) The basic $\triangle$P-Q relation for a given stenosis at rest flow changes only slightly at high flow during vasodilation of the normal artery on either side of the stenotic segment. Using the $\triangle$ P-Q analysis, the slight worsening of percent stenosis due to altered stenosis and geometry at high coronary flow caused only a 16% increase in pressure gradient over that gradient in the absence of vasodilation. Therefore, the $\triangle$P-Q relation, as compared to the $\triangle$P-V relation, conforms more closely to a quadratic equation over a wide range of flows and degrees of vasodilation without shifting or breaking as much to a steeper curve at higher flows. 2) The $\triangle$P-Q relation for a stenosis in a small artery is steeper, indicating greater hydraulic severity, as compared to a physiologically equal stenosis in a much larger artery because the small artery

transports less volume flow for any given pressure. Similarly, the △P-Q relation for a small artery with a given stenosis appears equal to the △ P-Q relation of a larger artery with a physiologically much more severe stenosis, because the more severe constriction of the larger artery reduces flow to the level of the less constricted smaller artery. Thus, if described hydraulically in terms of △P-Q relations, stenoses of equal physiologic severity in two arteries of different sizes appear unequal hydraulically and physiologically unequal lesions in two different arteries appear hydraulically equal. For these reasons the △P-Q relation is not useful or appropriate for comparing stenoses in different size arteries because misleading nonphysiologic comparisons result. 3) As a consequence of these characteristics, the △P-Q relation is the most appropriate and useful approach when comparing the geometric severity of a stenosis before an intervention to the same stenosis in the same artery after the intervention.

Inherent in such comparisons before and after an intervention is the underlying physiologic question of whether coronary volume flow and pressure to the distal coronary bed is effected by that intervention. As long as the end point of the intervention is a physiologic change of coronary blood flow and pressure to the distal coronary bed, the △P-Q relation is the most useful. Geometric stenosis severity as described by classical fluid dynamic △P-V relations, however, is not addressed by the △P-Q relation, which is dependent primarily on absolute stenosis diameter, not relative percent diameter, and is therefore highly specific for each artery. The △P-Q relation for a stenosis in a large artery therefore cannot be meaningful compared to the △P-Q relation of a small artery because the △P-Q relation is determined by the absolute volume flow in an artery as well as by the severity of stenosis.

Thus, the △P-V relation determined from either x-rays or direct pressure-flow velocity measurements provide information about stenosis severity per se as described by classic fluid dynamic equations (Binder, 1973), whereas the △P-Q relation determined from either x-rays or direct pressure-flow measurements provide information about the physiologic effects on pressure and flow seen by the distal vascular bed.

The results from this study of externally constricted normal coronary arteries in dogs conflict with results from studies in man where a decrease in stenosis severity occurred after nitroglycerin (Doerner et al., 1979). The explanation for these differences resides in the type of stenosis studied. For a circumferential, rigid stenosis with normal proximal and distal vasomotion, as in this model, the stenosis becomes modestly worse when distal vasodilation increases the percent narrowing. However, if part of the arterial wall of the stenotic segment is intact and capable of vasomotion, then vasodilation in the stenotic segment may make the narrowing less severe. Thus, our results and those of Doerner et al. do not conflict but rather demonstrate that different types of stenoses behave differently with coronary vasodilation, and no generalities can be made. Because Doerner et al. studied humans, their results would indicate that most patients have coronary lesions that are at least partially capable of vasomotion and improve after coronary vasodilators. Most patients probably do not have the type of lesion studied in this experimental preparation with a rigid circumferential stenosis. Therefore, although the animal model has provided important insights into our basic conceptual understanding of coronary stenoses, characterization of specific human coronary stenoses requires quantitative coronary arteriography in specific patients.

References

Berguer, R. and Hwang, N. H. C. 1974. Critical arterial stenosis: a theoretical and experimental solution. Ann Surg 180:39–50

Binder, R. C. 1973. *Fluid Mechanics.* Ed 5. Englewood Cliffs, N. J.: Prentice-Hall

Brown, B. G., Bolson, E., Frimer, M. and Dodge, H. T. 1977. Quantitative coronary arteriography. Circulation 55:329–337

Doerner, T. C., Brown, G. B., Bolson, E. Frimer, M. and Dodge, H. T. 1979. Vasodilatory effects of nitroglycerine and nitroprusside in coronary arteries—A comparative analysis (abs). Am J Cardiol 43:416

Gould, K. L., Lipscomb, K. and Calvert, C. 1975. Compensatory changes of the distal coronary vascular bed during progressive coronary constriction. Circulation 51:1085–1094

Gould, K. L. 1978. Pressure-flow characteristics of coronary stenoses in unsedated dogs at rest and during coronary vasodilation. Circ Res 43:245–253

Gould, K. L. 1980. Dynamic coronary stenosis. Am J Cardiol 45:286–292

Gould, K. L., Lee, D. and Lovgren, K. 1978. Techniques for arteriography and hydraulic analysis of coronary stenoses in unsedated dogs. Am J Physiol 235:H350–H356

Kelley, K. O. and Gould, K. L. 1981. Validation of computerized quantitative coronary angiography. Circulation 64:IV 107

Kreuzer, W. and Schenk, W. G. 1973. Effects of local vasodilation on blood flow through arterial stenoses. Eur Surg Res 5:233–242

Logan, S. E. 1975. On the fluid mechanics of human coronary artery stenosis. IEEE Trans Biomed Eng 22:327–334

Santamore, W. P. and Walinsky, P. 1980. Altered coronary flow responses to vasoactive drugs due to coronary arterial stenosis in the dog. Am J Cardiol 45:276–285

Shipley, R. E. and Gregg, D. E. 1944. Effect of external constriction of a blood vessel on blood flow. Am J Physiol 141:289–296

Swartz, J. S., Caryle, P. F. and Cohn, J. N. 1979. Effect of dilation of the distal coronary bed on flow and resistance in severely stenotic coronary arteries in the dog. Am J Cardiol 43:219–224

Walinsky, P., Santamore, W. P., Wiener, L. and Brest, A. N. 1979. Dynamic changes in the hemodynamic severity of coronary artery stenosis in a canine model. Cardiovasc Res 13:113–118

Walinsky, P., Santamore, W., Wiener, L., Cho, S. Y. and Brent, A. N. 1980. Effect of norepinephrine on coronary hemodynamics in a coronary stenotic canine model. Am Heart J 99:494–502

Young, D. F., Cholvin, N. R. and Roth, A. C. 1975. Pressure drops across artificially induced stenoses in the femoral arteries of dogs. Circ Res 36:735–743

Dynamics of Human Coronary Stenosis: Interactions Among Stenosis Flow, Distending Pressure and Vasomotor Tone

B. Greg Brown, Robert B. Petersen, Cynthia D. Pierce, Edward L. Bolson and Harold T. Dodge

Introduction

The early clinician, Sir William Osler, postulated transient coronary spasm as the basis for angina pectoris. However, subsequent pathologic teachings have been at variance with the perception of a flexible, vasoactive coronary stenosis. We have been taught that atherosclerosis or "hardening of the arteries" is a degenerative process involving cholesterol deposits, fibrosis and calcification. Medical students and heart surgeons alike know the palpably hard, nodular texture of an artery focally afflicted with an atheroma. The commonly accepted view of an arterial stenosis is that of a rigid, "fixed" constriction, reducing the normal diameter of the vessel lumen. Such a concept is consistent with the symptoms of a patient who can perform a predictable amount of effort before his angina pectoris appears. In this case, ischemia (pain) results when the myocardial oxygen demands exceed the capacity of the narrowed vessel to supply adequate perfusion. However, the fixed stenosis concept is at odds with certain common clinical observations: pain may occur at rest, or spontaneously even during sleep; pain may occur much more readily during effort in the early morning than it does in the afternoon (Yasue et al., 1979); the pain threshold may be lowered by cold exposure or emotional distress; angina may actually be precipitated by dipyridamole, one of the most potent of the known coronary arteriolar dilators. These common descriptions of angina challenge the simplistic model of a fixed coronary stenosis whose severity places an upper limit on the allowable oxygen consumption of the distal myocardium. Variable thresholds for angina in a given patient imply that coronary stenosis severity is changeable.

Until recently, there was no way to test this hypothesis in humans. However, recent technological advances in three disciplines now allow us to study the dynamic pathophysiology of human coronary stenosis. First, angiographic image quality has substantially improved in the past decade. Second, the principles of fluid flow in an arterial constriction have become better understood (May et al., 1963; Young et al., 1975; Gould et al., 1978; Gould, 1980; Logan, 1975). Third, methods to measure the severity of coronary stenosis in man have become more sophisticated (MacAlpin et al., 1973; Feldman et al., 1979; Sandor et al., 1979; Brown et al., 1977). In our laboratory a computer-assisted method used the clinical arteriogram to estimate absolute and relative dimensions in the coronary stenosis, the mass of the atherosclerotic plaque and the stenosis flow resistance, and to estimate change in these parameters with time and with different vasoactive interventions.

The purpose of this chapter is to present objective data from studies in patients with coronary disease. Certain dynamic phenomena in the coronary stenosis are illustrated. Some of the ways in which these dynamic responses may be used in the diagnosis and therapy of this disease process are discussed.

Morphologic and Physiologic Aspects of Stenosis Dynamics

The magnitude of pressure lost in transit through an arterial stenosis is predicted (Brown et al., 1981a) from classical fluid mechanics theory which, in principle, has been confirmed experimentally (Young et al., 1975; May et al., 1963; Gould, 1978):

$$\triangle P = \frac{30\mu Q}{d_{min}^4} L_e + 6\rho Q^2 (1/d_{min}^2 - 1/d_N^2)^2 \qquad (1)$$

Where: $\triangle P$ is the pressure loss in millimeters of mercury, Q is stenosis flow in millimeters per second, μ is blood viscosity in poise, d_{min} is minimum lumen diameter in the stenosis in millimeters, d_N is "normal" lumen diameter distal to the stenosis, ρ is blood density in grams per millimeter, and L_e is equivalent stenosis length in millimeter.

Table 1. Predicted Loss of Pressure for Blood Flowing Through Typical Human Coronary Lesions of Varying Severity.

Percent Stenosis (%)	Minimum Lumen Diameter in Stenosis (mm)	Predicted Flow Resistance (mm Hg/ml/sec)		Predicted Stenosis Pressure Loss (mm Hg)
		Viscous	Turbulent	
40	1.8	0.3	0.2	0.5
50	1.5	0.4	0.6	1.0
60	1.2	0.7	2.2	2.9
70	0.9	1.8	7.7	9.5
80	0.6	7.1	45.	52.
90	0.3	88.	812.	900.

Normal lumen diameter (3 mm) and flow (1 ml/sec) are assumed.

For "critical" human coronary lesions in the range 65–80% stenosis, the data of McMahon et al. (1979) fit the simplified expression:

$$\triangle P = \frac{3.2 + 6.8Q^2}{d_{min}^4} \quad (2)$$

Two points deserve mention. First, both the viscous and turbulent (orifice) terms of Expression 1 above contain $1/d_{min}^4$. The inverse fourth power of minimum lumen diameter is an exceptionally powerful factor in determining stenosis flow resistance, as Table 1 shows. Thus small changes in d_{min} have considerable effect on the hemodynamic impact of a coronary narrowing. Second, the dominant term in the $\triangle P$ expression, when coronary flow is in the usual 1–3 ml/sec range, is the Q^2 term. Thus increased coronary flow carries with it a Q^2 penalty in terms of stenosis pressure loss.

Stenosis pressure loss represents a waste of the energy available in arterial blood for coronary perfusion. To avoid myocardial ischemia, pressure distal to the stenosis must be sufficient to perfuse the subendocardium, the myocardial region that is most sensitive to reduced perfusion pressure (Hoffman and Buckberg, 1976; Buckberg et al., 1972). In practice, perfusion pressure beyond the stenosis must exceed 50–60 mm Hg in the resting state (Moir and DeBra, 1976; Wyatt et al., 1975). Figure 1 illustrates resting and exercise pressures in the central aorta, the poststenosis coronary artery and the left ventricle in a hypothetical patient with 70% coronary stenosis ($d_{min} = 0.88$ mm). The cross-hatched area under the aortic pressure waveform is the stenosis pressure loss. The pressure gradient for subendocardial perfusion is the stippled area between the poststenotic coronary pressure (dotted waveform) and diastolic left ventricular pressure. In the resting state, the stenosis

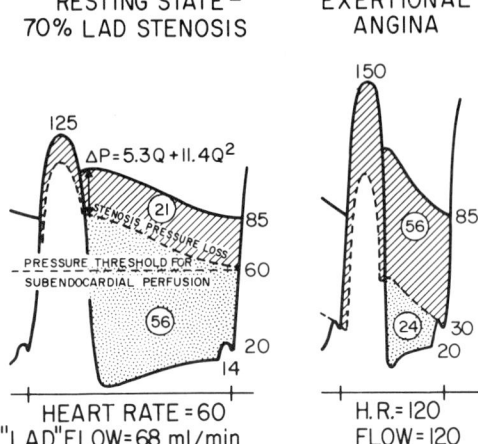

Fig. 1. Pressure waveforms in the central aorta and left ventricle, and in the coronary artery beyond a hypothetical 70% coronary stenosis (d_{min} = 0.88 mm). Predicted pressure loss at rest (Q = 1.13 ml/sec) is 21 mm Hg (the cross-hatched area). Pressure available for diastolic subendocardial perfusion is 56 mm Hg (the stippled area). During exercise, stenosis flow increases to the maximum (Q = 2 ml/sec); pressure loss is 56 mm Hg; and diastolic subendocardial perfusion pressure is an inadequate 24 mm Hg.

pressure loss is 21 mm Hg and the mean diastolic perfusion gradient is an adequate 56 mm Hg. The coronary arteriolar resistance bed has dilated partially to compensate for the added stenosis resistance and coronary flow is maintained at a normal level (Gould et al., 1975). With exercise, heart rate and blood pressure rise, coronary flow increases 68–120 ml/min in association with maximum dilation of the coronary resistance bed. At this rate of stenosis flow, $\triangle P$ calculates at 56 mm Hg and, with increased left ventricular filling pressure, the subendocardial diastolic pressure gradient averages 24 mm Hg, inadequate for the perfusion requirements associated with exercise. Ischemic pain results and persists until the resting state is resumed.

In addition to the stenosis diameter and its flow, the histologic structure of the stenosis is a third important determinant of the potential for dynamic behavior. Figure 2 illustrates schematically two commonly seen coronary histologic patters. Example a is the cross-section of an artery with an atheroma arising in one region of the intima. The remaining lumen is displaced eccentrically and is partially circumscribed by a flexible arc of relatively normal arterial wall. With this type of lesion architecture, stenosis lumen caliber may vary as a passive elastic response to alterations in intraluminal pressure, or vary as an active manifestation of alterations in coronary smooth muscle vasomotor tone. The potential for lumen caliber change in Section a is considerably greater than that in Section b, in which the centrally located lumen is surrounded by fibrotic, cholesterol-laden, calcified atheroma. As illustrated in Figure 2, a 10% shortening of the part of the outer arterial circumference that is still flexible results in a dramatic worsening of the lesion in Section a (49% → 76% stenosis); by comparison, the lesion in Section b is inflexible. While there are no good data on the relative frequency of occurrence of each of these lesion types, the flexible type is likely to be at least as common as the inflexible.

Coronary vasomotor tone is a loosely used term to describe the level of activity of various mechanisms responsible for the contraction of coronary vascular smooth muscle. At the most simplistic level consistent with current observations, one must distinguish between the smooth muscle tone of the arteriolar *resistance* vessels and that of the larger *conductance* vessels (arteries). The resistance bed receives sympathetic vasoconstrictor innervation, responds to vasoactive substances in arterial blood and to local tissue concentrations of the vasoactive metabolites of myocardial energy utilization (Berne, 1980). The conductance vessels also receive sympathetic innervation and respond to circulating vasoactive substances, but are not influenced by myocardial metabolites. Human coronary arteries undergo spontaneous, phasic, calcium-dependent vasoconstriction (Ross et al., 1980). The arterial stenosis, a focus for adherent thrombus, may also respond to locally released platelet vasoactive substances such as serotonin, potassium and thromboxane

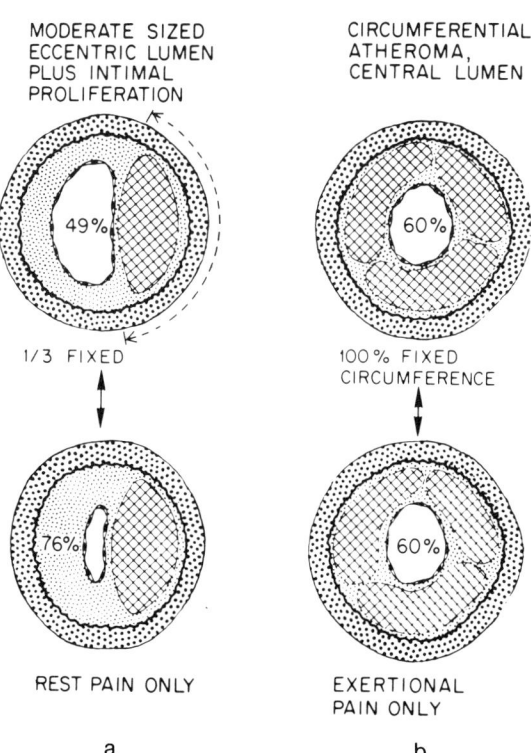

Fig. 2. Two of the observed histologic patterns in the morphologic spectrum of coronary atherosclerosis (top), and those two sections (bottom) during 10% vasomotor shortening of the still flexible part of the outer circumference. See text for details. The outer ring (coarse stippling) represents the original artery. The cross-hatched area represents the rigid atheroma. Fine stippling is intimal smooth muscle thickening. In a, lumen caliber may vary considerably with changes in intraluminal pressure, or as shown, increased vasomotor tone. In b, the lumen is circumscribed by atheromata and thus unaltered by vasomotor tone. With a mean diameter reduction of 49%, there are usually no ischemic symptoms; 60% results in exertional angina; and 76%, pain at rest.

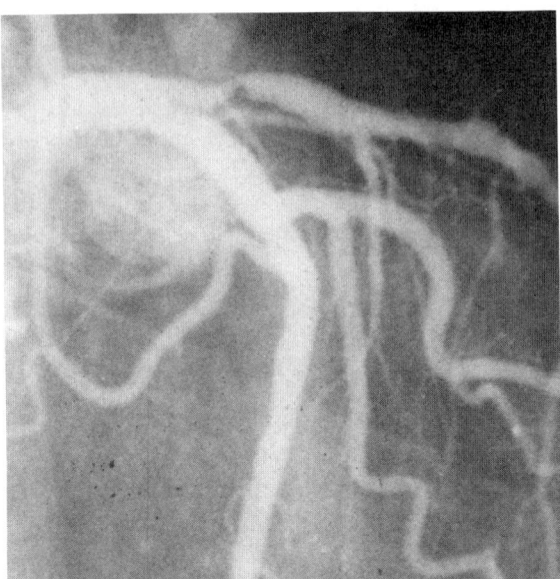

Fig. 3. Example of an arteriographic coronary image of sufficient quality for application of the quantitative method described. The left coronary artery is here entered by the 2.7-mm diameter catheter from the upper left. The anterior descending artery passes horizontally to the right and is 74% narrowed proximally. The left circumflex artery passes vertically downward giving marginal branches toward the right.

A_2 (Ellis et al., 1976). Electrophysiologic (Harder et al., 1979) and experimental coronary hemodynamic evidence (Winbury, 1971) together with the clinical data presented here provide convincing evidence that the coronary conductance and resistance vessels respond independently and sometimes in different directions to various physiologic and pharmacologic vasoactive interventions.

Patient Studies

At cardiac catheterization, 70 consenting male patients with symptomatic coronary artery disease were studied at rest and during a series of physical and pharmacologic stresses. In all cases, changes in coronary lumen caliber were measured from the arteriogram in "normal" and diseased segments, using the quantitative method described below. In 29 patients, coronary sinus flow was measured by a continuous thermodilution technique (Ganz et al., 1971).

Twenty-four patients (Group I) performed all or part of the following sequence. Baseline hemodynamic measurements, coronary sinus flow and arteriographic determinations were made. Isometric handgrip (HGP) was performed for 5 min at 25% of maximum grip strength; measurements were repeated between the 4th and 5th min of HGP. After return to baseline, dipyridamole (DP) was infused intravenously for 4 min to a dose of 0.56 mg/kg; measurements were repeated between the 5th and 6th min after the start of the DP infusion. Ten minutes after the start of DP, isometric handgrip was repeated; measurements were again obtained between the 4th and 5th min of handgrip. Ten minutes after release of this second HGP, sublingual nitroglycerin (NTG), 0.4 mg, was given; measurements were repeated 4 min after the NTG was dissolved.

Forty-six patients (Group II) were given nitroglycerin, 0.4–0.8 mg, sublingually after baseline hemodynamic and arteriographic determinations, which were repeated 4 min after NTG dissolved. Coronary sinus flow was measured in seven of these. Forty-nine diseased coronary segments were measured from the sequential arteriograms in the Group I patients. Seventy-six diseased segments were analyzed before and after NTG in the Group II patients.

Quantitative Coronary Arteriography

Analysis of these arteriograms was done with a computer-assisted method that produces a true scale, three-dimensional representation of any specified arterial segment (Brown et al., 1977). The method uses routine coronary cineangiograms, which are projected at about five-fold magnification in a dark room. Arteriographic images of the quality shown in Figure 3 are essential to the application of this method. Cineframes were selected from the two perpendicular angiographic projections (e.g., 40° right anterior oblique (RAO), 50° left anterior oblique (LAO)) in which a given lesion was best seen. The borders of the projected image of the diseased segment were traced from the "normal" proximal portion, through the stenosis to the "normal" distal" portion. A short length of catheter was also traced as a scaling factor. These traced border images were digitized from a tablet and terminal in Los Angeles, by telephone, into a PDP 11/45 digital computer in Seattle, Washington. The computer program reduces the lesion image to true scale by compensating for pincushion distortion, x-ray beam divergence and magnification. Figure 4 shows the true scale LAO and RAO images, which are combined in a three-dimensional characterization of the stenosis, from which are computed and printed the vessel diameters and cross-sectional areas in the "normal" ends and at the point of greatest narrowing. Percent diameter and area reduction in the stenosis are computed, in addition to lesion length, estimated atheroma mass and stenosis flow resistance. The accuracy of this

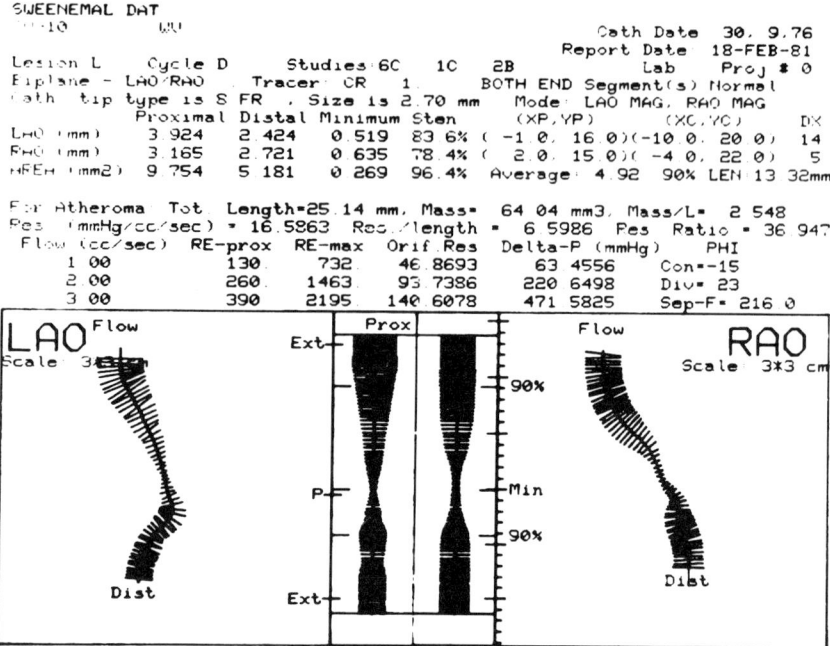

Fig. 4. Hard copy printout of computer analysis of a coronary stenosis. The left anterior oblique (LAO) and right anterior oblique (RAO) views of this segment are reduced to true scale in the 3 × 3-cm panels. These two views are matched at the point of greatest lumen narrowing and stretched mathematically to true length in the center panels. Absolute and relative lumen dimensions, atheroma mass and stenosis flow resistance are computed from this three-dimensional approximation of the diseased segment.

method averages within 0.08 mm for measurement of known dimensions. Its repeatability averages ±3% (SD) for estimates of "percent stenosis" and ±0.10 mm for estimates of minimum lesion diameter (Brown et al., 1977; McMahon et al., 1979; Koh et al., 1979).

In order to assess the effects of these physical and pharmacologic stresses on coronary lumen caliber, lesions from four cineframes were each traced by two experienced observers from the angiograms made during each of the serial stresses. These eight results were averaged to obtain the final lumen measurement for a given stress condition. Those doing the lesion analysis were blinded as to the condition being analyzed. For purposes of this report, we have measured the dynamic response of "normal" coronary lumen area, minimum lumen area and stenosis flow resistance to these different stresses.

Dynamic Coronary Response to a Vasoconstrictor Stress (HGP)

Sustained isometric handgrip (HGP) increases sympathetic nervous system activity with a resulting rise in heart rate, blood pressure and peripheral vasoconstrictor tone. Figure 5 illustrates the pertinent coronary vascular responses to HGP. Coronary lumen area in "normal" segments constricts by 9 ± 15% (SD) (P < 0.001); stenosis lumen area constricts by 13 ± 15% (P <0.001). On the average, predicted stenosis flow resistance increases 40 ± 51% (P < 0.001). Heart rate rises by 19% (P < 0.001), mean blood pressure by 24% (P < 0.001) and coronary sinus flow by 74% (P < 0.001), reflecting a 29% reduction in coronary vascular resistance. Thus the coronary microvascular bed dilates in response to the increased metabolic demands of HGP, but both "normal" and diseased portions of the epicardial conductance vessels constrict in response to increased sympathetic neurogenic activity. This

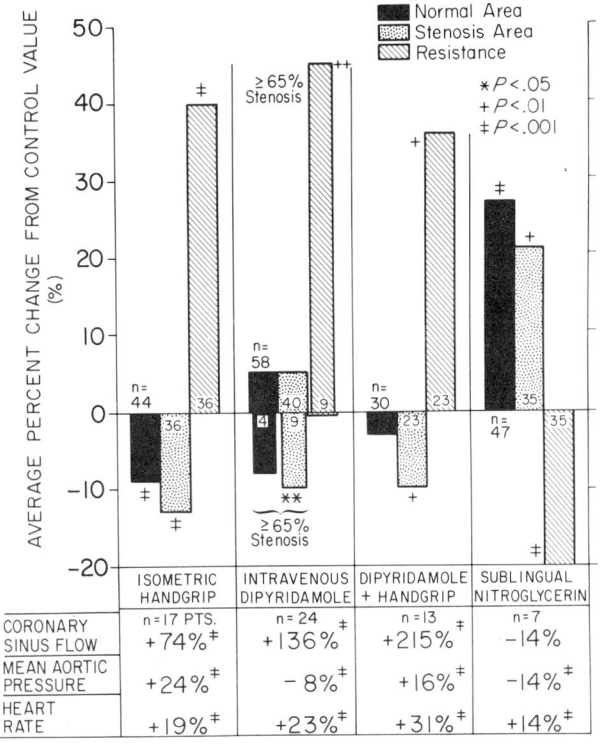

Fig. 5. Changes in hemodynamic parameters and coronary lumen measurements during certain vasoactive stresses. Results are expressed as a percentage change from the control state in a given variable during the given stress. Hemodynamic parameters include heart rate, mean aortic pressure and coronary sinus flow. Arterial measurements include "normal" lumen area, minimum lumen area in the stenosis, and predicted stenosis flow resistance. Vasoactive stresses include sustained isometric handgrip (HGP) for 5 min at 25% of maximum grip strength, intravenous dipyridamole (DP) at 0.56 mg/kg infused over 4 min, the combination of HGP and DP, and sublingual nitroglycerin (NTG) 0.4–0.8 mg.

	ISOMETRIC HANDGRIP	INTRAVENOUS DIPYRIDAMOLE	DIPYRIDAMOLE + HANDGRIP	SUBLINGUAL NITROGLYCERIN
	n=17 PTS.	n=24 ±	n=13 ±	n=7
CORONARY SINUS FLOW	+74%‡	+136%‡	+215%‡	−14%
MEAN AORTIC PRESSURE	+24%‡	−8%‡	+16%‡	−14%‡
HEART RATE	+19%‡	+23%‡	+31%‡	+14%‡

combination of stenosis constriction and flow increase would result in a 3.6-fold worsening of the pressure loss in a lesion having the characteristics given by Expression 2. If the resulting pressure loss were sufficiently great, angina could result. Angina occurs during HGP in 10-25% of patients with coronary disease (Siegel et al., 1972).

Dynamic Coronary Response to a Resistance Vessel Dilator (DP)

Dipyridamole (DP) is a dramatic and relatively selective dilator of the coronary resistance bed. Whereas near-maximal bicycle exercise increased coronary flow to 3.2 times baseline in normal subjects, i.v. DP raised it to 3.4 times baseline (Heiss et al., 1976). In our 24 Group I patients, as shown in Figure 5, DP increased heart rate 23% ($P < 0.001$), coronary flow 136% ($P < 0.001$) and lowered mean aortic pressure 8% ($P < 0.001$). *Resistance* bed dilation resulted in an average 61% ($P < 0.001$) reduction in coronary vascular resistance. DP, a potent arteriolar dilator, had little direct effect on the coronary *conductance* vessels, as shown in Figure 5. Forty lesions were of the less severe type (<65% stenosis). In these, DP induced a mild, nonsignificant dilation of the "normal" and stenotic coronary segments; there was no change in predicted stenosis resistance. In nine lesions with ≥65% stenosis, the minimum lumen area *constricted* by 10%, a response significantly different ($P < 0.05$) from that of the milder lesions; and the predicted resistance increased by 45%, also different from the milder lesion response ($P < 0.01$). Four "normal" segments distal to severe lesions constricted 8% after DP. In the resting state, these nine severe lesions had an average predicted pressure loss of 31 mm Hg at 1 ml/sec normal coronary flow. If these lesions were characterized by Expression 2, a 136% increase in stenosis flow would result in a 4.5-fold increase in stenosis pressure loss, or 140 mm Hg. Obviously a stenosis loss of this magnitude is impossible in a patient having only 100 mm Hg available for perfusion of the distal coronary bed. Consequently, in regions of significant coronary stenosis, the capacity to increase regional flow in response to hyperemic stresses (exercise, DP) is substantially curtailed. Figure 1 illustrates this principle in the setting of exercise hyperemia; the greatest part of available perfusion energy is wasted in stenosis loss, and the distal pressure is insufficient to perfuse the subendocardium. Predictably, ischemia would result; and, indeed, 41% of coronary disease patients given DP in this "diagnostic" dose experience some degree of chest pain.

In this context, we interpret the measured constriction of the stenosis lumen and distal normal lumen after DP to be a *passive* response to the reduced intraluminal coronary pressure associated with increased stenosis flow and pressure loss. An angina-mediated pain-reflex sympathetic vasoconstriction does *not* appear to explain our data for these nine severe lesions, because milder lesions in these same patients did not constrict following DP.

Dynamic Coronary Response to a Conductance Vessel Dilator (NTG)

Nitroglycerin (NTG) has distinctive effects on systemic hemodynamics that have been shown to reduce myocardial oxygen demand. Systemic pressure fell 14% (P < 0.001) in both our Group I and Group II patients (see Fig. 5). Heart rate increased 6% (P = not significant) in Group II. Seven patients receiving only NTG experienced a 14% mean reduction (P < 0.05) in coronary sinus flow. Reduced coronary flow is a reflection of reduced myocardial oxygen demand. Because precise arterial measurements have only recently become available (Gensini et al., 1971; Feldman et al., 1979; Brown et al., 1981b) it was previously concluded that the only beneficial effects of NTG were through its peripherally mediated effects on "preload" and "afterload." However, the

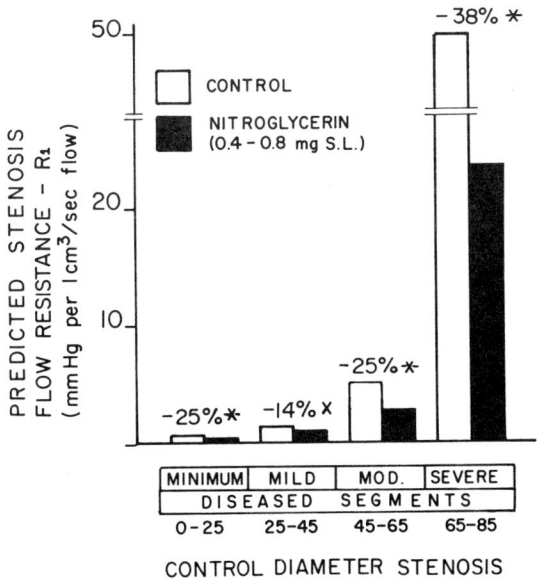

Fig. 6. Effect of nitroglycerin (NTG) on predicted stenosis flow resistance in 76 coronary lesions segregated into four groups on the basis of disease severity. Initially, the resistance in minimum lesions (0–25% stenosis) averaged 0.88 mm Hg/ml/sec; the average resistance reduction after NTG was 25% of controls. Initial resistance in 20 severe lesions (≥65% stenosis) averaged 48 mm Hg/ml/sec, which fell an average of 38% after NTG. Paired-t statistical comparison of pre- and post-NTG resistance values in each group: x = P < 0.05; * = P < 0.01.

data of Figure 6 demonstrate that NTG causes a statistically and physiologically significant dilation of *normal* and *diseased* portions of the coronary lumen. This dilation is a direct effect of NTG on the coronary smooth muscle, because it occurs despite a simultaneous reduction in arterial pressure. Predicted flow resistance in the average severe stenosis ($\geq 65\%$) fell 38% within 4 min after sublingual NTG. A careful review of the published data on other hemodynamic responses to NTG reveals that stenosis dilation is one of the greatest of the potentially beneficial effects of this drug (Brown et al., 1981b).

Thus the two "coronary vasodilators," DP and NTG, have diametrically opposite actions. DP dilates the resistance bed, but has no effect on the conductance vessels except to increase flow resistance by 45% in severe stenoses (which constrict passively in response to reduced intraluminal pressure). Clinically, in this large intravenous "diagnostic" dose, DP causes mild-to-significant angina in 41% of patients with coronary disease (Josephson et al., 1980).

Conversely, sublingual NTG dilates the conductance vessels, reducing flow resistance in severe stenoses by 38% without significantly affecting the ability of the coronary microvasculature to down-regulate coronary flow in response to reduced myocardial oxygen demand. And clinically, NTG is the most effective single drug we have for acute relief of angina.

Clinical Applications of Dynamic Stenosis Concepts

Diagnosis

Any stress that substantially increases stenosis flow has the potential for provoking subendocardial ischemia, as illustrated in Figure 1. Exercise is a stress that is used diagnostically to provoke chest pain or ischemic electrocardiographic abnormalities, or to induce ventricular contractile abnormalities (Borer et al., 1977). Dipyridamole also greatly increases flow to normally perfused myocardium; but a substantial regional hyperemic response is prevented by significant coronary stenosis. This principle is the basis for a method of myocardial perfusion imaging (Gould et al., 1978) in which thallium-201 or nitrogen-13 ammonium is given at the peak of DP-induced coronary hyperemia. These isotopes are taken up into myocardium in rough proportion to coronary flow; so a region that is perfusion-limited by a coronary stenosis shows as a regional defect on the cardiac scintigraphic image. DP- and exercise-induced hyperemia are of comparable utility for detection of $\geq 50\%$

coronary stenoses (Albro et al., 1978; Josephson et al., 1980) and coronary lesions as mild as 40% are frequently detected (Josephson et al., 1980).

When isometric handgrip is performed soon after the DP infusion, two potentially useful effects are observed (see Fig. 5). First, DP does not block the HGP-induced coronary arterial constriction; and second, coronary flow increases 68% more ($P < 0.02$) with the combined stresses than with DP alone. Thus the combined stresses further increase the disparities of regional myocardial perfusion (and regional isotope uptake) found in coronary disease and thus potentially improve the sensitivity for the scintigraphic detection of coronary stenosis.

Therapy

Based on the above principles, the ideal agent(s) for therapy of ischemic heart disease would dilate the coronary *conductance* vessels, and reduce the distal myocardial perfusion (oxygen) requirements by decreasing heart rate, myocardial contractility, diastolic preload and systolic afterload. In practice, the combination of beta-adrenergic blockade and long acting nitrates achieves these goals quite well. One must avoid too great a reduction in coronary perfusion pressure, because partial collapse of the stenosis under reduced intraluminal coronary pressure has been observed experimentally (Santamore and Walinsky, 1980; Schwartz et al., 1980) and clinically (see Fig. 5; Brown et al., 1981c; Feldman et al., 1978). This may explain the episodes of acute cardiovascular collapse sometimes seen after intravenous nitroglycerin in the coronary care unit (Come and Pitt, 1976).

The drugs dipyridamole and hydralazine have been associated with worsening angina in certain patients with coronary disease. Both drugs dilate the resistance bed rather than the conductance vessels. By the above principles they could worsen subendocardial perfusion in some patients with severe proximal stenosis. This possibility should be considered when using these drugs in patients with coronary disease.

Summary

Coronary artery lesions are not simply fixed impediments to coronary flow. Several aspects of the lesion behavior are sufficiently dynamic to be of importance in the interpretation of ischemic symptoms and their therapy. First, pressure lost in transit through any stenosis of 50%, or greater, is roughly determined by the *square* of stenosis flow. Hence, drugs or stresses that substantially increase regional myocardial flow requirements can jeopardize subendocardial perfusion distal to such a stenosis. Second, coronary stenoses commonly demonstrate active, sympathetically mediated vasoconstriction, or direct nitroglycerin-induced vasodilation. The physiologic impact of these vasoactive changes is of considerable magnitude. Third, severe stenoses demonstrate a passive elastic collapse in response to reduced intraluminal pressure, rendering the stenosis even more severe. These dynamic changes have important diagnostic and therapeutic implications, which are discussed.

Acknowledgment

Supported in part by Veterans' Administration Project 1102–01, in part by United States Public Health Service Grant HL 13517, HL 19451, HL 18805 and in part by American Heart Association-GLAA Grant-in-Aid 592. Dr. Brown is an Established Investigator of the American Heart Association.

References

Albro, P. C., Gould, K. L., Westcott, R. J., Hamilton, G. W., Ritchie, J. L. and Williams, D. L. 1978. Non-invasive assessment of coronary stenoses by myocardial imaging during pharmacologic coronary vasodilation. III. Clinical trial. Am J Cardiol 42:751–760

Berne, R. M. 1980. The role of adenosine in the regulation of coronary blood flow. Circ Res 47:807–813

Borer, J. S., Bacharach, S. L., Green, M. V. Kent, K. M., Epstein, S. E. and Johnston, G. S. 1977. Real-time radionuclide cineangiography in the non-invasive evaluation of global and regional left ventricular function at rest and during exercise in patients with coronary artery disease. N Engl J Med 296:839–844

Brown, B. G. 1981. Coronary vasospasm: Observations linking the clinical spectrum of ischemic heart disease to the dynamic pathology of coronary atherosclerosis. Arch Intern Med 41:716–722

Brown, B. G., Bolson, E. L., Frimer, M. and Dodge, H. T. 1977. Quantitative coronary arteriography: Estimation of dimensions, hemodynamic resistance, and atheroma mass of coronary artery lesions using the arteriogram and digital computation. Circulation 55:329–337

Brown, B. G., Bolson, E. L. and Dodge, H. T. 1981a. Coronary arteriography and the objective assessment of coronary artery pathology. In *The Coronary Artery*, ed. S. Kalsner, London: Croom-Helm, Ltd. in press

Brown, B. G., Bolson, E., Petersen, R. B., Pierce, C. D. and Dodge, H. T. 1981b. The mechanisms of nitroglycerin action: Stenosis vasodilation as a major component of the drug response. Circulation 64:1089–1097

Brown, B. G., Josephson, M. A., Petersen, R. B., Pierce, D. C., Wong, M., Hecht, H. S., Bolson, E. and Dodge, H. T. 1981c. Intravenous dipyridamole combined with isometric handgrip for near-maximal acute increase in coronary flow in patients with coronary disease. Am J Cardiol 48:1077–1085

Buckberg, G. D., Fixler, D. E., Archie, J. P. and Hoffman, J. I. E. 1972. Experimental subendocardial ischemia in dogs with normal coronary arteries. Circ Res 30:67–81

Come, P. C. and Pitt, B. 1976. Nitroglycerin-induced severe hypotension and bradycardia in patients with acute myocardial infarction. Circulation 54:624–628

Ellis, E. F., Oelz, D., Roberts, L. J., Payne, N. A., Sweetman, B. J., Nies, A. S. and Oates, J. A. 1976. Coronary arterial smooth muscle contraction by a substance released from platelets; evidence that it is thromboxane A_2. Science 193:1135–1137

Feldman, R. L., Pepine, C. J. and Conti, C. R. 1978. Unusual vasomotor coronary arterial responses after nitroglycerin. Am J Cardiol 42:517–519

Feldman, R. L., Pepine, C. J., Curry, R. C. and Conti, C. R. 1979. Quantitative coronary arteriography using 105-mm photospot angiography and an optical magnifying device. Cathet Cardiovasc Diagn 5:195–201

Feldman, R. L., Pepine, C. J., Curry, R. C. and Conti, C. R. 1979. Coronary arterial responses to graded doses of nitroglycerin. Am J Cardiol 43:91–97

Ganz, W., Tamura, K., Marcus, H. S., Donoso, R., Yoshida, S. and Swan, H. J. C. 1971. Measurement of coronary sinus blood flow by continuous thermodilution in man. Circulation 54:181–195

Gensini, G. G., Kelly, A. E., DaCosta, B. C. B. and Huntington, P. P. 1971. Quantitative angiography: The measurement of coronary vasomobility in the intact animal and man. Chest 60:522–530

Gould, K. L. 1978. Pressure-flow characteristics of coronary stenoses in unsedated dogs at rest and during coronary vasodilation. Circ Res 43:242–253

Gould, K. L. 1980. Dynamic coronary stenosis. Am J Cardiol 45:286–292

Gould, K. L., Lipscomb, K. and Calvert, C. 1975. Compensatory changes of the distal coronary vascular bed during progressive coronary constriction. Circulation 51: 1085–1094

Gould, K. L., Westcott, R. J., Albro, P. C. and Hamilton, G. W. 1978. Non-invasive assessment of coronary stenoses by myocardial imaging during pharmacologic coronary vasodilation. II. Clinical methodology and feasibility. Am J Cardiol 41: 279–287

Harder, D. R., Belardinelli, L., Sperelakis, N., Rubio, R. and Berne, R. M. 1979. Differential effects of adenosine and nitroglycerin on the action potentials of large and small coronary arteries. Circ Res 44:176–182

Heiss, H. W., Barmeyer, J., Wink, K., Hell, G., Cerny, F. J., Keul, J. and Reindell, H. 1976. Studies on the regulation of myocardial blood flow in man. Basic Res Cardiol 71:658–675

Hoffman, J. I. E. and Buckberg, G. D. 1976. Transmural variation in myocardial perfusion. In *Progress in Cardiology*, eds. P. N. Yu and J. F. Goodwin, pp. 38–52. Philadelphia: Lea & Febiger

Josephson, M. A., Brown, B. G., Hecht, H. S. Hopkins, J., Pierce, C. D. and Petersen, R. B. 1980. Detection and localization of ≥40% coronary stenosis in patients: Comparison of exercise and dipyridamole thallium-201 myocardial imaging. Am J Cardiol 45(abs):399

Koh, D., Mitten, S., Stewart, D., Bolson, E. and Dodge, H. T. 1979. Comparison between computerized quantitative coronary angiography and clinical interpretation. Circulation 60(Suppl II):II–160

Logan, S. E. 1975. On the fluid mechanics of human coronary artery stenosis. IEEE Trans Biomed Eng 22:327–334

MacAlpin, R. N., Abbasi, A. S., Grollman, J. H., Jr. and Eber, L. 1973. Human coronary artery size during life. A cinearteriographic study. Radiology 108: 567–576

May, A. G., Van den Berg, L., DeWeese, J. A. and Rob, C. G. 1963. Critical arterial stenosis. Surgery 54:250–259

McMahon, M. M., Brown, B. G., Cukingnan, R. A., Rolett, E. L., Bolson, E., Frimer, M. and Dodge, H. T. 1979. Quantitative coronary angiography: Measurement of the "critical" stenosis in patients with unstable angina and single-vessel disease without collaterals. Circulation 60:106–113

Moir, T. W. and DeBra, D. W. 1967. Effect of left ventricular hypertension, ischemia, and vasoactive drugs on myocardial distribution of coronary flow. Circ Res 21:65–74

Ross, G. S., Stinson, E., Schroeder, J. and Ginsburg, R. 1980. Spontaneous phasic activity of isolated human coronary arteries. Cardiovasc Res 14:613–618

Sandor, T., Als, A. V. and Paulin, S. 1979. Cine-densitometric measurement of coronary arterial stenoses. Cathet Cardiovasc Diagn 5: 195–201

Santamore, W. P. and Walinsky, P. 1980. Altered coronary flow responses to vasoactive drugs in the presence of coronary arterial stenosis in the dog. Am J Cardiol 45:276–285

Schwartz, J. S., Carlyle, P. F. and Cohn, J. N. 1980. Effect of coronary arterial pressure on coronary stenosis resistance. Circulation 61:70–76

Siegel, W., Gilbert, C. A., Nutter, D. O., Schlant, R. C. and Hurst, J. W. 1972. Isometric handgrip and treadmill exercise in atherosclerotic heart disease. Am J Cardiol 30:48–54

Winbury, M. M. 1971. Redistribution of left ventricular blood flow produced by nitroglycerin. Example of integration of the macro- and microcirculation. Circ Res 28 (Suppl I):140–147

Wyatt, H. L., Forrester, J. S., Tyberg, J. V., Goldner, S., Logan, S. E., Parmley, W. W. and Swan, H. J. C. 1975. Effect of graded reductions in regional coronary perfusion on regional and total cardiac function. Am J Cardiol 36:185–192

Yasue, H., Omoto, S., Takizawa, A., Magao, M., Miwa, K. and Tanaka, S. 1979. Circadian variation of exercise capacity in patients with Prinzmetal's variant angina: Role of exercise-induced coronary arterial spasm. Circulation 59:938–948

Young, D. F., Cholvin, N. R. and Roth, A. C. 1975. Pressure drop across artificially induced stenoses in the femoral arteries of dogs. Circ Res 36:735–743

Young, D. F. and Tsai, F. Y. 1973. Flow characteristics in models of arterial stenosis. I. Steady flow. J Biomech 6:395–410

Discussion

Dr. Gould: Could you comment on your stenotic model? I believe that the intraluminal construction will greatly amplify some of the responses you are observing.

Dr. Santamore: The balloon catheter has a tremendous advantage because it allows both vasoconstrictor and changes in the intraluminal pressure to be analyzed in the same stenosis while an external snare eliminates the vasoconstriction. The price you pay for this advantage is some amplification or increased responsiveness of the vessel. In comparison with my own data (I have also used the external snare in open chest preparation), we get about twice the response to changes in distal pressure with intraluminal obstruction. So it is a little more sensitive, but the balloon catheter does have the advantage that you can examine vasoconstriction and passive characteristics all in the same animal. You are also able to instrument an animal without touching the coronary vessels.

Dr. Thomas: Dr. Santamore, you mentioned that in your in vitro prep you used both coronaries and carotid arteries. Did you have any differences in response?

Dr. Santamore: Qualitatively, the coronary and carotid arteries had similar responses. The major difference is the carotids are much more muscular and they constrict more.

Dr. Maseri: Dr. Santamore, this is a very nice series of experiments you have whereby, vasodilating, either by pacing or by adenosine, you can get a zero flow. If I remember correctly, perfusion pressure remains exactly the same. So, in spite of the perfusion pressure, because you reduce distal pressure, you reach the point where you have a critical closing pressure. Are we going to stay like that?

Dr. Santamore: Yes. First of all, this paradoxical flow response is only going to occur with severe underlying stenosis; also the vessel has to be compliant and able to respond to changes in pressure. The flow reduction itself would be maintained if we had kept the pacing up. If we turn the pacer off, there is generally a recovery period where the animal would reestablish his normal hemodynamics.

Dr. Maseri: But if you keep pacing or if you keep giving adenosine, the flow remains depressed. (Yes.) In spite of the fact that you produced ischemia with an S-T segment elevation.

Dr. Santamore: The flow would stay down. At least we have observed pacing for 20 min and the flow is still depressed.

Dr. Maseri: Well, it is interesting because about 5 years ago we observed coronary blood flow to go down with pacing. There was a long dispute with Paul Cannon and Paul Lintlan. They never observed this because they were using the technique the other way around. But in our technique of injecting the xenon, then doing the pacing, we were seeing the flow stop completely. This passive collapse could be the explanation for this flow response you just reproduce in our experiments.

Dr. Santamore: There are a couple of other clinical studies that have reported a slight reduction in flow with pacing.

Dr. Maseri: Selwyn observed this with pacing.

Dr. Ginsburg: In angioplasty you are dilating the coronary artery, which we do, and giving a calcium antagonist and dilating it further, giving systemic nitroglycerin and dropping the systemic blood pressure. Despite dropping the distal pressure by a variety of substances, we have never seen the vessel collapse. As a matter of fact, the uniform experience is that the vessel is larger and the geometry of the stenosis, especially the diameter, is considerably bigger. Do you have any comments on that?

Dr. Santamore: Nitroglycerin is a very potent larger coronary artery vasodilator. In the in vitro preparation there were no drugs, we were looking purely at pressure-dependent phenomenon. Clinically, you have a pressure-dependent phenomenon plus a drug-dependent mechanism. Maybe if you used another dilator that didn't affect the large coronary vessels, you might see that type of vessel collapse.

Dr. Gould: Do you think that intracoronary nitroglycerin is not vasodilator? I understand from the animal literature that, systematically, nitroglycerin does not increase coronary flow. But intracoronary does.

Dr. Santamore: My point was that intracoronary nitroglycerin is primarily a large coronary artery vasodilator. According to my theory, anything that increases the proximal coronary diameter size is beneficial. So you give nitroglycerin to cause the large proximal coronary artery to dilate, which should be beneficial. We would expect to see the results that Dr. Ginsburg mentioned.

Dr. Pepine: We have made thermodilution coronary venous measurements in the angioplasty setting across a partially dilated stenosis, and given nitroglycerin distally through the balloon catheter and flow goes up. It would seem that according to your model, you got the opposite effect.

Dr. Santamore: It depends upon the level of stenosis.

Dr. Pepine: These are patients with gradient of 30–40 mm Hg across the stenosis.

Dr. Santamore: In compliant stensoses that can respond to changes in intraluminal pressure, we always observe an increase in the hemodynamic severity of the stenosis after distal coronary arteriolar dilation. Always. The coronary flow response is variable and depends upon the total coronary resistance. If the stenotic resistance increase is more than the distal coronary resistance decrease, then coronary flow decreases. If the stenotic resistance increase is less than the distal coronary resistance decrease, then coronary blood flow increases.

Dr. Brown: Dr. Gould, your data is for group data, and I wondered if you saw that extremely tight stenoses did collapse distally in response to vasodilators. In other words, if it was an increase flow and a much greater pressure drop across this stenosis, was that pressure drop even greater enough to cause a passive collapse distal to the stenosis.

Dr. Gould: The answer is complex. The vasodilator changes occur in two phases. After vasodilators at maximum flow there is a mild collapse, a slight decrease in stenosis of the narrow segment, but later as the flow comes down a bit and the proximal and distal arteries vasodilate, it reverts to its normal size. The distal coronary arteriolar bed vasodilates with a different timing than of the proximal arteries. The distal arteriolar bed dilates quickly and it goes away quickly. The proximal artery vasodilates slower and it persists longer and there are the consequences. The minimal cross-sectional area of the stenosis decreases very slightly, then it immediately gets a bit larger and then the same as it is in the beginning. The cross-sectional area of the proximal and distal segments get progressively larger during this period of time. The viscous resistance doesn't change between early and late for the following reasons. Because the stenosis is a little bit less at the stenotic segment, everyone would expect the viscous loss to be greater. It isn't, because the proximal and distal part of the artery vasodilates and reduces the viscous resistance term that it is in fact passive, because of it going away immediately, and one is left then with the fixed geometrical changes 60 sec later that I described to you. According to Bernoulli the pressure in the stenotic segment here will be a bit less because the velocity is higher. There is a very mild passive change, but one cannot argue then that the stenosis is worst at this point in the primary sense, because it is entirely passive, and that as the rest of the artery vasodilates, the rest of the changes occur that revert back to normal and are not in fact self-propagating changes.

Dr. Maseri: You didn't tell us what sort of dilator you used.

Dr. Gould: In these cases I used intracoronary papaverine in the distal coronary arteries. I can also reproduce the same changes within ADP, dipyramidol or contrast media. All deliver distally, so they are not direct on the proximal coronary artery. The proximal artery vasodilates as a function of an increase in flow to the arteriolar bed. There is an intracoronary reflex from the distal bed to the proximal. It happens regardless of the agents you used when it was given distally.

Dr. Maseri: Expanding on the first point: To give it distally, the dilation that you had in the proximal segment, as you said, is reflex because pressure proximally remains the same.

Dr. Gould: That is correct. There is no change in aortic pressure.

Dr. Maseri: So you assume it is an axil reflex—the proximal dilation.

Dr. Gould: It is very complex. Hill showed that shear forces can probably vasodilate arteries. Whether it is neural reflex or mediated by some of the vasoactive compounds that we discussed this morning or whether it is the vibration of high shear forces, no one knows. Roche says it is vibration, but that is extremely complex. We are in the process of trying to sort it out.

Dr. Maseri: Thank you for the answer. Another thing I want to know is that you had a stenosis which was reducing the lumen, the cross-section, to about 10% of the original lumen. So there was a very severe stenosis.

Dr. Gould: Yes.

Dr. Maseri: Now, when you increased flow, the stenotic lumen did not collapse, although you had decreased pressure.

Dr. Gould: That is correct.

Dr. Maseri: How low was the pressure distally? Because you only showed gradients, you didn't show the actual pressure. How low did it go?

Dr. Gould: In these experiments it went down to 20 mm Hg, 15–20. That first slide I showed you showed a very low pressure. But even with distal pressures of that magnitude, the distal coronary artery clearly gets bigger. So the artery doesn't collapse as a consequence of pressure, but rather it changes the pressure in the consequences of primary vasomotion with changes in flow.

Dr. Maseri: Dr. Brown, I wish to compliment you for this very nice method that you set up to assess the stenosis very accurately. However, I think that proper interpretation of angiography is one of the very important parts of the investigation of the patient. It is hard to tell, however, what is the functional significance of that stenosis in your patient because you have no way of assessing the collaterals, which are not always visible on angiography, because they are below 100 μm. And yet there may be many of them and they may be significant. What I mean to say is that I think I was impressed by the fact that that nice stenosis that you removed from your patient was very tight, and yet the patient had a normal stress test, as you say. And there are very many patients like that. So an accurate assessment of one stenosis should go hand-in-hand with an overall evaluation of the coronary flow reserve of that patient. Putting all things together, this is the balance between severity of the stenosis and efficacy of collateral vascularity, be it visible at angiography or not visible (because most of it is not often visible).

Dr. Brown: Thank you for your observation. I have always been impressed by the importance of collaterals. In spite of its apparent severity, we would predict that the lesion that you saw in that patient would not cause clinical symptoms. It was 1½ mm^2, and usually we get clinical symptoms when we get down around 1.2–1.3 mm^2. So that although it looked severe as a percentage of diameter, it was a big artery and the percent stenosis that was on the order of 60% left a 1½ square mm^2 lumen measured from the angiogram and also measured from the histological specimen. It points out that the difference between subjective angiography and the ability to quantitate lesions in terms of what we know about the hemodynamic behavior of the stenosis. Thus, if we measure things, we can perhaps be a little more precise about predicting the importance of the stenosis. But I agree entirely that you can see a completely occluded vessel supplied by collaterals in a patient that has no infarct or even symptoms.

Section V

Current Clinical Aspects of Coronary Artery Disease

James F. Spann, *Chairperson*

Coronary Artery Spasm and Atherosclerosis

Attilio Maseri

Introduction

There is growing evidence that the clinical manifestations of ischemic heart disease result from a variable combination of fixed organic stenosis and of transient functional changes in the coronary lumen, resulting from vasoconstriction and intravascular obstruction by blood elements. The interest in "variant" angina, the revival of coronary spasm and the recent appraisal of the close interaction between substances released by aggregating platelets and vasomotor tone indicates that the epicardial coronary arteries should not be viewed any longer as a system of rigid tubes forming the plumbing system of the heart, but as a very dynamic system modulated by nervous impulses and constantly interacting with the blood it carries. This dynamic concept applies also to segments severely involved by atherosclerosis and is opening new avenues for research, diagnosis, therapy and prevention.

Coronary Anatomy and Physiology Revisited

Postmortem casts of coronary arteries (Baroldi and Scomazzoni, 1967) reveal a number of vessels and collaterals that look quite impressive when compared with the best in vivo coronary angiograms. In particular, the number of collaterals in the presence of stenoses or obstructions is surprisingly greater and larger in postmortem casts than in angiographic studies. This suggests that a large number of coronary vessels is not fully dilated in vivo, not only at the level of capillaries and resistive vessels, but also at the level of larger branches. Thus a modulation of coronary caliber occurs in vivo and inappropriate constriction may lead to, or worsen, acute myocardial ischemia. Studies in conscious dogs indicate that collaterals can compensate large vessel occlusions in a few days (Hregg and Bedynek, 1978) and provide good compensation some time later, also during severe exercise (Lambert et al., 1977). In animals constriction of epicardial arteries can be produced by alpha-adrenergic stimulation (Gross and Feigl, 1975), in particular, after induction of hypercholesterolemia (Rosendorff et al., 1981), by serotonin (Brazenor and Angus, 1981), by thromboxane A_2 (Ellis et al., 1977). In patients, spasm can be induced by histamine (Ginsburg, 1981) and constriction and dilation even at the site of severe atherosclerotic stenosis can be produced, respectively, by handgrip and by nitroglycerine (Brown et al., 1981).

Clinical Clues

It is well established that coronary atherosclerosis begins at birth and increases with age so that by the 5th decade about 50% of the population has one or more severe atherosclerotic coronary narrowings. Yet clinical manifestations of ischemic heart disease occur only in a few percent of the population; they usually, but not necessarily, occur in the individuals with more severe lesions, suddenly and unexpectedly, and exhibit unpredictable spontaneous periods of waxing and waning of symptoms. However, the severity of angiographic lesions is similar in stable and unstable angina (Fuster et al., 1975; Neill et al., 1977) and does not change when the acute phase of the disease is over (Neill et al., 1980), suggesting waxing and waning of functional factors transiently interfering with coronary blood supply rather than sudden worsening of organic lesions and subsequent gradual development of collaterals. This conclusion is in agreement with the observation that angina at rest is not caused by increased demand (Maseri et al., 1975; Guazzi et al., 1975; Chierchia et al., 1980; Figueras et al., 1979a, b) but by a transient reduction of supply (Maseri et al., 1976; Chierchia et al., 1980a, b; Ricci et al., 1978).

Coronary spasm appears to be a proven hypothesis for "variant" angina (Meller et al., 1976), for other forms of angina (Hillis and Braunwald, 1978) and it seems a possible initiating mechanism of myocardial infarction (Maseri et al., 1978). It can cause sudden death (Maseri, et al., 1981) and may contribute to the development of organic lesions in the coronary arteries (Maseri et al., 1980).

Coronary Vasomotion and Spasm

Vasomotion at the site of an organic coronary artery obstruction, categorically denied by Keefer and Resnik (1928), was considered possible by Blumgart et al. (1940). Leary (1934) observed that coronary arteries with narrowings could retain remarkable flexibility and a normal smooth muscle medium to allow spasm to play a role in angina and sudden death. Preservation of elasticity in atherosclerotic coronary arteries with eccentric stenoses was subsequently confirmed by Vlodaver and Edwards (1971).

Computerized measurement of coronary artery caliber on high quality biplane angiography has convincingly proved the possibility of a considerable coronary artery constriction and dilation, even at the site of severe organic narrowings (Brown et al., 1981). Therefore, it becomes important to discuss the relation between coronary vasomotion and acute myocardial ischemia.

Passive Changes in Vessel Caliber

A recent series of studies (Schwartz et al., 1979; Walinsky et al., 1979; Santamore et al., 1980) focused the attention on passive rather than active changes in caliber at the site of coronary stenosis in response to changes in transmural distending pressure. In collapsible vessels and tubes a reduction of outflow pressure does not result in cessation of flow because a waterfall or sluice phenomenon takes place. Thus, the difference between inflow pressure and extravascular pressure at the site of the collapsible vessels becomes the driving pressure and the level of outflow pressure becomes irrelevant when lower than extravascular pressure. Under these conditions, at constant inflow and extravascular pressure, when outflow pressure is progressively decreased below extravascular pressure, calculated flow resistance remains constant if taken as the difference between inflow and extravascular pressure, but increases progressively when calculated as inflow minus outflow pressure. However, in experimental studies with external constriction of a coronary artery, severe enough to abolish reactive hyperemia, a reduction in flow was demonstrated during peripheral coronary vasodilation (Schwartz et al., 1979; Walinsky et al., 1979). Accordingly, in large arteries without active tone with a severe external constriction, decrease in flow was observed when distal pressure was reduced to low levels (Santamore et al., 1980). Although the validity of these observations in patients remains to be proven, a passive wall collapse in an elastic coronary stenosis secondary to a fall in distending pressure was recently postulated by Ganz (1981) to explain vessel closure during spontaneous and exertional angina documented at angiography. This proposition assumes a critical fall of systemic arterial pressure or of distal perfusion pressure as the initiating event. However, if the mechanisms of vascular occlusion were caused only by purely passive hydrodynamic phenomena, ischemic episodes should occur predictably every time perfusion pressure is lowered and every time peripheral coronary dilation is produced in any given patient. Common clinical experience indicates that this is not the case, and active increase in vasomotor tone up to a level where critical closing pressure becomes higher than inflow pressure must be postulated for the genesis of coronary occlusion.

Changes in Normal Vasomotor Tone

As clearly pointed out by Prinzmetal et al. (1959) and theoretically discussed by MacAlpin (1980a, b), a small increase of smooth muscle tone is required to impair flow in a coronary artery branch at the site of a subintimal plaque that critically encroaches upon the lumen. This theory was elegantly verified experimentally (Santamore et al., 1980). On the basis of this consideration, MacAlpin suggests that normal changes in vasomotor tone may be responsible for impairment in flow at the site of large subintimal plaques, whereas spasm would be responsible for reduction or impairment in lumen in arteries without appreciable subintimal obstructions.

The hypothesis that physiological changes in vasomotor tone can be, per se, a general mechanism responsible for the onset of spontaneously transient ischemic attacks, is difficult to accept for the reasons discussed in the next paragraph. However, physiological changes in vasomotor tone may: 1) become important in the presence of local vascular hypersensitivity to abnormal constrictive stimuli; 2) modulate the susceptibility to abnormal constrictive stimuli; 3) modulate the maximal increase in flow across a stenosis at any given time.

Increased vasomotor tone appears to lower the threshold for spasmogenic stimuli in the early morning (Yasue et al., 1979). It may contribute to the variablity of effort tolerance observed in some patients and for the "walk-through" phenomenon.

Coronary Artery Spasm

In spontaneous angina transient impairment of coronary blood supply appears to be caused by abnormal constrictive stimuli or by local hypersensitivity to physiological stimuli rather than by passive changes in vessel lumen or by physiological changes in vasomotor tone alone, for the following reasons.

1. The alternans of severe recurrence of anginal attacks with relative asymptomatic phases of the disease, so often observed in patients with angina at rest, suggests waxing and waning of some transient pathological mechanism rather than passive changes in lumen or physiological variations in coronary vasomotor tone as the cause of transient ischemic episodes.
2. Should passive changes in lumen or increase in *normal* vasomotor tone play a major role, per se, in patients with atherosclerotic narrowings, "spontaneous" anginal attacks should be much more frequent than usually observed, considering that coronary artery diameter may decrease on the average about 15% after ergonovine (Curry et al., 1977), or handgrip (Brown et al., 1981). However, the positivity of these provocative tests is observed only in a few patients, independently of the severity of their organic coronary artery narrowings.
3. In the same patient transient occlusion of the vessels is not always localized at the site of the most severe stenosis (MacAlpin, 1980a, b) and the response to vasoconstrictive stimuli varies considerably in different phases of the disease.
4. Angiographic as well as visual observations at open heart surgery show diffuse and intense constriction of the vessel, also proximally and distally to the site of the organic stenosis.

Therefore, we propose a broad, provisional definition of coronary artery spasm as "*inappropriate, active constriction, focal or diffuse, of one or more large conductive coronary arteries.*"

Spasm and the Vessel Wall

There is a close, dynamic interaction among coronary smooth muscle tone, endothelium, vasoactive substances carried by blood and blood components. On the one hand increased sympathetic tone, as well as thromboxane A_2, serotonin and histamine, constrict epicardial arteries to a moderate extent in quiescent phases of the disease, but to the point of causing acute ischemia in susceptible vessels during active phases of the disease. Ischemic episodes with or without pain may occur repeatedly during the day and last from a few to 20–30 min. On the other hand, experimental constriction of coronary arteries was shown to cause early endothelial damage (Joris and Majno, 1981) and result in thrombus formation (Gertz et al., 1981). This hypothesis is consistent with the endothelial injury hypothesis of the genesis of atherosclerosis (Ross, 1981), which indicates that substances released at the site of injury by platelets, leukocytes and macrophages, stimulate smooth muscle cell migration into the intima and proliferation to form a plaque. Accordingly, clinical observations lead one to propose a possible causal effect of spasm on the formation of plaques (Maseri et al., 1980; Marzilli et al., 1980).

The loop of a vicious circle leading to worsening of the disease closes with decreased production of prostacyclin and of other substances maintaining the homeostasis at the vessel wall, platelet adhesion and increased diffusion of constrictive substances into the media. Finally, prolonged and repeated constriction may cause blood stagnation, plaque rupture and hemorrhage, resulting in thrombus formation. The thrombus can subsequently be lysed or become organized depending on the prevailing equilibrium between fibrinolytic and clotting mechanisms. If the thrombus becomes organized, then spasm contributes to the genesis of atherosclerosis according to the Rokitansky theory. The specimens removed during coronary endarterectomy, which appear like casts of the artery, indeed, appear to be the result of organized thrombi.

Atherosclerosis, Spasm, Syptoms and Prognosis

The severity of atherosclerotic lesions is similar in stable and unstable angina despite the worse prognosis of the latter. However, the clinical manifestations of ischemic heart disease are obviously influenced by the severity of atherosclerosis and of impairment of ventricular function.

The poor correlation between severity of symptoms and coronary atherosclerosis may not be contradictory if transient "functional" factors, such as coronary vasospasm and possibly platelet aggregation, play a major role in the development of the clinical manifestations of ischemic heart disease. While spasm can occur and cause ischemia and symptoms in patients with extremely variable severities of coronary atherosclerosis, in turn, the severity of coronary obstructions only conditions the threshold of myocardial demand that the patient can never exceed without developing ischemia.

While not necessarily closely correlated with the severity of symptoms, the extent to which the coronary circulation is jeopardized by the presence of atherosclerosis and the impairment of left ventricular function certainly influences prognosis. The effects of spasm are more devastating in a patient with multiple severe stenosis than in one with an otherwise normal heart; however, the presence of plaques favors the development of intimal damage, plaque rupture or hemorrhage, with a consequent tendency to prolonged or permanent occlusions. Thus, prognosis appears to be influenced by the presence and severity of acute transient functional factors such as spasm and by the extent to which the coronary circulation and the myocardium are already chronically jeopardized.

References

Baroldi, G. and Scomazzoni, G. 1967. Coronary circulation in the normal and pathologic heart. Washington, D.C.: American Registry of Pathology, Armed Forces Institute of Pathology, Government Printing Office.

Blumgart, H. L., Schlesinger, M. J. and Davis, D. 1940. Studies on the relation of the clinical manifestations of angina pectoris, coronary thrombosis and myocardial infarction to the pathological findings. With particular reference to the significance of the collateral circulation. Am Heart J 19:1–91

Brazenor, R. M. and Angus, J. A. 1981. Ergometrine contracts isolated canine coronary arteries by a serontonergic mechanism: no role for alpha-adrenoceptors. J Pharmacol Exp Ther 218: 530–536

Brown, B. G., Petersen, R. B., Pierce, C. D., Bolson, E. L. and Dodge, H. T. 1981. Dynamics of human coronary stenosis: interactions among stenosis flow, distending pressure and vasomotor tone. Presented at the Philadelphia Physiological Society Symposium, May 7–8

Chierchia, S., Brunelli, C., Simonetti, I, Lazzari, M. and Maseri, A. 1980a. Sequence of events in angina at rest: primary reduction in coronary flow. Circulation 61:759–768

Chierchia, S., Lazzari, M., Simonetti, I. and Maseri, A. 1980b. Haemodynamic monitoring in angina at rest. Herz 5: 189–198

Curry, R. C., Jr., Pepine, C. J., Sabom, M. B., Feldman, R. L., Christie, L. G. and Conti, C. R. 1977. Effects of ergonovine in patients with and without coronary artery disease. Circulation 56:803–809

Ellis, E. F., Oelz, O., Roberts, I. J., Payne, N. A., Sweetman, B. J., Nico, A. S. and Oates, J. A. 1977. Coronary arterial smooth muscle contraction by a substance released from platelets: evidence that it is thromboxane A_2. Science 193:1135–1137

Figueras, J., Singh, B. N., Ganz, W., Charuzi, Y. and Swan, H. J. C. 1979a. Mechanisms of rest and nocturnal angina: Observations during continuous haemodynamic and electrocardiographic monitoring. Circulation 59:955–961

Figueras, J., Singh, B. N., Ganz, W. and Swan, H. J. C. 1979b. Haemodynamic and electrocardiographic accompaniments of resting postprandial angina. Br Heart J 42: 402–409

Fuster, V., Frye, R. L., Connolly, D. C., Danielson, M. A., Elvesack, L. R. and Kurland, L. T. 1975. Arteriographic patterns early in the onset of the coronary syndromes. Br Heart J 37:1250–1255

Ganz, W. 1981. Coronary spasm in myocardial infarction: fact or fiction? Circulation 63:487–488

Gertz, S. D., Uretsky, G., Wajnberg, R. S., Navot, N. and Gotsman, M. S. 1981. Endothelial cell damage and thrombus formation after partial arterial construction: Relevance to the role of coronary artery spasm in the pathogenesis of myocardial infarction. Circulation 63:476–486

Ginsburg, R. 1981. Drug effects on human coronary arteries. Presented at the Philadelphia Physiological Society Symposium, May 7–8

Gregg, D. E. and Bedynek, J. L., Jr. 1978. Compensatory changes in the heart during progressive coronary artery stenosis. In *Primary and Secondary Angina Pectoris,* eds. Attilio Maseri, Gerry Klassen and Michael Lesch, pp. 3–11. New York: Grune & Stratton

Gross, G. J. and Feigl, E. O. 1975. Analysis of coronary vascular beta receptors in situ. Am J Physiol 228:1909–1913

Guazzi, M., Polese, A., Fiorentini, C., Magrini, F., Olivari, M. T. and Bartorelli, C. 1975. Left and right heart haemodynamics during spontaneous angina pectoris. Comparison between angina with ST segment depression and angina with ST segment elevation. Br Heart J 37:401–413

Hills, L. D. and Braunwald, E. 1978. Endothelial changes induced by arterial spasm. Am J Physiol 102: 346–358

Hillis, L. D. and Braunwald, E. 1978. Coronary artery spasm. N Engl J Med 299: 695–702

Joris, I. and Majno, G. 1981. Endothelial changes induced by arterial spasm. Am J Pathology 102:346–358

Keefer, C. S. and Resnik, W. H. 1928. Angina pectoris: a syndrome caused by anoxemia of the myocardium. Arch Intern Med 41: 769–807

Lambert, P. R., Hess, D. S. and Bache, R. J. 1977. Effect of exercise on perfusion of collateral-dependent myocardium in dogs with chronic coronary artery occlusion. J Clin Invest 59:1–7

Leary, T. 1934. Coronary spasm as a possible factor in producing sudden death. Am Heart J 10:338–344

MacAlpin, R. N. 1980a. Contribution of dynamic vascular wall thickening to luminal narrowing during coronary arterial constriction. Circulation 61:296–301

MacAlpin, R. N. 1980b. Relation of coronary arterial spasm to sites of organic stenosis. Am J Cardiol 46:143–153

Marzilli, M., Goldstein, J., Trivella, M. G., Palombo, C. and Maseri, A. 1980. Some clinical considerations regarding the relationship of coronary vasospasm to coronary atherosclerosis: A hypothetical pathogenesis. Am J Cardiol 45:882–887

Maseri, A., Chierchia, S. and L'Abbate, A. 1980. Pathogenetic mechanisms underlying the clinical events associated with atherosclerotic heart disease. Circulation 62: (suppl)3–13

Maseri, A., L'Abbate, A., Baroldi, G., Chierchia, S., Marzilli, M., Ballestra, A. M., Severi, S., Parodi, O., Biagini, A., Distante, A. and Pesola, A. 1978. Coronary vasospasm as a possible cause of myocardial infarction. A conclusion derived from the study of "preinfarction" angina. N Engl J Med 299:1271–1278

Maseri, A., Mimmo, R., Chierchia, S., Marchesi, C., Pesola, A. and L'Abbate, A. 1975 Coronary artery spasm as a cause of acute myocardial ischemia in man. Chest 68:625–633

Maseri, A., Parodi, O., Severi, S. and Pesola, A. 1976. Transient transmural reduction of myocardial blood flow, demonstrated by thallium-201 scintigraphy, as a cause of variant angina. Circulation 56:280–288

Maseri, A., Severi, S. and Marzullo, P. 1981. Role of coronary artery spasm in sudden coronary ischemic death. Presented at the New York Academy of Sciences, May 7–9, 1981, New York

Meller, J., Pichard, A. and Dack, s. 1976. Coronary arterial spasm in Prinzmetal's angina: A proven hypothesis. Am J Cardiol 37:938–940

Neill, W. A., Ritzmann, L. W. and Selden, R. 1977. The pathophysiologic basis of acute coronary insufficiency. Observations favoring the hypothesis of intermitten reversible coronary obstruction. Am Heart J 94:439–444

Neill, W. A., Wharton, T. P., Jr., Fluri-Lundeen, J. and Cohen, I. S. 1980. Acute coronary insufficiency. Coronary occlusion after intermittent ischemic attacks. N Engl J Med 302:1157–1162

Prinzmetal, M., Kennamer, R., Merliss, R., Wada, T. and Bor, N. 1959. Angina pectoris. 1. A variant form of angina pectoris. Am J Med 27:375–388

Ricci, D. R., Orlick, A. E., Doherty, P. W., Cipriano, P. R. and Harrison, D. C. 1978. Reduction of coronary blood flow during coronary artery spasm occurring spontaneously and after provocation by ergonovine maleate. Circulation 57: 392–395

Rosendorff, C., Hoffman, J. I. E., Verrier, E. D., Rouleau, J. and Boerboom, L. E. 1981. Cholesterol potentiates the coronary artery response to norepinephrine in anesthetized and conscious dogs. Circ Res 48:320–329

Ross, R. 1981. Pathogenesis of coronary artery disease. Classic theories. Presented at the Philadelphia Physiological Society Symposium, May 7–8

Santamore, W. P., Walinsky, P., Bove, A. A., Cox, R. H., Carey, R. A. and Spann, J. F. 1980. The effects of vasoconstriction on experimental coronary artery stenosis. Am Heart J 100:852–858

Schwartz, J. S., Carlyle, P. F. and Cohn, J. N. 1979. Effect of dilation of the distal coronary bed on flow and resistance in severely stenotic coronary arteries in the dog. Am J Cardiol 43:219–224

Vlodaver, Z. and Edwards, J. E. 1971. Pathology of coronary atherosclerosis. Prog Cardiovasc Dis 14:256–259

Walinsky, I., Santamore, W. P., Weiner, L. and Brest, A. N. 1979. Dynamic changes in the haemodynamic severity of coronary artery stenosis in a canine model. Cardiovasc Res 13:113–118

Yasue, H., Omote, S., Takazawa, A. and Tanaka, S. 1979. Circadian variation of exercise capacity in patients with Prinzmetal's variant angina: Role of exercise induced coronary arterial spasm. Circulation 59:938–948

Diagnosis and Treatment of Coronary Artery Spasm

Carl J. Pepine, Robert L. Feldman and C. Richard Conti

Introduction

Identification of coronary artery spasm as the basis of transient myocardial ischemia, and its management, have become extremely important issues in clinical cardiology over the past decade (Pepine and Conti, 1980). The purpose of this chapter is to review the approach to these issues used at our institution.

Certain historical, electrocardiographic (ECG), and other noninvasive test findings can be suggestive of coronary spasm (Table 1). However, the definitive diagnosis can be made only by coronary angiography performed during an ischemic episode. Additionally, the precise angiographic appearance of the coronary artery or arteries before, during and after relief of spasm can provide useful information that may be important in management and prognosis of a given patient. For instance, in patients with coronary artery

Table 1. Diagnostic Criteria for Coronary Artery Spasm.

Suspect
    Rest angina syndrome
        Minimal change in heart rate and BP at onset
        Transient S-T elevation or arrhythmias
    Effort angina variable threshold
Definite
    Transient coronary narrowing of physiologic importance associated with evidence for ischemia

disease, it is important to know if spasm involves the region of atherosclerotic narrowing alone or occurs diffusely along the entire course of that vessel or another coronary artery. It is important to know whether spasm involves one or multiple arteries with or without atherosclerotic coronary disease. Such questions can only be answered by coronary angiography performed during an ischemic episode.

In our experience, most cases of coronary spasm are identified by performing angiogram during spontaneous pain. When episodes of ischemia do not occur spontaneously during the angiographic study, it is often desirable to attempt to provoke them. Although provocative tests designed to evoke spasm can be performed outside the catheterization laboratory, we believe that the initial test in any patient should be performed during catheterization (Pepine et al., 1980a). This practice allows hemodynamic as well as electrocardiographic evaluation of the course of the ischemic episode. Overall, this practice ensures the safest approach to recognize and handle potentially serious effects such as heart block, ventricular arrhythmia and prolonged ischemia secondary to spasm. A number of provocative tests have been used, but only ergonovine remains useful.

Criteria for Coronary Artery Spasm during Testing

Before discussing specifics of ergonovine provocative testing, it is important to try to decide what constitutes a response indicative of spasm (i.e., a "positive" test). We propose that 1) consistently detectable *coronary diameter reduction* after a low dose of ergonovine ($\leq$ 0.2 mg) accompanied by 2) *objective evidence for ischemia* with or without chest pain, but 3) without important increases in heart rate or blood pressure, that 4) *can be promptly reversed by intracoronary nitroglycerin,* fulfill criteria for coronary spasm. Objective evidence for myocardial ischemia include: 1) transient ECG changes such as

Table 2. Specific Indications for Provocative Testing for Coronary Spasm.

Transient nonspecific ECG abnormalities during angina
Ventricular arrhythmias or syncope during angina
Normal ECG during "ischemic" cardiac pain
Rest pain with an ECG pattern of conduction abnormality that prohibits interpretation of the S-T segment (pacer, Left Bundle Branch Block, Wolf-Parkinson-White)
Rest angina when no ECG's have been obtained during pain
Rest angina with little or no change in heart rate or blood pressure at onset
To attempt to predict efficacy of therapy or spontaneous remission
Angina recurring after coronary bypass surgery

Table 3. Contraindications to Provocative Testing for Coronary Spasm.

Recent myocardial infarction
Uncontrolled angina
Uncontrolled ventricular arrhythmias
Amenorrhea in a premenopausal female
Severe hypertension
Severe left ventricular dysfunction
Severe aortic stenosis
Significant left main coronary stenosis

S-T shifts, normalization of previously depressed S-T segments and peaking of T waves; 2) exaggerated rise in left ventricular end and diastolic pressure. The rise in left ventricular end diastolic pressure must be greater than expected from the loading effects due to increased aortic pressure and venoconstriction; 3) decrease in regional coronary flow of thallium-201-uptake associated with deterioration in regional wall mounting; 4) abnormal changes in regional lactate extraction or other metabolic indicators.

Indications and Contraindications to Testing

The general indication for ergonovine testing is the need to know whether or not coronary spasm is contributing to a patient's chest pain syndrome in the absence of contraindications. To be more specific, some common indications in patients with normal or near normal coronary arteries that we have identified appear in Table 2.

The above indications also apply to patients with more severe coronary atherosclerosis if suspicion of spasm is high, e.g., the patient with rest angina and relatively well preserved or variable effort tolerance. We also recommend ergonovine testing in patients who have test angina with transient S-T elevation (variant angina) in whom spontaneous angina does not occur during catheterization. Here clinical indications for testing are to: 1) confirm the presence of spasm; 2) define the location and degree of spasm, number of vessels involved and relationship to atherosclerotic coronary narrowing (i.e., at the site, proximal, distal, etc.) and 3) provide baseline data for later evaluation of therapy or course of disease (i.e., spontaneous remission). Information obtained in these variant angina patients is important in terms of prognosis, drug selection and potential for cardiac surgery, i.e., bypass, plexectomy, denervation, etc. Contraindications to ergonovine testing are shown in Table 3. The first three listed in Table 3 are relative contraindications. In some instances, we have found it necessary to test patients with these problems. The latter five are absolute.

Protocol for Provocative Testing with Ergonovine

At the University of Florida, we use a "lot-total cumulative dose" protocol. Tests are performed in the catheterization laboratory. No premedication, atropine or nitrates are given. Both nitroprusside and nitroglycerin are on hand for parenteral use. If nitroglycerin is not available through the pharmacy at your hospital, a solution for emergency use can be prepared as follows. Crush two 0.4-mg "fresh" tablets and place in a 10-cc glass syringe. Add 8 cc of saline and shake. Inject mixture through a millipore filter into another 10-cc syringe. Final solution yields approximately 100 μg of nitroglycerin/cc.

Baseline angiographic, hemodynamic and multiple lead ECG recordings are obtained in a pain-free period. If the patient does not have spontaneous angina during the course of the catheterization study, ergonovine 0.025 or 0.05 is injected i.v. as a bolus. The choice of initial dose is based on clinical findings and presence of coronary artery disease. Heart rate, blood pressure, ECG and possible onset of symptoms are observed for 3–5 min. If no changes occur, an additional 0.05 mg of ergonovine is administered. This procedure is repeated until a total dose of 0.2 mg is reached. Should symptoms occur or hemodynamic or ECG changes result, recordings are repeated and both left and right coronary angiograms are performed. Nitroglycerin is given promptly. If hypotension occurs or spasm does not reverse promptly, intracoronary nitroglycerin should be given immediately. Recently we have been using intracoronary nitroglycerin (50–100 μg) immediately after spasm is identified. This dose, injected into the coronary artery involved, immediately reverses ischemic findings without producing hypotension (Pepine et al., 1982).

Others have employed higher dose protocols. However, because the majority of patients with coronary spasm who respond to ergonovine do so at a dose less than 0.2 mg and because of our concern for safety, we limit the total dose to 0.2 mg. Another reason to limit the dose is to avoid possible provocation of an ischemic or angiographic response not due to spasm (i.e., "false positive" response) in patients with angiographically severe coronary stenosis. In a patient with subtotal obstructive coronary atherosclerosis, larger doses of a vasoconstrictor, like ergonovine, could produce total occlusion. If one believes the hypothesis that patients with coronary spasm have "hypersensitive" coronary artery responses to vasoconstrictor stimuli, the clinical importance of this type of pharmacologically induced total occlusion is unclear.

Hazards of Provocative Testing with Ergonovine

Major risks are ventricular arrhythmias, heart block, myocardial infarction and death. Fortunately, the incidence of either death or myocardial infarction is very low. Ventricular arrhythmias are not uncommon and are generally easily reversed by nitroglycerin. Heupler (1980) summarized experience of 852 patients undergoing ergonovine testing in 12 institutions, including ours. No deaths or infarctions were reported. In our patients (greater than 400) we have not had a death or myocardial infarction. However, a recent collective report of three deaths in patients undergoing provocative testing indicates that the test is not benign (Buxton et al., 1980). These deaths related to ergonovine-induced spasm occurred in patients who received either higher initial or total doses of ergonovine than we use. Use of intracoronary nitroglycerin was limited to only one of these three cases and apparently after a long period of ischemia.

It should be emphasized that ergonovine testing is more hazardous in patients with a positive test than those with a negative test. For example, Waters and colleagues (1980) report using ergonovine in 100 consecutive patients, with 4 episodes of ventricular arrhythmia in 64 patients with a negative test compared to 18 ventricular arrhythmias in 36 patients with a positive test. No other complications were reported in patients with a negative test. But in the 36 with a positive test, 4 experienced severe hypotension, 1 had severe recurrent angina, and another subendocardial infarction.

Results of Provocative Testing with Ergonovine

At the University of Florida Hospitals, bolus injection of 0.025–0.2 mg of ergonovine has been shown to produce chest pain with S-T segment elevation in essentially all patients with the clinical syndrome of variant angina who are in an active phase of their disease and in 2–5% of patients with classical effort angina syndrome (Pepine et al., 1980a). Localized reversible severe dynamic coronary narrowing occurred in all of these patients usually at a lower dose range, i.e., approximately 0.05–0.15 mg. In other patients presenting with chest pain syndromes, not thought to be classical or variant angina, this protocol has only rarely (2% of tests) provoked chest pain, S-T segment and coronary angiographic changes of importance. In these patients, subsequent follow-ups, ranging from several months to years, yielded additional clinical findings to implicate coronary spasm as the basis for a component of their angina syndrome. These findings included episodic periods of S-T elevation or

Table 4. Treatment of Coronary Artery Spasm.

Control-precipitating or aggravating factors
Drugs
  Vasodilators
  Slow-channel Ca^{2+} blockers
  Adrenergic blockers
  Platelet-aggregation inhibitors
IAPB - Intra Aortic Balloon Pump
CABG - Coronary Artery Bypass Graft
Cardiac denervation

T wave peaking, arrhythmias, pain at rest or very low levels of activity, etc. Patients failing to respond to ergonovine (cumulative dose 0.2 mg) have neither subsequently developed a variant angina syndrome nor have been found to have coronary spasm at a later date. Similar findings have been reported by other investigators (Chaine, 1980).

Other Tests

The cold pressor test (i.e., hand immersion in iced water), histamine and exercise may be useful in a few selected cases to provoke coronary artery spasm. However, the experience with these tests is limited. At present, we use these tests only when a patient's history suggests that these conditions are likely to evoke chest pain due to coronary spasm.

Management of Patients with Myocardial Ischemia Resulting from Coronary Artery Spasm

The rationale for use of various pharmacologic agents in patients with ischemic heart disease has been reviewed elsewhere in this symposium. Therefore, this section is limited to results of treatment of patients with coronary artery spasm as the basis for a component of their clinical findings due to ischemia. The agents available for use in these patients are summarized in Table 4.

Nitrates

As with other forms of ischemic heart disease, nitrates remain the cornerstone of pharmacologic management of transient myocardial ischemia due to coronary artery spasm. Their actions include dilation of both arteriolar and venous (capacitance) vascular beds. These changes tend to result in reduction in myocardial oxygen demand. Nitroglycerin also has a more direct influence on the coronary circulation. Nitroglycerin is a potent dilator of the large epicardial coronary arteries (Feldman et al., 1978) and is extremely useful when given to patients with coronary artery spasm (Pepine et al., 1982). In addition, nitroglycerin dilates coronary artery collateral channels; and evidence has been presented to indicate that blood flow to ischemic myocardium increases after nitroglycerin (Mehta and Pepine, 1978). These beneficial effects of nitroglycerin tend to make this agent extremely useful in patients with coronary spasm. Many include this direct coronary response to nitroglycerin in the definition of coronary spasm.

The relative amount of dilation in these vascular beds seems to be dependent upon the rate at which the drug is administered, the site of administration and the dose. For example, when a small dose (100 g) is administered directly into a coronary artery, intense coronary artery dilation occurs almost immediately. Little systemic effect is observed, and the major benefit is to patients with coronary spasm where this route of administration provides almost immediate relief of obstruction and increases blood flow (Pepine et al., 1982).

When nitrates are administered into the sytemic circulation rapidly and in large doses, as occurs with amyl nitrite inhalation or bolus nitroglycerin injection, intense systemic vasodilation predominates. When nitrates are given more slowly into the systemic circulation, as occurs with slow i.v. infusion, sublingual or topical administration, there is predominant dilation of the venous capacitance bed and only minimal to moderate arterial dilation. Using continuous intravenous infusion of isosorbide dinitrate, Distante and co-workers (1976) found that most episodes of ischemia in a group of patients with proven coronary spasm could be prevented.

Calcium Antagonists

A new pharmacological approach to coronary artery spasm is offered by a group of drugs collectively termed calcium antagonists or slow channel blockers (Fleckenstein, 1977). Knowledge of the importance of Ca^{2+} in vascular smooth muscle contraction is essential to the understanding of the action of calcium antagonists in coronary spasm. Based on current information, it appears that this new class of agents provides considerably greater flexibility for management of patients with coronary spasm.

They should be used either alone or in combination with other drugs on the basis of sound physiologic observations, i.e., what is responsible for the ischemic cardiac pain? It is essential to know the contribution made by important atherosclerotic and dynamic obstruction to the etiology of myocardial ischemia in any given patient. Beta blockers are known to be effective in patients with atherosclerotic coronary artery obstruction and relatively reproducible stress-induced angina, whereas coronary vasodilators should be the initial therapy in patients with angina pectoris due to coronary spasm, or coronary atherosclerosis or the combination of both, because oxygen demand and supply are beneficially altered.

The calcium blockers uniformly increase coronary flow primarily by decreasing coronary vascular resistance and increasing epicardial coronary artery size. In this regard, they are similar to the nitrates but dissimilar to beta blockers, which generally increase coronary artery resistance and decrease epicardial coronary artery size.

Results of Treatment with Calcium Blockers

Results of Treatment with Perhexiline

We treated 21 variant angina pectoris patients with the calcium blocker, perhexiline, at the University of Florida between 1975 and 1978 using 200–800 mg/day (Conti et al., 1979). These patients were referred for treatment of recurrent angina after trial with nitrates and propranolol. Each patient had angiographically documented coronary spasm. Thirteen of the 21 patients had hemodynamically important coronary atherosclerotic disease. Mean follow-up was approximately 1 year. During perhexiline treatment, reduction in nitroglycerin consumption paralleled reduction in angina frequency. Five of the 21 patients (24%) were asymptomatic. Ten of the 21 (48%) had a 50% decrease in angina frequency. Six of the 21 (28%) had less than a 50% reduction in angina. Five of these six patients had important coronary artery disease. Thus, from this *uncontrolled* evaluation, 72% of these patients with coronary spasm appeared to respond satisfactorily to perhexiline.

During follow-up, we withdrew perhexiline in 5 of the 13 patients with coronary disease and in 5 of 8 patients without coronary disease. Angina frequency and nitroglycerin consumption in the five coronary disease patients never returned to either pretreatment or perhexiline-treatment frequency. In the patients without coronary artery disease, angina frequency did not return to pretreatment level but did increase above the level observed during perhexiline treatment. It appeared that patients with normal coronary arteries were more likely to respond to this drug therapy. Because of the wide and unpredictable variation in symptom frequency in patients with coronary spasm, it is apparent that controlled trials are essential for evaluation of medical therapy.

Results of Treatment with Diltiazem

The next calcium blocking agent that we studied was diltiazem. Based upon favorable preliminary reports by Yasue (1979), we did a double-blind evaluation using 120 and 240 mg/day dosage schedules in 12 patients with variant angina (Pepine et al., 1981). Three of these patients had coronary artery disease. One of the 12 patients developed ventricular fibrillation during placebo. He was resuscitated and is not included in analysis of data. He was given open label diltiazem and has been asymptomatic since. Seven of the remaining 11 patients became asymptomatic or had 50% decrease in angina on diltiazem. Four remaining patients had less than 50% decrease in symptoms compared to placebo. One of these patients had coronary disease. Therefore, it appeared that diltiazem was effective in most patients tested. Similar effects in 15 patients with coronary artery spasm were found by Rosenthal and co-workers (Rosenthal et al., 1980). In both studies, diltiazem appeared remarkably free of side-effects over short term trial. No patients showed evidence for rebound or increase in symptoms upon withdrawal of diltiazem. In our study, there was a suggestion that diltiazem had some "carry-over" effect relative to continued suppression of angina. This suggestion was derived by comparing angina frequency in placebo periods that followed placebo to placebo periods that followed diltiazem. Comparison of these data showed placebo periods that followed diltiazem had significant reduction in angina frequency compared to placebo periods that followed placebo. If these results can be duplicated in more patients and are applicable to the larger group of patients with coronary artery disease and spasm, this agent will be a major advance in management.

Results of Treatment with Nifedipine

Based upon preliminary results reported in 26 patients with variant angina by Endo et al. (1978), nifedipine was evaluated in a large, open label trial in this country. Antman et al. (1980) reported results of therapy in 127 patients with either angiographically documented coronary spasm, angina at rest with reversible S-T elevation or both. Patients were treated with nifedipine in doses ranging from 40–160 mg/day. Follow-up averaged 9 months, and 87% of these patients had at least a 50% reduction in angina frequency, and in 63% angina was abolished.

We undertook a double-blind, randomized, controlled study to evaluate the effectiveness of nifedipine, compared to that of isosorbide dinitrate, in patients with coronary artery spasm.

Results of this trial in 15 patients indicate that frequency of angina and nitroglycerin requirements decreased with both nifedipine and isosorbide dinitrate (ISDN) (Hill et al., 1981). Intolerance necessitating drop-out occurred in two patients with ISDN and in none with nifedipine. One patient died suddenly while taking nifedipine. A greater than 50% decrease in angina frequency occurred in 8 of the remaining 12 patients on nifedipine and in 5 on ISDN. Although group responses were similar comparing the lead-in phase, nifedipine, and ISDN phases, certain patients appeared to have a particularly beneficial response to either nifedipine or ISDN. These findings in a limited number of patients suggest that both nifedipine and ISDN are similarly effective in a group of patients with coronary spasm. However, nifedipine may be better in certain patients, while ISDN may be better in others. Again, these results emphasize the need for controlled trials in evaluating therapy of patients with coronary artery spasm. Furthermore, comparison trials are important to attempt to identify what characteristics predict the response to a particular agent in any given patient.

Results of Treatment with Verapamil

Severi et al. (1980) followed 138 patients who had ECG changes during angina at rest. The majority of these patients had abnormal coronary arteries. Medical therapy consisted of isosorbide dinitrate and verapamil ("standard dose" 240 mg/day). In the first month of follow-up, 28 patients developed a nonfatal myocardial infarction and 5 died. Between 1 and 4 years after therapy, seven additional patients died and four developed an acute myocardial infarction. The authors note that after 4 years about 50% of patients were asymptomatic. The tendency to remission of symptoms was generally greater in those patients with less severe coronary artery disease. These, of course, are uncontrolled observations.

We have examined effects of verapamil in 15 patients with rest angina associated with ECG changes using a randomized double-blind trial. Thirteen of the 15 patients responded to verapamil. One responded to placebo and never reached the verapamil phase, while another did not respond to either verapamil or placebo. Except for the development of first degree A-V block in two patients, no other important adverse effects were observed. These results suggest the oral verapamil is effective as initial therapy for preventing episodes of ischemia in patients with rest angina (Schang and Pepine, 1977).

Beta Blockers

Controversy arises regarding use of propranolol in patients with coronary spasm. Propranolol has been found to be effective, occasionally effective, and even harmful in patients with coronary spasm (Pepine and Conti, 1980). One may want to discontinue beta blocking agents if symptoms increase or are not controlled by this agent or if the patient has normal coronary arteries with coronary spasm. The basis for this lack of effect resides in the finding that propranolol increases coronary resistance in certain settings (Schang and Pepine, 1977). Propranolol may block beta-adrenergic coronary dilator receptors, while leaving alpha-adrenergic constrictor receptors unopposed. This situation could theoretically result in more pronounced coronary artery constriction. Despite this objection to use of propranolol in patients with coronary spasm, propranolol may be worth trying in an individual patient. We have shown that addition of nitrates should counteract propranolol-related vasoconstriction (Schang and Pepine, 1978). Propranolol also has other effects that may be advantageous in ischemic heart disease, such as effects on arrhythmias, platelet aggregation and redistribution of myocardial blood flow. Some newer beta blocking agents also possess intrinsic sympathomimetic activity. These agents depolarize the beta receptor while blocking responses to sympathetic stimulation. Thus, heart rate tends to remain unchanged or may even increase at rest, but exercise-induced increases are attenuated. These agents may provide the vasodilating stimulus necessary to prevent coronary spasm and may warrant trial.

A new class of beta-adrenergic blocking agents also possesses alpha blocking activity. Labetolol is the prototype agent of this class. In a recently published preliminary trial (Halprin et al., 1980), labetolol was reported effective in significantly reducing or abolishing frequency of "spontaneous angina."

Platelets and Prostaglandins

Recently, the role of prostaglandins in the pathogenesis of vascular spasm and myocardial ischemia has been actively investigated (Pepine and Conti, 1980). One substance released by aggregating platelets is thromboxane A_2, a potent platelet-aggregating stimulator and vasoconstrictor. Arachidonic acid, in the presence of cyclooxygenase, produces endoperoxides, which in turn are modified by specific synthetase to form either prostacyclin (PGI_2) or thromboxane. PGI_2 formed within vascular walls is a potent vasodilator and inhibits platelet aggregation. Thus, PGI_2 acts to increase regional myocardial blood flow. In contrast, thromboxane A_2 synthesized by platelets is a potent vasoconstrictor and stimulates platelet aggregation. It has been suggested that, within a vascular bed, platelet aggregation, vasoconstriction and vasodilation can be altered by the relative balance between PGI_2 and thromboxane A_2 production. With either reduced PGI_2 or increased thromboxane production, the balance is shifted to favor vasoconstriction. Some investigators have proposed that such a mechanism may provoke "coronary vasospasm" that could trigger an acute ischemic crisis." Recently, marked elevation of thromboxane B_2, the major metabolite of thromboxane A_2, was found in patients with coronary spasm.

The observation that coronary spasm occurs frequently at sites of minimal atherosclerosis has led to the suggestion that vascular endothelium produces deficient amounts of PGI_2 in these atherosclerotic areas. Under conditions in which platelet adhesion and aggregation are increased, release of thromboxane A_2 would result in vasoconstriction. Because of these findings, treatment with antiplatelet agents has been suggested; but early results have not been successful. Preliminary, acute studies found that aspirin, given in doses that reduced platelet-thromboxane production to negligible levels, did not prevent episodes of spontaneous angina in a small group of patients. Continuous intravenous infusion of PGI_2 in six patients with angina due to coronary artery spasm induced systemic vasodilation and reduced platelet aggregation but did not prevent ischemic episodes in five of these six patients (Maseri et al., 1980). Nonetheless, a variety of other methods to inhibit either platelet aggregation or prostaglandin pathways are possible. These include other nonsteroidal anti-inflammatory agents, stable PGI_2 analogs, PGI_2-releasing agents and specific inhibitors of thromboxane A_2. It should also be mentioned that some calcium blocking agents, in particular verapamil and diltiazem, have potent effects acting to inhibit platelet aggregation. Results of studies using more specific platelet aggregation or thromboxane inhibitors are expected to shed new light on mechanisms of coronary constriction and may provide avenues for future treatment. At present, however, these agents are not recommended in the usual management of patients with coronary spasm.

Summary and Conclusions

Our current understanding of the pathophysiology of restricted coronary artery blood flow includes both anatomic and dynamic mechanisms. The relative contribution made by hemodynamically important atherosclerotic obstruction and dynamic coronary artery obstruction to the pathophysiology of ischemia in any given patient should be delineated. This information appears to be extremely useful to identify patients likely to achieve major benefit from vasodilators on one hand or beta-adrenergic blocking agents on the other hand. A number of agents are now available within these two pharmacologic classes. There are some differences in the action of these agents that require a thorough familiarity with the effects of these drugs so that their action can be optimized.

Practically speaking, the large majority of patients with syndromes related to coronary spasm respond to nitrates. Nitrates are extremely safe, thus use for relief or prevention of the acute ischemic episode remains the initial treatment of choice. When symptoms are more than mild to moderate in severity or unacceptably controlled in frequency using nitrates alone, other pharmacologic measures are needed. In patients who also have effort angina, suggesting a hemodynamically important atherosclerotic type obstruction in addition to spasm, beta-adrenergic blocking drugs can be helpful. If effort angina remains unacceptably controlled or adverse effects occur, a calcium antagonist may be added or substituted. These agents do not exacerbate bronchospasm or peripheral vascular disease and offer a distinct advantage over beta-adrenergic blocking agents in patients with angina who have such disorders. Additionally, no withdrawal or rebound phenomena have been described with calcium antagonists; yet these phenomena occur regularly with beta-blocking agents. Where the predominant symptom is rest angina or the patient has other evidence suggesting coronary artery spasm, a calcium antagonist may result in a very favorable response. This therapy should be extended to patients in whom spasm not only occurs spontaneously but to those in whom it can be provoked by stimuli such as effort or cold. When spasm is superimposed upon hemodynamically important atherosclerotic obstruction, the favorable response does not seem to be as great as that seen when spasm exists alone. In these cases, coronary artery bypass surgery, plexectomy and other nonpharmacologic approaches may have to be added to the pharmacologic regimen. Recommendations for the latter nonpharmacologic approaches, however, require demonstration that spasm is occurring in and about the area of fixed atherosclerotic obstruction and not occurring in other vessels or over the entire course of the mild and distal vessel.

References

Antman, E., Muller, J., Goldberg, S. et al. 1980. Nifedipine therapy for coronary artery spasm. Experienced in 127 patients. N Engl J Med 302:1269

Buxton, A., Goldberg, S., Hirschfeld, J. et al. 1980. Refractory ergonovine induced coronary vasospasm: Importance of intracoronary nitroglycerin. Am J Cardiol 46: 329–334

Chaine, R. A. 1980. The provocation of coronary artery spasm. Cardiac Cathet Cardiovasc Diagn 6:1–5

Conti, C. R., Pepine, C. J. and Curry, J. C. 1979. Coronary artery spasm: An important mechanism in the pathophysiology of ischemic heart disease. Curr Probl Cardiol IV:4,56

Distante, A., Severi, S., Biagini, A. and Maseri, A. 1976. Clinical results with nitrates in patients with "primary" angina at rest. In: *Primary and Secondary Angina Pectoris.* Proceedings of International Symposium held in Pisa. eds. A. Maseri, G. A. Klassen and M. Lesch, pp. 389–395. New York: Grune and Stratton

Endo, M., Kanda, I., Hosada, S. et al. 1978. Prinzmetal's variant form of angina pectoris: Re-evaluation of mechanisms. Circulation 52:137

Feldman, R. L., Pepine, C. J., Currcy, R. C. and Conti, C. R. 1978. A case against the routine use of glycerin-tinitrate before coronary angiography. Br Heart J 40:992–997

Fleckenstein, A. 1977. Specific pharmacology of calcium in myocardium, cardiac pacemakers, and vascular smooth muscle. Ann Rev Pharmacol Toxicol 17:149–166

Halprin, S., Frishman, W., Kirschner, M. and Strom, J. 1980. Clinical pharmacology of the new beta-adrenergic blocking drugs. Part II. Effects of oral labetalol in patients with both angina pectoris and hypertension. Preliminary experience. Am Heart J 99:388–396

Heupler, F. 1980. Provocative testing for coronary arterial spasm: Risk, method and rationale. Am J Cardiol 46:335–337

Hill, J. A., Feldman, R. L., Pepine, C. J. et al. 1981. Randomized double blind comparison of nifedipine and isosorbide dinitrate in patients with coronary spasm. Clin Res 29:206A

Maseri, A., Chierchia, S. and L'Abbate, A. 1980. Pathogenetic mechanisms underlying the clinical events associated with atherosclerotic heart disease. Circulation 62:6, V-8

Mehta, J. and Pepine, C. J. 1978. Effect of sublingual nitroglycerin on regional coronary flow in patients with and without coronary disease. Circulation 58:803–807

Pepine, C. J. and Conti, C. R. 1980. Acute and chronic heart disease—coronary artery spasm: An important pathophysiologic consideration. In *Current Cardiology,* Vol. 2, ed. Rosen, K. M., pp. 295–329. Mass.: Houghton Mifflin

Pepine, C. J., Feldman, R. L. and Conti, C. R. 1980a. Recommendations for use of ergonovine to provoke coronary artery spasm. Cardiac Cathet Cardiovasc Diagn 6:423–426

Pepine, C. J., Feldman, R. L. and Conti, C. R. 1982. Action of intracoronary nitroglycerin in refractory coronary artery spasm. Circulation 65: 500–503

Pepine, C. J., Feldman, R. L., Whittle, J., Currcy, R. C. and Conti, C. R. 1981. Effects of the calcium antagonist diltiazem in patients with variant angina. Am Heart J 101: 719–725

Rosenthal, S. J., Ginsburg, R., Lamb, I. 1980. Efficacy of diltiazem for control of symptoms of coronary arterial spasm. Am J Cardiol 46:1027–1032

Schang, S. J. and Pepine, C. J. 1977. Effects of propranolol on coronary hemodynamic and metabolic responses to tachycardia stress in patients with and without coronary disease. Cathet Cardiovasc Diagn 3:47–57

Schang, S. J. and Pepine, C. J. 1978. Coronary hemodynamic and metabolic effects of nitroglycerin in patients pretreated with propranolol. Br Heart J 40: 1221–1228

Severi, S., Davies, G., Maseri, A. et al. 1980. Long term prognosis of variant angina with medical treatment. Am J Cardiol 46:226–232

Waters et al. 1980. Ergonovine testing in a CCU. Am J Cardiol 46:922–930

Yasue, H. 1979. Exertional angina pectoris by coronary arterial spasm: Effect of various drugs. Am J Cardiol 43:3, 647

Thromboxane A_2 in Coronary Artery Disease

*Paul Walinsky, Mark Lebenthal,
J. Bryan Smith and Alan M. Lefer*

The discovery by Samuelsson, Svensson and Hamberg of a prostaglandin derivative that has the potential to significantly affect coronary artery tone has resulted in interest and speculation regarding the role of this compound and related compounds in coronary artery pathophysiology (Hamberg et al., 1975). Thromboxane A_2 has been demonstrated to cause coronary artery constriction and also has been demonstrated to enhance platelet aggregation. Both of these phenomena could result in exacerbation of coronary artery insufficiency. These phenomena, however, have been demonstrated in vitro and a clear understanding of the role of these compounds in clinical events remains to be elucidated.

Thromboxane A_2 is generated from activated platelets. Phospholipids on the platelet membrane are cleaved by phospholipases (Needleman and Kaley, 1978) (Fig. 1). This results in the generation of arachadonic acid. Arachadonic acid is then metabolized to a variety of compounds having differing vascular effects. Arachadonic acid is converted to intermediate endoperoxides by the action of the enzyme cyclooxygenase. These intermediate endoperoxides, PGG_2 and PGH_2 are subsequently converted to thromboxane A_2 by an enzyme thromboxane synthetase or to PGI_2 (prostacyclin) by the enzyme prostacyclin synthetase. The intermediate peroxides are also converted to PGE_2, which also has vascular effects, via additional enzymatic pathways.

Thromboxane A_2 is only short lived in aqueous solution, having a half-life of approximately 30 sec. Thromboxane A_2 is converted to thromboxane B_2, which is stable in aqueous solution and which can be measured by radioimmunoassay (Ferraris et al., 1977). Similarly, while PGI_2 may not be measured

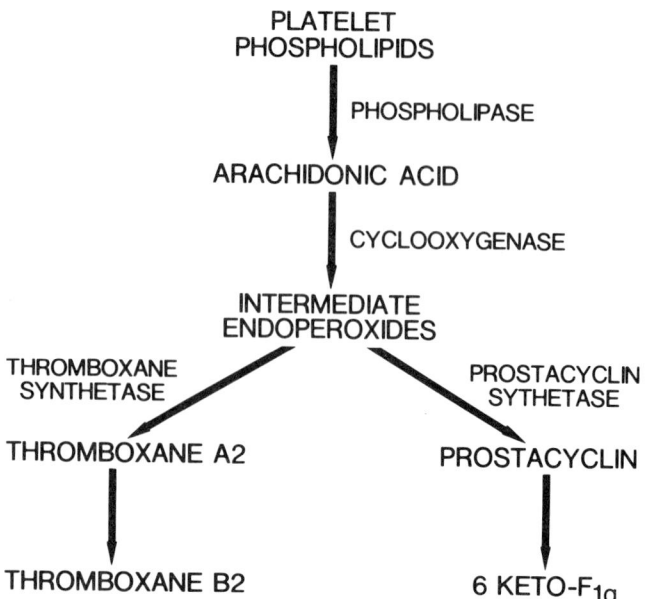

Figure 1.

directly, its metabolic byproduct $PGF_{1\alpha}$ may be measured by radioimmunoassay. Thromboxane A_2 and PGI_2 have recently been characterized as the "goodie" and the "baddie" compounds (Mitchell, 1981). This is understandable because thromboxane A_2 has been demonstrated in vitro to have the effects mentioned above of inducing vascular, specifically coronary, vasoconstriction and of enhancing platelet aggregation. PGI_2 has been demonstrated to have the opposite effects of vasodilation and of decreasing the propensity to platelet aggregation. Thromboxane A_2 is produced by platelets, while PGI_2 is produced by the vascular wall. Modulation of coronary artery tone has been postulated as the result of a dynamic balance between these related prostaglandin compounds. Because additional prostaglandin metabolites can effect vascular tone, they also may have a role in vascular dynamics.

Although thromboxane A_2 has intriguing potential as a significant factor in coronary artery disease its specific role remains to be elucidated. As of this time studies have been reported demonstrating the presence of thromboxane B_2 in the presence of coronary artery spasm, acute myocardial infarction and classical angina pectoris. We reported on a group of eight patients with Prinzmetal's angina who had elevated peripheral levels of thromboxane B_2 (Lewy et al., 1979). In our laboratory the limits of detection are 0.5 pmol/ml. Normals have no detectable thromboxane within the limits of our testing procedure. The eight patients with Prinzmetal's angina had resting levels of thromboxane B_2 that were elevated (1.57 ± 0.34 pmol/ml). During spontaneous angina, samples were drawn and demonstrated a further increase in thromboxane B_2 level to 2.83 ± 0.56 pmol/ml. The highest levels were demonstrated 5–10 min after relief of angina by nitroglycerin when the mean level was 6.41 ± 1.46 pmol/ml.

Whether thromboxane A_2 was causal or secondarily generated in the patients with spasm remained unclear on the basis of this study. Subsequent reports would suggest that the latter is true. Robertson has reported the results of a study in which serial samples were drawn from the coronary sinus and systemic artery during and after S-T segment elevation in patients with Prinzmetal's angina (Robertson et al., 1981). Arterial levels of thromboxane B_2 did not rise before the development of S-T segment elevation. Additionally, samples taken from the coronary sinus from 2 min before the start of pain up to 30 sec after the start of pain were not elevated above the baseline. The highest levels, as in our study, were obtained after resolution of S-T segment elevation. In another study Chierchia and co-workers administered low dose aspirin to seven patients with Prinzmetal's angina (Chierchia and Maseri, 1980). Aspirin was given intravenously in a dose of 2 mg/kg Serum thromboxane B_2 was measured before and after aspirin. The number of ischemic episodes was not altered by the administration of aspirin, although the serum thromboxane B_2 level decreased from 250 ± 12–4.6 ± 1.5 ng/ml after the aspirin. These data suggested that thromboxane A_2 is not a necessary component in the development of coronary artery spasm. These conclusions must be tempered, however, by the fact that aspirin is a cyclooxygenase inhibitor and hence may decrease generation of both PGI_2 and thromboxane A_2. Although it has been suggested that low dose aspirin in contrast to higher dose aspirin would selectively inhibit thromboxane A_2 rather than PGI_2 production, a recent report has demonstrated that both PGI_2 and thromboxane A_2 are inhibited by a single dose of 150 mg of aspirin (Preston et al., 1981). Thus, it is possible that both prostacyclin and thromboxane A_2 were inhibited in the dosage administered.

Thromboxane B_2 has also been demonstrated in the presence of nonvasospastic coronary artery disease. Hirsh and co-workers (1981) recently reported on a study in which samples of blood were aspirated from the coronary sinus and from the aorta at the start of elective cardiac catheterization. There was no significant association between the absolute values of coronary sinus and aortic levels and clinical status. However, when the ratio of coronary sinus to aortic levels was studied it was found that patients who had angina within 24 hours of sampling had a higher ratio than patients who had pain greater than 24 hours previously or who had no anginal pain. In this study there was no association between PGI_2 levels and pain status and no association between PGI_2 levels and thromboxane levels.

In a recent report Hirsh has also reported preliminary results in a group of patients with unstable angina in whom arterial pacing was performed (Hirsh et al., 1981). They were unable to demonstrate a relationship between transcardiac thromboxane B_2 ratios as expressed as the ratio of coronary sinus to aortic levels in patients with coronary artery disease in whom atrial pacing was performed. This differs from our experience in a group of patients with coronary artery disease of a nonvasospastic nature in whom atrial pacing was performed (Lewy et al., 1980). In 14 patients atrial pacing was performed to a rate of 140 beats/min for 4 min. Samples were aspirated from both aorta and coronary sinus before and after pacing. All 14 patients had significant coronary artery disease. Mean thromboxane B_2 levels rose from 0.77 ± 0.13 and 0.53 ± 0.16 pmol/ml in the coronary sinus and aorta to 2.34 ± 0.88 and 1.23 ± 0.36 pmol/ml, respectively. Severe myocardial ischemia postpacing was indicated by the demonstration of lactate production of 74.28 ± 20.32 in the postpacing period. Thus, in our experience thromboxane B_2 is elevated after the induction of myocardial ischemia in patients with significant coronary artery disease.

We are also in the process currently of evaluating peripheral samples of blood in a series of patients admitted to our cardiac care unit for evaluation of unstable angina or because of suspicion of acute myocardial infarction. In 15 patients admitted for evaluation of unstable angina, 50 samples of blood were aspirated from a peripheral vein during a pain-free period. There were 15 samples with thromboxane B_2 present in detectable levels. During or immediately after pain 17 out of 24 samples were found to demonstrate the presence of greater than 0.5 pmol/ml. In contrast, in nine patients admitted to rule out acute myocardial infarction, who subsequently were demonstrated not to have acute myocardial infarction or active coronary artery disease, 0 out of 29 samples had greater than 0.5 pmol/ml. In acute myocardial infarction in four patients who had samples drawn within 2 hours after the onset of pain all four had thromboxane B_2 elevations greater than 0.05 pmol/ml.

In summary, significant levels of thromboxane B_2 have been demonstrated in the presence of coronary artery spasm, pacing-induced myocardial ischemia and acute myocardial infarction. In patients with unstable angina, there seemed to be an association between the presence of anginal episode and the presence of thromboxane B_2.

Although additional observations will be needed to substantiate these preliminary findings, generation of thromboxane A_2 must be taken into account as one of the pathophysiologic alterations of myocardial ischemia and likely myocardial infarction. A number of questions remain to be fully understood. First, what is the source of the thromboxane that has been demonstrated? It seems likely that thromboxane is generated in some intravascular site related to the atherosclerotic coronary vessel. Presumably this process involves the activation and involvement of platelets at the atherosclerotic site. Other vascular sites as source of the generation of thromboxane have not been ruled out. In particular, the pulmonary artery has been demonstrated to have the potential to produce thromboxane.

Secondly, what is the diagnostic significance of the demonstration of thromboxane B_2? It initially seemed that the presence of thromboxane B_2 might be a marker for the presence of coronary artery spasm (Lewy et al., 1979). Because we have additionally demonstrated the presence of thromboxane B_2 in the presence of other coronary artery syndromes this view is no longer tenable. Thromboxane B_2, however, may be a good index of the presence of platelet activation in addition to some of the other biochemical indicators of platelet activity that have been used for that purpose.

Thirdly, what is the pathophysiologic significance of thromboxane A_2 in the initiation and continuation of myocardial ischemia? The study of thromboxane A_2 in clinical situations is methodologically quite difficult. It is not possible to leave indwelling catheters in various sites of interest for aspiration of samples during clinical events. Any catheters left indwelling would be suspect for the development of platelet aggregates or thrombus and hence might result in artifactual values. Thus, it is only fortuitous that we may have the ability to sample from the coronary sinus or from arterial sites during the acute events that we would like to further understand. One must address individually three subsets of coronary pathology: vasospastic angina, nonvasospastic angina and acute myocardial infarction with regard to understanding the role of thromboxane A_2 in initiating or potentiating the event. As mentioned above there is currently no evidence that suppression of thromboxane A_2 generation by aspirin or indomethacin in vasospasm angina has decreased the frequency of ischemic events (Robertson et al., 1981; Chierchia and Maseri, 1980). We have had an occasional patient who has had some improvement with aspirin. That has been the exception rather than the rule. There is thus no evidence that thromboxane A_2 initiates the spastic epidsode. The measure limitation in this conclusion is that we are able to sample only crudely even at the time of pain. It is possible that local concentrations of thromboxane may be generated that are able to initiate the ischemic episode. In addition, it is possible that a deficiency in the generation of prostacyclin may result in symptomatology as well. Our sampling of 6-keto $F1\alpha$, the metabolic product of prostacyclin, has not provided us any useful information, however, in this regard.

With regard to pacing-induced angina the significance of thromboxane generation is also unclear. The potential to compromise collateral flow is certainly evident. Alternatively, the vasoconstrictive effect of thromboxane A_2 may be of value in preventing a coronary steal type physiology. It may also be of homeostatic value in maintaining distal perfusion pressure and preventing any adverse alteration in stenotic resistance induced by excessive vasodilation (Walinsky et al., 1979; Santamore and Walinsky, 1980).

With regard to acute myocardial infarction our observations are inadequate to assess the potential role of thromboxane A_2 in initiation of the events related to myocardial infarction. However, thromboxane A_2 may have an adverse effect by compromising collateral flow or flow in normal vessels. It has been demonstrated in animal studies after myocardial infarction, there is a superimposed vasospasm (Hellstrom, 1971). Animal studies have also demonstrated release of Thromboxane B_2 after acute coronary ligation (Sakai et al., 1980). Thromboxane A_2 is thus a potential cause of that generalized vasospastic response. By administration of a specific thromboxane synthetase inhibitor, after experimental myocardial infarction a reduction in infarct size was able to be demonstrated in one study (Schror et al., 1980). Conversely, in experimental myocardial infarction administration of CTA_2, a synthetic analog of thromboxane A_2, resulted in an increase in infarct size (Smith et al., 1981). Thromboxane has also been demonstrated by some investigators to be associated with the development of arrhythmias after myocardial infarction.

Further study of thromboxane should yield additional information regarding its role in the various vascular syndromes associated with coronary artery pathology. There are several specific thromboxane synthetase inhibitors that are available and which have been used in animal studies (Schror et al., 1980). A recent report has additionally described such an agent given to human subjects without any short term side-effects (Tyler et al., 1981). Further clinical trials with such inhibitors of thromboxane generation, or of thromboxane receptor blockers, will offer us a more clear understanding of the role of thromboxane in coronary artery disease and, it is hoped, any therapeutic advantage from its inhibition.

References

Chierchia, S. and Maseri, A. 1980. Low dose aspirin prevents thromboxane A_2 synthesis by platelets but not attacks of Prinzmetal's angina. Circulation Suppl III:111–215

Ferraris, V., Smith, J. B. and Silver, M. J. 1977. Radioimmunoassay of thromboxane B_2. Thromb Haemostas 38:20

Hamberg, M., Svensson, J. and Samuelsson, B. 1975. Thromboxanes: A new group of biologically active compounds derived from prostaglandin endoperoxides. Proc Natl Acad Sci USA 72:2294–2298

Hellstrom, H. R. 1971. Coronary artery stasis after induced myocardial infarction in the dog. Cardiovasc Res 5:371–375

Hirsh, P. D., Firth, B. G., Campbell, W. B., Dehmer, G. J., Willerson, J. T. and Hillis, L. D. 1981. Transcardiac thromboxane and prostacyclin during provocation in patients with ischemic heart disease. Clin Res 29:206A

Hirsh, P. D., Hillis, L. D., Campbell, W. B., Firth, B. G. and Willerson, J. T. 1981. Release of prostaglandins and thromboxane into the coronary circulation in patients with ischemic heart disease. N Engl J Med 304:685–691

Lewy, R. I., Wiener, L., Smith, J. B., Walinsky, P., Silver, M. J. and Saia, J. 1979. Comparison of plasma concentrations of thromboxane B_2 in Prinzmetal's variant angina and classical angina pectoris. Clin Cardiol 2:404–406

Lewy, R. I., Wiener, L., Walinsky, P., Lefer, A. M., Silver, M. J. and Smith, J. B. 1980. Thromboxane release during pacing-induced angina pectoris: Possible vasoconstrictor influence on the coronary vasculature. Circulation 61:1165–1171

Mitchell, J. R. A. 1981. Prostaglandins in vascular disease: A seminal approach. Br Med J 282:590–594

Needleman, P. and Kaley, G. 1978. Cardiac and coronary prostaglandin synthesis and function. N Engl J Med 20:1122–1128

Preston, F. E., Whipps, S., Jackson, C. A. French, A. J., Wyld, P. J. and Stoddard, C. J. 1981. Inhibition of prostacyclin and platelet thromboxane A_2 after low-dose aspirin. N Engl J Med 304:76–79

Robertson, R. M., Robertson, D., Roberts, L. J., Maas, R. L., Fitzgerald, G. A., Friesinger, G. C. and Oates, J. A. 1981. Thromboxane A_2 in vasotonic angina pectoris. N Engl J Med 304:998–1003

Sakai, K., Ito, T., Ogawa, K., Enomoto, I., Kai, I. and Satake, T. 1980. Increased levels of prostaglandins and thromboxane after acute coronary occlusion. Circulation 62:111–241

Santamore, W. P. and Walinsky, P. 1980. Altered coronary flow responses to vasoactive drugs due to coronary artery stenosis in a canine model. Am J Cardiol 45: 276–285

Schror, K., Smith, E. F., Bickerton, M., Smith, J. B., Nicolaou, K., Magolda, R. and Lefer, A. M. 1980. Preservation of ischemic myocardium by pinane thromboxane A_2. Am J Physiol 238: H87–H92

Smith, E. F., Lefer, A. M., Aharony, D., Smith, J. B., Magolda, R. L., Claremon, D. and Nicolaou, K. C. 1981. Carbocyclic thromboxane A_2: Aggravation of myocardial ischemia by a new synthetic thromboxane A_2 analog. Prostaglandins 21:443–456

Tyler, H. M., Saxton, C. A. and Parry, M. J. 1981. Administration to man of Uk-37, a selective inhibitor of thromboxane synthetase. Lancet 1: 629–632

Walinsky, P., Santamore, W. P., Wiener, L. and Brest, A. N. 1979. Dynamic changes in the hemodynamic severity of coronary artery stenosis in a canine model. Cardiovasc Res 13:113–118

Intracoronary Thrombolysis: A New Treatment For Myocardial Infarction

James F. Spann

The mortality from acute myocardial infarction averages 10–15% during hospitalization and 20% in the following year (Pitt, 1976). Over the past decade there have been major efforts to develop techniques for reduction of the size of myocardial infarction and thus decrease mortality due to acute power failure and chronic congestive heart failure (Maroko et al., 1971).

Regardless of the initiating event that causes the myocardial infarction, a thrombus generally forms in the occluded artery at a high grade atherosclerotic obstruction (Fletcher and Sherry, 1968; DeWood et al., 1980). Once formed, the thrombus precludes flow through the vessel. Therefore, therapies designed to remove the thrombus may potentially reduce the infarct size and, it is hoped, reduce mortality.

Animal experiments show that rapidly instituted reperfusion of totally ischemic myocardium results in increased animal survival (Baughman et al., 1981). When reperfusion is accomplished by ultrarapid coronary vein bypass grafting it appears that the acute infarction can sometimes be interrupted in man (DeWood et al., 1979). Unfortunately, it is rarely possible to mobilize and accomplish surgical reperfusion in the required period of less than 3 hours. As a consequence, other avenues of reperfusion of the ischemic myocardium have been sought.

It is well known that streptokinase infusion results in rapid lysis of intra-arterial clots. Fletcher, Sherry and colleagues (Fletcher et al., 1959) first used streptokinase in myocardial infarction. Subsequently, more than a dozen large clinical trials of thrombolytic therapy in acute myocardial infarction were completed (Simon et al, 1973; Van de Loo and Verstraete, 1974; Aber et al.,

1976). While results were mixed, the majority of trials revealed a trend toward reduced mortality in patients treated with streptokinase. For example, the 1979 report from the European Cooperative Study Group of 512 medium risk patients who received streptokinase within 12 hours of the onset of symptoms showed a statistically significant reduction in mortality. The overall mortality rates were 15.6% in the streptokinase group and 30.6% in the control group ($P < 0.01$). While bleeding complications were more frequent in the streptokinase group, only two bleeding complications were clinically important. At least four other studies have shown statistically significant positive results (Simon et al., 1973). However, several studies have shown only trends towards positive results with streptokinase, which lacked statistical significance or similar mortality in the treatment and control groups (Simon et al., 1973). Unfortunately, however, a major problem is present in each of these studies; the time that was allowed to elapse between the onset of symptoms and the institution of thrombolytic therapy was 12–24 hours. The maximum duration of complete ischemia from which the myocardium can recover is thought to be 1–3 hours (Baughman et al., 1981).

Very recently the concept of intracoronary infusion of streptokinase has been studied in at least five centers (Rentrop et al., 1981; Mathey et al., 1981; Ganz et al., 1981; Gold and Leinbach, 1980; Rutsch et al., 1980). Intracoronary infusion of streptokinase provides a high concentration of thrombolytic agent at the site of the thrombus and avoids the potential problem of systemic bleeding. In each study the infusion of intracoronary streptokinase was begun 3–6 hours or less after the onset of the symptoms of acute myocardial infarction.

Rentrop et al. (1981) reported 29 patients with acute myocardial infarction treated by intracoronary infusion of streptokinase at a rate of 1000–2000 units/min. The coronary artery was reopened in 22 patients within 15–90 min of the initiation of infusion. The initiation of study averaged 5.6 ± 4 hours after the onset of pain. Coronary flow was reestablished by intracoronary nitroglycerin in only 4 of the 29 patients. It would appear from these and other data that coronary spasm is relatively rare as the sole cause of myocardial infarction. These data, however, do not exclude the possibility that spasm may initiate a process that is followed by myocardial thrombosis. In one other patient, sublingual nifedipine allowed some blood flow through an initially total obstruction of the coronary artery and in one patient, antegrade flow was reestablished by a guide wire passed through the occlusion. However, in all six of these patients who responded to nitroglycerin, nifedipine or guide wire perforation, there was additional improvement in lumen diameter during streptokinase infusion. In each of the 22 patients in whom intracoronary lysis of thrombus was successful, lesions of 80–90% obstruction of the coronary artery were demonstrated at the site of thrombus removal. Premature ventricular complexes appeared in 7 of the 22 patients at the time of reperfusion and no arrhythmias were observed in the remaining 15 patients. Change in symptoms could be evaluated in 19 patients. Five of these 19 patients became asymptomatic after intravenous or intracoronary nitroglycerin. Thirteen of 14 patients who had chest pain at the start of intracoronary streptokinase infusion were asymptomatic after streptokinase infusion. These improvements in symptoms occurred either immediately before or within 10 min after the achievement of reperfusion. In 16 of 17 patients with S-T elevation, the S-T segment either was reduced or returned to baseline after the streptokinase infusion. Ejection fraction increased from 50.5 ± 12–$54.6 \pm 9\%$ ($P < 0.05$) in the 14 patients in whom it was determined before and after streptokinase. Poststreptokinase therapy consisted of intravenous heparin for 4–7 days and long term anticoagulation with warfarin. Aortocoronary bypass surgery had been carried out in six of the patients at the time of the report and was scheduled in an additional four. In 9 of these 10 patients, the indication for surgery was persistent angina. Intraoperative observation of the segment supplied by the previously obstructed blood vessel showed active contraction of the myocardium in the area at risk. Two patients required femoral artery surgery due to hemorrhage at the site of femoral artery puncture. One patient died 3 hours after reperfusion. An additional patient died 31 days later after a repeat infarction. A third patient died 10 weeks later of vein graft occlusion 1 week after coronary bypass surgery. The remaining 26 of the original 29 patients were alive at a maximum of approximately 7 months of follow-up.

Mathey et al. (1981) studied 41 patients with acute myocardial infarction within 3 hours after onset of symptoms. They preceded streptokinase infusion, 2000 units/min, by intracoronary injection of nitroglycerin, an attempt to recanalize the vessel by flexible guide wire and intracoronary injection of plasminogen. Nitroglycerin opened the coronary artery in 1 patient, the guide wire succeeded in 4 of 15 patients and contrast injection alone was successful in 7 patients. In 18 patients, the occluded coronary artery was recanalized by streptokinase infusion alone. When reperfusion was established by nonthrombolytic means, streptokinase infusion significantly further reduced the degree of stenosis and resulted in the disappearance of angiographically visible thrombi. The occluded coronary artery was successfully opened in 30 of the 41 patients (73%) with an average time to recanalization of 29 min. Successful recanalization was always associated with relief of chest pain and significant reduction of S-T segment elevation. New Q waves or R wave reduction did, however, appear in 24 of 34 patients with successful recanalization. Twenty patients who were successfully recanalized were subsequently treated medically. Three of these patients had reinfarction 10 days to 8 weeks after recanalization and 2 developed unstable angina. The remaining 15 patients have been asymptomatic for 3–12 months. After observing the three patients with reinfarction, these workers instituted early bypass surgery as a routine procedure for recanalized patients. An additional 10 patients have undergone coronary bypass surgery without difficulty within the week after recanalization. In these 10 patients, no hemorrhagic infarct was seen at the time of surgery. In 11 successfully recanalized patients, the global left ventricular ejection fraction rose significantly from $37 \pm 5\%$–$47 \pm 5\%$. In all five unsuccessful patients, the ejection fraction fell. Seven of the 41 patients (17%) had ventricular fibrillation during the angiographic or recanalization procedure. Five of these episodes of fibrillation occurred during reperfusion, while two of the episodes immediately followed contrast injection. In every case, defibrillation established normal sinus rhythm. No bleeding complications were observed. None of the 30 successfully recanalized patients died. Three of the patients who survived after recanalization were initially in cardiogenic shock with severe hypotension, signs of peripheral hypoperfusion and an elevated pulmonary capillary wedge pressure.

Ganz et al. (1981) used a mixture of streptokinase and plasmin in a dose of 4000 units/min until opening of the coronary artery and then 2000 units/min for an additional 60 min. Twenty patients were studied 1.5–3.2 hours after the onset of chest pain. Intracoronary nitroglycerin caused faint visualization of the distal coronary artery in 2 of the 20 patients. This effect persisted for 5–10 min. Infusion of thrombolysin resulted in opening of the coronary artery in 19 of the 20 patients within 8–43 min (average, 21). The coronary artery was completely occluded in 18 of the 20 patients before the infusion. In the two patients with subtotal occlusion, expansion of the lumen was observed during infusion with thrombolysin. Coronary reperfusion was accompanied by gradual relief of chest pain and a gradual return of the S-T segments to the isoelectric line. The reperfusion was frequently accompanied by premature ventricular contractions, bigeminy or isorhythmic dissociation, which usually responded to 50–75 mg of lidocaine intravenously. In one patient, the isorhythmic dissociation deteriorated into ventricular tachycardia that required electrical conversion. The one patient, in whom thrombolytic therapy failed to open the right coronary artery, died after rupture of the intraventricular septum and surgical repair of the defect. Of the 19 patients with successful reperfusion, 12 were subsequently treated medically. In each of these 12 patients, heparin was initiated as soon as the partial thromboplastin time fell to twice normal control and warfarin was substituted for heparin before discharge and maintained for at least 3 months. In 7 of the 19 patients, elective coronary bypass surgery was done because of severe stenosis of major coronary arteries.

All seven have survived. At the time of operation there was no evidence of intramyocardial bleeding in the thrombolysin-treated patients. Thallium-201 and left ventricular regional wall motion (determined by contrast ventriculography, two-dimensional echocardiography and multiple gated blood pool scintigraphy) showed improvement in regional wall motion abnormalities 10–12 days after reperfusion. Quantitative data was not presented regarding either the thallium, angiographic, echocardiographic or multiple gated blood pool scintigraphy studies.

Gold and Leinbach (1980) have briefly reported treating 12 patients having acute myocardial infarction resistant to intravenous propranolol and nitroglycerin with intracoronary streptokinase 3 ± 1.4 hours after pain of myocardial infarction. All patients had complete coronary occlusion before institution of streptokinase. Antegrade coronary flow was restored in 10 of 12 patients within 30 min. S-T segment elevation fell 58%. No severe arrhythimias occurred. Severe coronary stenosis averaging 86% was observed after reestablishing antegrade coronary flow. No mention was made of whether heparin or warfarin was used. Four of the 10 patients had reocclusion of the coronary artery. Three additional patients required emergency coronary bypass surgery for recurrent pain. There was a significant reduction of akinesis in jeopardized segments of myocardium reexamined 1 week later ($P < 0.02$). Thirty percent of the jeopardized area remained akinetic after 1 week in patients with patent recanalization. Conversely, in the patient with resistant occlusion and the three with repeat occlusion 83% of the jeopardized segments remained akinetic.

Rutsch et al. (1980) have briefly reported 50 patients with impending myocardial infarction who were treated within 3 hours of the onset of angina and stated that recanalization was achieved in "almost all." Ventriculography performed 3 weeks after infarction demonstrated a 40% reduction in length of the akinetic segment and a 58% increase in regional wall motion. These workers reported a mortality of 3%.

If one combines the three studies (Rentrop et al., 1981; Mathey et al., 1981; Ganz et al., 1981) that have been reported in full, there is a remarkable similarity among data from each study (Table 1). Intracoronary infusion of streptokinase with or without plasmin in patients admitted within 3 hours of the onset of the symptoms resulted in reperfusion of in 71 of 90 patients (79 %). The average time to reperfusion was 26 min. Conversely, intracoronary nitroglycerin was successful in reestablishing perfusion in only 6 of 90 patients (7%) and this reestablishment appeared transitory. Ventricular irritablity was frequent at the time of successful reperfusion. The incidence of ventricular fibrillation or ventricular tachycardia requiring cardioversion was 5%, 9% and 23% in the three studies. Only two bleeding complications, both hematomas requiring surgical repair of the femoral artery, were reported. In all patients, chest pain was relieved and S-T segment elevation was reduced or abolished. Global ejection fraction increased in all 3 studies and this increase in ejection fraction was significant, averaging 10% and 26% increase in the two studies in which quantitative data were reported. There were no intrahospital deaths reported in the 71 patients who achieved successful recanalization. The acute and short term follow-up mortality (estimated to be 3–6 months of follow-up) combined was 7% in the total group of 90 patients. Of 71 successful

Table 1. Thrombolytic Therapy in Acute Myocardial Infarction.

Data	Average	Rentrop et al. (1981)	Mathey et al. (1981)	Ganz et al. (1981)
Number of Patients	90	29	41	20
Benefit by Intracoronary Nitroglycerin	6%	3	1	2
Number Recanalized by Thrombolysis	71	22	30	19
Percent Recanalized	79%	76	73	95
Minutes of Infusion Needed to Recanalize	26	22	30	19
Rapid Relief of Chest Pain and S-T elevation	yes	yes	yes	yes
Reocculsion—Total with Medical Follow-up Treatment	6%	1/19	3/20	0/12
Bleeding	2%	2	0	?
Ventricular Tachycardia or Fibrillation Requiring Cardioversion at Time of Reperfusion	14%	2/22	7/30	1/19
No Symptoms During 3–6 Month Follow-up	70%	11/22	15/20	12/12
Coronary Bypass Surgery Done Empirically or for Symptoms	37%	9/22 (For symptoms)	10/30 (Done empirically)	7/19 (Done empirically)
Increase of Ejection Fraction in Recanalized Patients	yes	yes	yes (10% significant)	yes (26% significant)
Mortality in Recanalized Patients, Acute and 3–6 months	1/71	1/22	0/30	0/19
Mortality in Total Group, Acute and 3–6 months	7/90	3/29	3/41	1/20

recanalizations, the subsequent treatment was medical in 54 (76%). All patients received heparin immediately after thrombolytic therapy and then oral anticoagulants for at least 3 months. Thirty-nine (72%) of the 54 medically treated patients remained asymptomatic, four (7%) had reinfarction or demonstrated reocclusion of the coronary artery and 11 (21%) had angina pectoris requiring coronary bypass surgery. Coronary bypass grafting was done in 26 patients (37%). This surgery was done in 9 patients due to angina, in 7 patients due to severe stenosis of major vessels and in 10 patients after coronary bypass surgery was instituted as a routine postrecanalization procedure. When the heart was inspected at surgery there was no hemorrhagic infarction present and the myocardium at risk from the previously occluded vessel was contracting normally.

Intracoronary streptokinase is an exciting and promising new therapy. In addition, these studies strongly support the concept that coronary thrombosis is a major factor in acute myocardial infarction. A number of very substantial questions, however, remain for future research to answer (Muller et al., 1981). The extent of myocardial salvage is only partially known. The high incidence of ventricular fibrillation during either coronary angiography or at the time of reperfusion is a potential problem, although rapid defibrillation appears to be possible. The overall effect of this therapy on mortality due to acute myocardial infarction cannot be established from the studies done to date. Carefully controlled randomized trials are essential to establish this very important information. It is difficult to institute the relatively complex therapy of acute coronary visualization and intracoronary infusion of streptokinase in large numbers of patients within 3 hours of the onset of their chest pain. If it is determined that this exciting and promising new therapy should be widely applied to the more than 1 million new infarctions occurring in the United States per year, major additional advances must be made. The patients will have to be educated to come to the hospital more rapidly after the onset of chest pain and teams will have to be on standby if these acute and relatively complex procedures are to be done in such a short time. Alternatively, a more simple method for causing recanalization may be needed.

References

Aber, C. P., Bass, N. M., Berry, C. L., Carson, P. H. M., Dobbs, R. J., Fox, K. M., Hamblin, J. J., Haydu, S. P., Howitt, G., MacIver, J. E., Portal, R. W., Raftery, E. B., Rousell, R. H. and Stock, J. P. P. 1976. Streptokinase in acute myocardial infarction: a controlled multicentre study in the United Kingdom. Br Med J 2:1100–1104

Baughman, K. L., Maroko, P. R. and Vatner, S. F. 1981. Effects of coronary artery reperfusion on myocardial infarct size and survival in conscious dogs. Circulation 63:317–323

DeWood, M. A., Spores, J., Notske, R. N., Lang, H. T., Shields, J. P., Simpson, C. S., Rudy, L. W. and Grunwald, R. 1979. Medical and surgical management of acute myocardial infarction. Am J Cardiol 44:1356–1364

DeWood, M. A., Spores, J., Notske, R., Mouser, L. T., Burroughs, R., Golden, M. S. and Lang, H. T. 1980. Prevalence of total coronary occlusion during the early hours of transmural myocardial infarction. N Engl J Med 303:897–902

European Cooperative Study Group for Streptokinase Treatment in Acute Myocardial Infarction. 1979. Streptokinase in acute myocardial infarction. N Engl J Med 301:797–802

Fletcher, A., Sherry, S., Alkjaersig, N., Smyrniotis, F. and Jick, S. 1959. Maintainence of a sustained thrombolytic state in man II. Clinical observations on patients with myocardial infarction and other thromboembolic disorders. J Clin Invest 38:1111–1119

Fletcher, A. P. and Sherry, S. 1968. Thrombolytic therapy in acute myocardial infarction. In *Symposium on Coronary Heart Disease,* ed. H. L. Blumgart, pp 95–103. New York: American Heart Association, Inc.

Ganz, W., Buchbinder, N., Marcus, H., Mondkar, A., Maddahi, J., Charuzi, Y., O'Connor, L., Shell, W., Fishbein, M. C., Kass, R., Miyamoto, A. and Swann, H. J. C. 1981. Intracoronary thrombolysis in evolving myocardial infarction. Am Heart J 101:4–13

Gold, H. K. and Leinbach, R. C. 1980. Coronary flow restoration in myocardial infarction by intracoronary streptokinase. Circulation Suppl III 62(Abs):III–161

Maroko, P. R., Kjekshus, J. K., Sobel, B. E., Watanabe, T., Covell, J. W., Ross, J. and Braunwald, E. 1971. Factors influencing infarct size following experimental coronary artery occlusions. Circulation 43:67–82

Mathey, D. G., Kuck, K.-H., Tilsner, V., Krebber, H.-J. and Bleifeld, W. 1981. Nonsurgical coronary artery recanalization in acute transmural myocardial infarction. Circulation 63:489–497

Muller, J. E., Stone, P. H., Markis, J. E. and Braunwald, E. 1981. Let's not let the genie escape from the bottle—again. N Engl J Med 304:1294–1296

Pitt, B. 1976. Natural history of myocardial infarction and its prodromal syndromes. Circulation 53:I-132–I-140

Rentrop, P., Blanke, H., Karsch, K. R., Kaiser, H., Kostering, H. and Leitz, K. 1981. Selective intracoronary thrombolysis in acute myocardial infarction and unstable angina pectoris. Circulation 63:307–317

Rutsch, W., Weber, H., Paeprer, H., Dorow, P., Schartl, M. and Schmutzler, H. 1980. Recanalization of coronary arteries in impending myocardial infarction by means of intracoronary streptokinase infusion. Circulation Suppl III 62(Abs):III-80

Simon, T. L., Ware, J. H. and Stengle, J. M. 1973. Clinical trials of thrombolytic agents in myocardial infarction. Ann Int Med 79:712–719

Van de Loo, J. and Verstraete, M. 1974. Fibrinolytic treatment of acute myocardial infarction: A question still open. Throm Diath Haemorrh 59 (Suppl): 203–212

Lifestyle Patterns As A Defense Against Coronary Heart Disease

Ralph S. Paffenbarger, Jr.

Introduction

The pathological changes underlying coronary heart disease (CHD) begin in early childhood and are influenced by personal characteristics and patterns of living that exert their force over long periods before the clinical recognition of the disease. Among the characteristics and lifestyles associated with an increased risk of the disease are cigarette smoking, increased body weight-for-height, psychological stress, higher levels of blood pressure, certain patterns and levels of blood lipids, dietary indiscretions, diabetes and lower levels of physical activity. The presence of these characteristics in combination strengthens the association, demonstrates a further increased risk of CHD, and implies the multifactorial nature of its cause. Moreover, actuarial statistics implicate such characteristics in shortening the life span, largely through the development of CHD.

With the exception of cigarette smoking and hypertension, in which lapsed smokers and adequately treated hypertensives promptly lose most of their excess risk, there is only limited evidence that the correction of the other high risk characteristics is followed by reduction in the incidence of CHD. Although the value of more extensive intervention procedures are not proven, the collected implications are so strong that numerous preventive programs are already underway.

Correction of three high risk characteristics, namely, cigarette smoking, hypertension and sedentary lifestyle, offer promise of achievement, perhaps more than attempted control of other high risk characteristics. Accordingly the influence of these three in affecting CHD risk, and the anticipated percent reduction in such risk with their control, are emphasized.

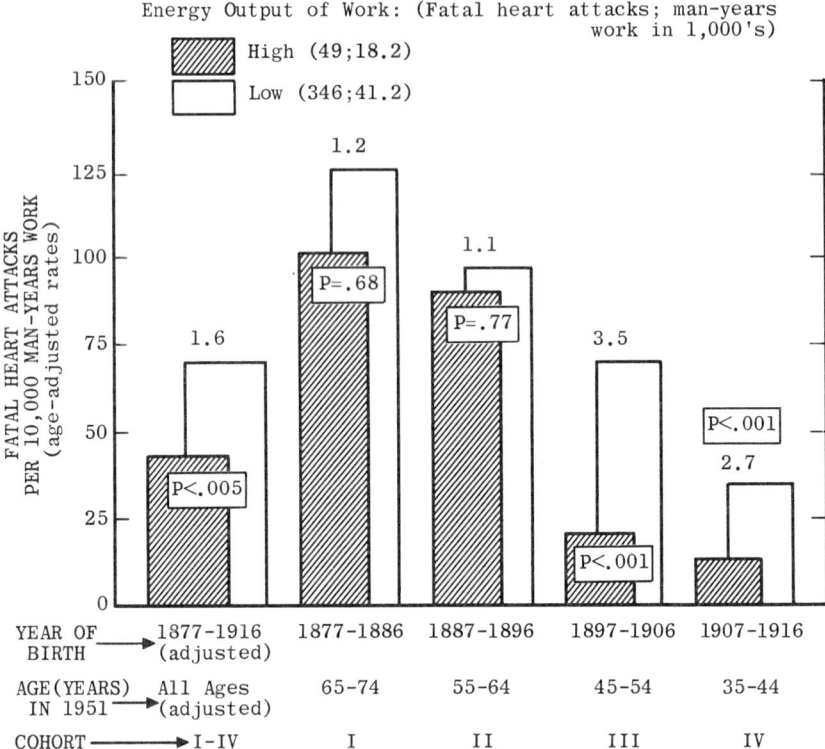

Fig. 1. Death rates from coronary heart disease (heart attacks) among birth cohorts of longshoremen in a 22-year follow-up, by high (8500+ kcal/week) and low levels of work energy output.

Lifestyles of Longshoremen

The work activity and fatal CHD records of San Francisco longshoremen are of interest because they cover a wide range of energy expenditures, based on physical measurements taken in actual on-the-job situations, and they have afforded a 22-year follow-up of work assignments and heart attacks since an initial multiphasic screening examination of several thousand cargo handlers and dock workers (Paffenbarger and Hale, 1975). Cigarette habits were assessed and many physical and physiological measurements were made at the beginning of this follow up period.

Figure 1 displays rates of fatal CHD among birth cohorts of 3686 San Francisco longshoremen during the years 1951–1972, as expressed per 10,000 man-years of work, by age at death and job energy output status. Energy output calculations were based on actual observations and measurements of various longshoring tasks on the job, and allowances were made for rest periods and slack moments between heavy work episodes. Job assignments were checked annually to adjust for transfers, but those changes did not greatly alter the findings. About 11% (395) of the longshoremen died of CHD during the 22-year period. Men who expended 8500 or more kcal/week at work (32% of the man-years of follow-up) had less risk of fatal CHD, particularly at younger ages, than men whose jobs required less exercise.

The older longshoremen may have been allowed to ease their work effort even on heavy jobs, or experience may have taught them to work more efficiently or casually, reducing the distinction between their energetic and less energetic classifications. Or, the younger cohorts may be presenting a new and different pattern of risk that was unknown to the older cohorts who in youth performed

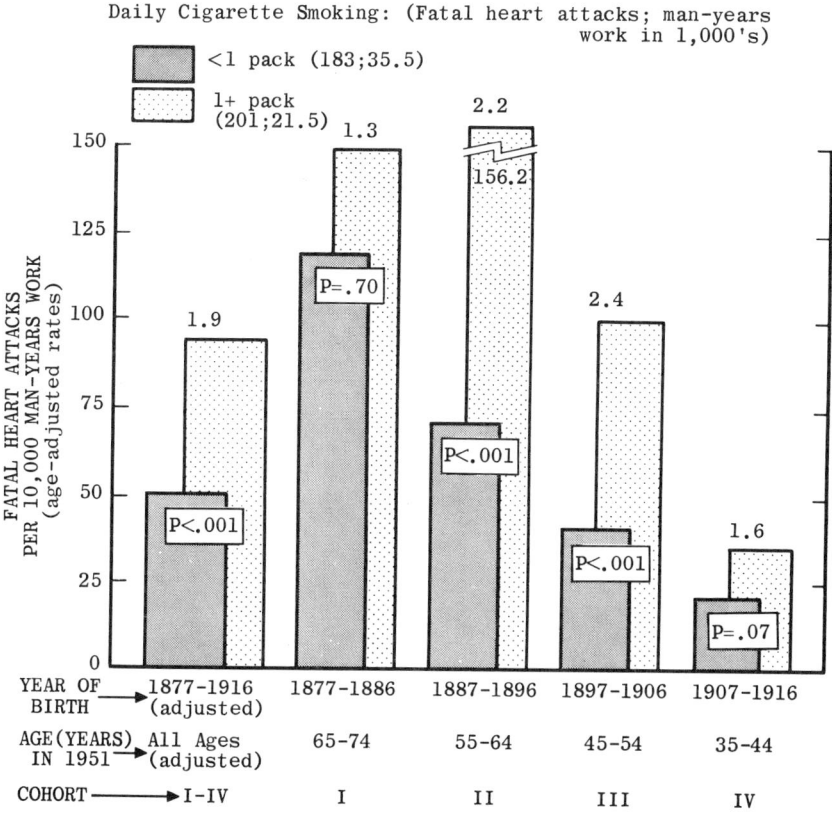

Fig. 2. Death rates from coronary heart disease (heart attacks) among birth cohorts of longshoremen in a 22-year follow-up by cigarette smoking habit.

much manual labor in all jobs. Yet, the older cohorts may represent what the younger cohorts will become; the young groups may include men at high risk of fatal CHD, whose counterparts had already vanished from the older cohorts before the study began. Because cargo handling now relies more on machinery than on muscle power, the younger cohorts have been losing opportunity for high energy output on their jobs, and the need for vigorous exercise in leisure time activities has become as important for longshoremen as for more sedentary populations.

CHD risks were nearly double among longshoremen who were heavy cigarette smokers or had higher than average systolic blood pressure for their age. For both of these characteristics, the increased risks were evident in each birth cohort (Figs. 2 and 3).

By means of a multiple logistic regression analysis it is possible to set aside the effects of age, follow-up interval and the other two characteristics to delineate the

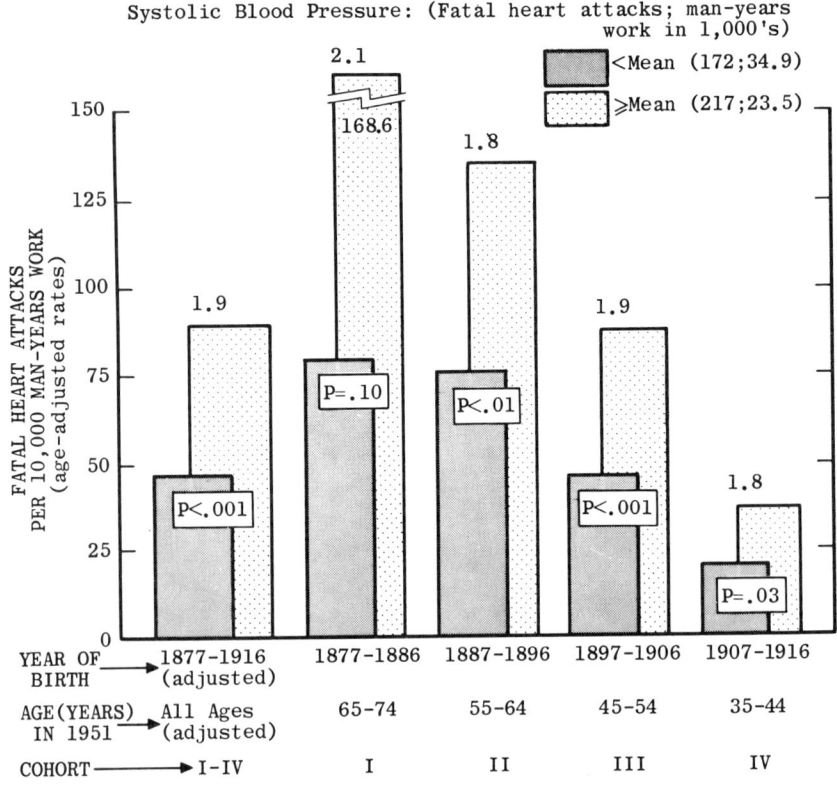

Fig. 3. Death rates from coronary heart disease (heart attacks) among birth cohorts of longshoremen in a 22-year follow-up by systolic blood pressure level.

Table 1. Death Rates and Attributable Risks of Coronary Heart Disease Among San Francisco Longshoremen by Specific Combinations of Work-energy Output, Cigarette Smoking and Blood Pressure Level in a 22-year Follow-up.

Characteristic	Man-years in 1000s	Death Rate (In 10,000 Man-years)	Attributable Risk (%)
1. Low energy output*	41	70	49
2. Heavy cigarette smoking†	21	94	28
3. Higher systolic blood pressure‡	23	89	29
1, 2 or both	15	96	65
1, 3 or both	16	92	74
2, 3 or both	8	162	50
1, 2, 3 or combination	4	152	88

Rates and risks are adjusted for differences in age and follow-up interval.
* Physical activity represented by <8500 kcal/week in job performance.
† One or more packs per day.
‡ Equal to or greater than mean for age.

role of the third characteristic in establishing CHD risk. In doing so it is evident that each characteristic made an independent contribution to CHD risk.

It might be anticipated that in the absence of low energy output, heavy smoking, and higher blood pressure from the longshoremen population, the death rates from CHD would have been substantially lower over the 22-year period of follow-up. Table 1 gives attributable risk percentages, i.e., the estimated reductions in rates of fatal CHD that would have been changed from high to low risk levels. If all longshoremen had worked at the level of 8500 or more kcal/week, the death rate from CHD might have been reduced by about 49%. If all men had worked at high energy levels, smoked less than a pack of cigarettes per day or not at all, and had systolic blood pressures less than average for longshoremen of their age, the corresponding total reduction might have approximated 88%, a substantial salvage over the actual experience. These estimates, of course, are theoretical in that they assume a causal and dose-response relationship between each characteristic and fatal CHD, that the characteristics can be modified to the low risk level and that any other influences on CHD risk are equally distributed between high and low risk groups. In the longshoring population the attributable risk connected with low energy expenditure is larger than the corresponding risk for the heavy cigarette habit or high systolic blood pressure level.

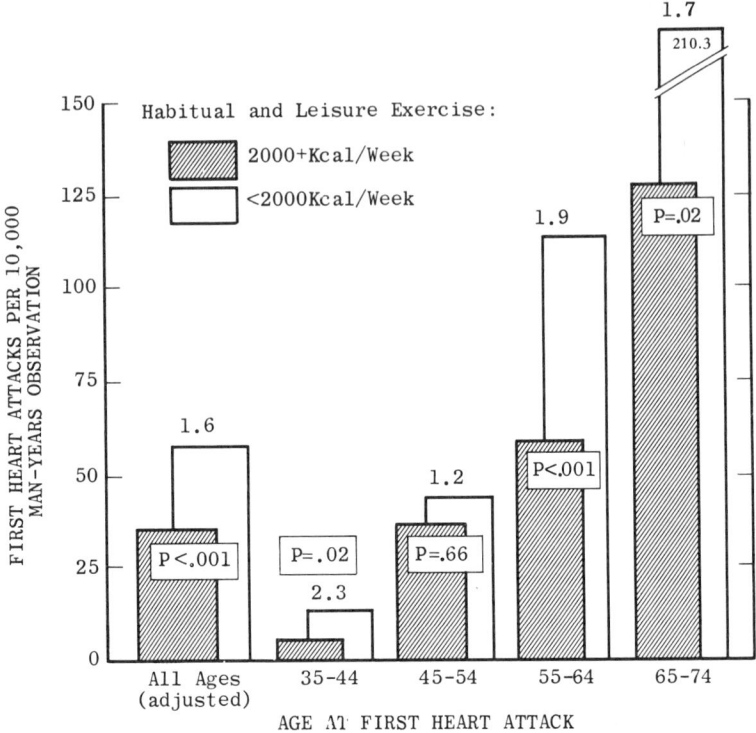

Fig. 4. Age-specific and age-adjusted rates of coronary heart disease (heart attacks) among Harvard alumni in a 6- to 10-year follow-up by level of leisure-time energy output.

Lifestyles of College Men

Study of the habitual leisure-time exercise patterns in relation to health status among a group of college alumni has helped to clarify the role of past and contemporary exercise in relation to CHD risk (Paffenbarger et al., 1978). Figure 4 shows age-specific rates, age-adjusted rates and relative risks of first CHD attacks among 16,936 Harvard University alumni over a 6- to 10-year period (1962 or 1966 through 1972) per 10,000 man-years of habitual and leisure-time physical activity patterns, expressed as a composite index. The index was compiled from stair climbing (10 per day = 28 kcal/week) city block walking (1 per day = 56 kcal/week), and participation in light sports (5 kcal/min) and vigorous sports (10 kcal/min). Men whose index was less than 2000 kcal/week comprised 60% of the total and were at 64% greater risk of heart attack than men who reported exercising more. The effect was consistent at each 10 year age class available for study, 35–74. Also, patterns were similar in relation to fatal and nonfatal attacks.

Although the range of energy output for the college men in leisure-time activity seemed considerably lower than for longshoremen on the job, findings ran parallel for CHD risk. In the alumni study, no allowance was made for energy expended other than through walking, climbing stairs, and sports play. To compare the alumni with the longshoremen, an additional 4500–5000 kcal/week should be added to the alumnus leisure-time energy expenditure to allow for energy output during a 40-hour work week.

An analysis of age-adjusted first CHD attacks by cross-tabulation of Harvard student and alumni physical activity rankings is given in Table 2. Student exercise is assessed as varsity or casual sports, and alumni exercise as kilocalories expended per week in stair climbing, walking and sports play. Thus CHD rates are given for men who were rated less active as students but more active as alumni, or vice versa, or who showed little or no change in physical activity level. Fifty-six percent of the former varsity players have maintained their active status in vigorous sports or high output exercise; evidently they had developed ingrained habits of being energetic and sports oriented. On the other hand, athletes who gave up their former routines tended to be at even greater risk of CHD than alumni who had never been active. About 38% of the nonvarsity alumni reported sufficient exercise to place themselves in the upper range of energy output (2000+ kcal/week), and they experienced substantially lower CHD rates than their less active alumni classmates regardless of their student exercise rating. Thus, the inverse gradient patterns of risk and alumni exercise show plainly that only a physically active adulthood is associated with lower CHD rates. These parallels

Table 2. Attack Rates of Coronary Heart Disease Among Male Harvard Alumni by Student and Alumnus Physical Activity Patterns in a 6- to 10-year Follow-up.

Student Physical Activity Rating	Alumnus Physical Activity Index in kcal/week		
	<500	500–1999	2000+
Varsity athlete			
No	71	54	35
Yes	93	45	35
Sports play, hours/week (excludes varsity athletes)			
<5	86	55	33
≥5	61	49	28

Rates in 10,000 man-years adjusted for differences in age and follow-up interval.

of experience signify that continued vigorous activity such as aerobic sports play in adult life is independent of early physical or physiological endowment or youthful activity in predicting lower CHD risk.

The relationships of the cigarette smoking habit and a history of physician-diagnosed hypertension to CHD risk were examined among the alumni. As in most other populations where such relationships have been studied, there was a twofold higher risk of CHD morbidity and mortality among subjects with these characteristics taken separately, as compared with their former classmates without them. Again differences were evident in all age classes in the 6- to 10-year period of follow-up.

The potential saving effect of elimination of any or all of these three characteristics can be expressed as attributable risk percent, that is, the estimated percentage reductions that could have been anticipated over the follow-up period if all alumni had achieved an adequate physical activity index (2000+ kcal/week), abstained from cigarettes and controlled hypertension. Avoidance of an inactive lifestyle might have reduced CHD risk by 26%. Similarly, the estimates from elimination of cigarettes are 25%, and for control of hypertension they represent a 16% reduction. Avoidance of combinations of any two characteristics might have reduced risk by 31%. Finally, if all three adverse characteristics had been abolished, the alumni might have spared themselves 48% of their CHD risk.

Attributable risk estimates for specific combinations of these three characteristics, together with corresponding prevalence figures, are given in Table 3.

Table 3. Attack Rates and Attributable Risks of Coronary Heart Disease Among Male Harvard Alumni by Specific Combinations of Sedentary Lifestyle, Cigarette Smoking and Hypertension in a 6- to 10-year Follow-up.

Sedentary lifestyle* (+ = present; − = absent)	Cigarette Smoking†	Hypertension‡	Prevalence (%)	Attack Rate (In 10,000 Man-years)	Attributable Risk (%)
+	+	+	2	203	88
+	+	−	22	66	60
+	−	+	3	102	76
−	+	+	1	79	68
+	−	−	32	35	28
−	+	−	14	50	48
−	−	+	2	42	41
−	−	−	23	26	

Rates and risks are adjusted for differences in age and follow-up interval.
* Physical activity represented by expenditure of <2000 kcal/week in walking, climbing, and sports play.
† Any amount.
‡ Physician diagnosed.

Table 4. Relative Attack Risks and Clinical Attributable Risks of Coronary Heart Disease Among Male Harvard Alumni by Specific Characteristics in a 6- to 10-year Follow-up.

Characteristic	Prevalence (%)	Relative Risk* (%)	Attributable Risk (%)
Sedentary lifestyle †	61	49	33
Cigarette smoking ‡	52	30	23
Hypertension §	9	134	57
Obesity ‖	38	32	24
Parental CHD #	39	28	22

Rates and risks are adjusted for differences in age, follow-up interval and each of the other characteristics listed.
* Excess risk (%) with characteristic.
† Physical activity represented by expenditure of <2000 kcal/week in walking, climbing, and sports play.
‡ Any amount.
§ Physician diagnosed.
‖ Twenty percent or more over ideal weight for height.
Father, mother or both.

As for longshoremen shown in Table 1, similar theoretical considerations (cause and effect, proportional changes, risk alterability and equivalent distributions of other risk factors) are applied to the three most prominent risk characteristics—sedentary lifestyle, cigarette smoking and hypertension.

Broadening the approach to include other risk factors of CHD, a multiple logistic regression analysis, controlling for all the other characteristics, assesses the effect of each of the following: sedentary lifestyle, cigarette smoking, hypertension, obesity (20% or more over the ideal weight for height), and a history of parental CHD. The last named probably denotes a complex of genetic and environmental influences. As seen in Table 4, the relative risk of CHD among men who expended less than 2000 kcal/week in walking, climbing stairs and participating in sports was 49% higher than the risk in more active men, and this sedentary lifestyle may have accounted for 33% of CHD attacks in sedentary men. The risk of CHD was 30% higher in smoking than nonsmoking men and 23% of the added risk may have been due to this cause. The risk of CHD was 134% higher in hypertensive than in normotensive men, and 57% of the added risk may have been due to hypertension. Corresponding rates and risks for obesity were 32% and 24% and for a parental history of CHD, 28% and 22%. Thus each of these five characteristics makes an independent and statistically significant contribution to CHD risk. Hypertension seems to be the most potent of these risk factors in a clinical sense, but because of its high prevalence, a sedentary lifestyle (as defined here) would represent the most potent risk factor in a community or public health sense.

Other Lifestyles

Among other lifestyle patterns associated with an increase risk of CHD, an atherogenic diet and psychosocial stress deserve special mention. Together with sedentary living, smoking, hypertension and obesity, an imprudent diet and time-urgent competitiveness round out a list of six villains in our lifestyle melodrama. We hardly need to be told that these habits of living are hazardous to health, if not conducive to hypertensive-atherosclerotic disease.

While only a few studies of American populations have shown a relationship between dietary intake and CHD risk (Shekelle et al., 1981; Glueck and Connor, 1978), cross-cultural comparison, metabolic ward studies and animal experimentation (Keys, 1980) implicate long term consumption of saturated fat, cholesterol and excess calories as contributing to hypercholesterolemia. Moreover, vegetarian diets and those low in saturated fat and cholesterol when established as new eating practices often lead to weight reduction, which in turn affects favorably several other CHD risk factors (hypertension, diabetes and blood lipid, glucose and uric acid levels). Also, of course, it is considered well to keep salt intake low. In excess, alcohol may damage the myocardium leading to dysrhythmia or it may induce hypertension. Yet in moderation it is associated with favorable blood lipid patterns. Exercise has some useful associations with diet, especially by helping to control obesity—or, as one happy expression has it, "eat more and weigh less through exercise."

Psychosocial stress is a more difficult item to assess, as nearly everyone is subject to it at one time or another, especially the type of stress associated with time-oriented anxiety, anger, impatience, frustration, competitiveness and similar assaults on the psyche (Haynes et al., 1980). This may be one reason why stress is the most uncertain of these risk factors to study with definite conclusions, as the very same problem may bother one person greatly and another not at all. Thus the real psychological risk factor is not the problem or stimulus but the *distress* or reaction aroused in the enervated—the failure to cope. It is difficult to remain patient in a traffic jam, or to keep calm in the midst of an office crisis, yet we know that things usually go better if we can manage to do so. Such an adjustment of our adult lifestyle pattern may be what we should expect to work for, instead of raging against the external circumstances that have disturbed us.

Psychological benefits that accompany general fitness include increased self-confidence, self-awareness, improved mental recall heightened mood or "affect." These are all attitudes that should tend to counteract stress, or stand by the individual in dealing with stressful situations.

Returning to the topic of exercise, we note that it has many beneficial effects, both physiological and biochemical: it increases maximal oxygen uptake, slows the resting heart rate, lowers the casual blood pressure, enlarges coronary artery bore, improves the efficiency of cardiac action, increases cardiac output and enhances physical work capacity. Exercise alters the blood-lipid profile favorably, as it does fibrinolytic activity, platelet aggregation, carbohydrate metabolism, appetite and even sleep patterns (Astrand and Rodahl, 1970; Wood and Haskell, 1979). In this sense, exercise is a risk factor that touches everyone, no matter what other risk factors they may have, and no matter what their age, sex, rate, heredity, education or other personal characteristics may be.

A further consideration is that exercise has favorable effects on other risk factors such as cigarette smoking, obesity, dietary habits and hypertension. As for stress, many dedicated joggers, aerobic dancers or spirited tennis players testify that their bouts of exercise bring them a new peace of mind or even a sense of euphoria. And it seems obvious that an individual who takes up vigorous habitual running, swimming or the like, will probably give up cigarette smoking if he has had the habit. So if smoking is hazardous to health and increases risk of CHD, it follows that any lifestyle alteration that leads to a cessation of smoking reduces such risk accordingly. Thus exercise not only exerts its own direct training effect on the cardiovascular system, but it reduces CHD risk still further by helping to abolish the cigarette smoking risk as well.

Modern day societies find themselves facing a complex of problematic dichotomies in lifestyles: the sedentary versus the vigorous, the obese versus the trim, the feeble versus the stalwart, the chain smoker versus the chain breaker, the boozer versus the self-controlled imbiber, the hypertensive versus the normotensive, the omnivorous glutton versus the prudent feeder, the uptight versus the relaxed, the depressed versus the contented. Intervention through reductions of hazards and attention to lifestyles should lead society to self-preservation by improving the quality of daily life as well as preventing or forestalling the onset of CHD.

References

Astrand, P.-O. and Rodahl, K. 1970. *Textbook of Work Physiology*. New York: McGraw-Hill

Glueck, C. J. and Connor W. E. 1978. Diet: Coronary heart disease relationships reconnoitered. Am J Clin Nutr 31:727

Haynes, S. G., Feinleib, M. and Kannel, W. B. 1980. The relationship of psychosocial factors to coronary heart disease in the Framingham study. III. Eight-year incidence of coronary heart disease. Am J Epidemiol 111:37–58

Keys, A. 1980. *Seven Countries. A Multivariate Analysis of Death and Coronary Heart Disease*. Cambridge: Commonwealth Fund. Harvard University

Paffenbarger, R. S., Jr. and Hale, W. E. 1975. Work activity and coronary heart mortality. N Engl J Med 292:3–8

Paffenbarger, R. S., Jr., Wing, A. L. and Hyde, R. T. 1978. Physical activity as an index of heart attack risk in college alumni. Am J Epidemiol 108:161–175

Shekelle, R. B., Shryock, A. M., Paul, O. et al. 1981 Diet, serum cholesterol, and death from coronary heart disease. N Engl J Med 304:65–70

Wood, P. D. and Haskell, W. L. 1979. The effect of exercise on plasma high density lipoproteins. Lipids 14:417–427

Discussion

Dr. Naramay: Dr. Maseri, you mentioned that 33% of the people had old myocardial infarction. What were the criteria used—whether anybody saw those changes on an electrocardiogram? And, if you used an angiogram, whether you saw the hypokinesis or akinesis in that area?

Dr. Maseri: Well, if I say it was myocardial infarction, it was just myocardial infarction because it meets a criterion of history, EKG and hypokinesis. I don't think this was a selective population. They had myocardial infarction because they had a clinical myocardial infarction that was diagnosed from the history, the EKG and ventriculography. And some had one or more myocardial infarctions.

Dr. Walinsky: Dr. Maseri, I am not sure if I saw your slide correctly, the next-to-last slide demonstrating the percentage of patients that were symptomatic or asymptomatic. It looked like the normals were lowest on that curve; were they the most symptomatic or least symptomatic with the passage of time?

Dr. Maseri: The patients who had normal coronary arteries at 4 years were all asymptomatic. So when the line went down to zero, it went down to zero symptoms. When the line went down to 60%, 60% of the patients did have symptoms and 40% did not, which is the percentage of patients with double and triple disease where approximately 40% of them did not have symptoms during the last year. No angina.

Dr. McKenzie: I have two questions for Dr. Maseri. You showed there was a decrease in the oxygen content in coronary sinus blood. You looked at myocardial metabolites, specifically lactate; does that increase with coronary spasm?

Dr. Maseri: Yes, on occasions where we have measured lactate and also potassium increase.

Dr. McKenzie: Another question: During an ergonovine-produced spasm, have you ever tried infusing adenosine intracoronary?

Dr. Maseri: No, we have not. Adenosine is not supposed to relax the large coronary arteries, not to my knowledge. We have tried to prevent ergonovine attacks with prostacyclin infusion, unsuccessfully, with regitine infusion 2 mg/min, unsuccessfully, and we were only able to block them with high doses of nitrates.

Dr. Baum: I would like to ask a question of Dr. Pepine. Do you have any data on the use of calcium antagonists in patients with angina in which the angina is less clearly defined as vasospastic, in which there is an overlay of exercise-induced angina?

Dr. Pepine: No. These agents are investigational in this country and our protocols required that the patients have either documented spasm at the time of catheterization or rest angina with S-T elevation highly suspect for spasm. We specifically avoided other subsets of patients with ischemic heart disease.

Dr. Watkins: In your study comparing nifedipine and isosorbide dinitrate, you indicated that you have five patients who either did not benefit at all by nifedipine or their condition actually became worse. I wonder if those patients had an exaggerated tachycardia response to nifedipine?

Dr. Pepine: Please let me clarify our results. Two of our 18 patients taking nifedipine had no change and 3 had less than 50% decrease in angina frequency. We did not see the type of exaggerated tachycardia response seen in some Japanese patients. For the purpose of time, I tried to make the details of the protocol brief. The nifedipine and isosorbide dinitrate phases were each 5 weeks long. The first week of each phase was for dose titration, starting at 10 mg of either agent, four times daily. The patients were hospitalized in the Clinical Research Center and each patient's dose was titrated to the maximal tolerated dose. If side-effects occurred, we reduced the dose. Subsequently, we evaluated antiangina responses over the next 4 weeks using that dose. No patient had an exaggerated tachycardia response during the 4 weeks of follow-up treatment. The only side-effects that we saw, other than lightheadedness, was edema in two patients during nifedipine.

Dr. Wolf: Dr. Pepine, could you comment on using intracoronary nitroglycerin or ergonovine in patients with multivessel significant or apparently "fixed" coronary disease? In such patients, do you recommend using ergonovine or intracoronary nitroglycerin?

Dr. Pepine: I have avoided the term "fixed" because we believe that many atherosclerotic lesions are dynamic. When I perform coronary angiography on a patient with three-vessel disease who has rest pain with a history of a variable angina threshold or S-T segment elevation, I will consider ergonovine stimulation if the patient did not have an episode of spontaneous angina during the study. The importance of opacifying the coronary arteries during angina cannot be over-emphasized if one is to identify spasm. Complete occlusion at the site of the previously observed 90% narrowing is not the uniform finding. Occasionally, we find occlusion downstream from high grade atherosclerotic narrowings, or dynamic narrowings in other vessels remote from the atherosclerotic narrowing. Of course, we are concerned about the possibility of a nonspecific vasoconstriction response making a 90% atherosclerotic narrowing 100% over ergonovine. But we use very low doses (0.025–0.15 mg) in these patients. We use low dose intracoronary nitroglycerin as a diagnostic test. In our experience, 50 or 100μg of nitroglycerin given into the artery under question relieves coronary spasm within a few seconds with little to no systemic effect at the onset of relief.

Dr. Brown: It is known that people have increased platelet consumption or shortened platelet survival in coronary disease with stable angina. Have you done or do you know of any correlation where the level of venous thromboxane B_2 is compared with the rate of platelet consumption? Or is there a much easier way to determine which of the coronary disease patients are in fact consuming platelets?

Dr. Walinsky: We haven't done any correlations and I am not aware of any having been reported. However, the observations in the literature are certainly consistent with what we see in the setting of coronary artery disease. I would basically assume that we are seeing different markers of the same kind of phenomena, but I am not aware of any study that has been done to correlate thromboxane with other indices of platelet function.

Dr. Tuma: You postulated that thromboxane may be of some benefit in preventing myocardial steal syndrome and I can't conceptually follow that, because this is thought to be due to a loss of vasodilating capabilities in the ischemic area. I don't see how thromboxane being present in that area could help the situation.

Dr. Walinsky: I think that it has been shown that if there is a vasodilator administered intracoronary in a vessel that has normal flow and a vessel that has impaired flow, because of a differential alteration in the resistance in those two vascular beds, there can be a decrease in collateral flow or a shunting of flow from the bed of the impaired vessel to the normal bed. So all I am saying is that if you get excess vasodilation, you may have a coronary steal physiology develop. If there is some modulation of that vasodilation, it might conceivably have some role in preventing or modifying that kind of response.

Dr. Tuma: You pointed out that some vasodilators do not have the effect of causing a coronary steal, but it is because they produce vasodilation in the healthier, nonischemic areas. Thromboxane could only overcome that if it was having its effect in the nonischemic areas rather than in the ischemic areas. This could only happen if the thromboxane had an effect on the healthy tissue and not on the ischemic tissue. That is what I have difficulty in understanding.

Dr. Walinsky: It is not really clear to me what happens to this substance, once it is formed. We see it in the coronary sinus and we see it in the arterial samples as well. So, once it is formed locally it is distributed, I would presume, not only to the ischemic but also to the nonischemic bed.

Dr. Nanarday: When you measure the potassium, or lactate or prostaglandin level after acute myocardial infarction or unstable angina, you see an increase in the level of those substances. Still we don't postulate that they cause myocardial ischemia on infarction. Why do you postulate that regarding thromboxane?

Dr. Walinsky: I didn't postulate that thromboxane was the causative agent. I said that because it has vasoconstrictor properties that this is a possibility. I think the one interesting thing about thromboxane is that it has vasoactive properties. This is in contrast to many of the other biochemicals that may efflux from myocardium during ischemia, and is also in contrast to other platelet factors that are released such as beta thromboglobulin and platelet factor 4. These agents do not have vasoactive properties. That is the only reason for making that suggestion.

Dr. Nanarday: What is the response to nitrates? When you give patients nitrates does thromboxane come down as the patient becomes asymptomatic?

Dr. Walinsky: With regard to coronary spasm, when you give nitrates and you have relief of spasm, as I mentioned previously, the levels that are measured are highest. This suggests that there is washout effect occuring. You have a build-up of the substance during spasm and then when you dilate the vessel you have a washout of thromboxane.

Dr. Santamore: How much is 2000 kcal/week or what additional exercise would be needed?

Dr. Paffenbarger: The "jogging quotient" of 2000 kcal energy expenditure approximates 2½ hours of running at a pace of 8½–9 min/mile. Of course anyone who would spend that much time jogging weekly might be expected to do considerable walking and stair climbing as well, so that his weekly energy expenditure would greatly exceed 2000 kcal.

Dr. Wendling: What evidence is there for the role of caffeine or coffee drinking increasing heart disease? This is an area of controversy.

Dr. Paffenbarger: Although some of the earlier epidemiologic studies of potential risk factors of coronary heart disease, notably Oglesby Paul's observations on employees of the Hawthorne works of the Western Electric Company, implicated coffee as a predictor of increased coronary risk; most other prospective studies have denied such a relationship. Many investigators believe there to be no important association between coffee or caffeine consumption and atherosclerotic processes. However, the question continues under active investigation.

Dr. Vanner: You mentioned dose response with respect to activity in your alumni study. If you were to write an exercise prescription, what would it be in order to achieve in shortest possible time the maximum protection that you saw in your highly active alumni?

Dr. Paffenbarger: I believe Dr. Kenneth Cooper at the Institute for Aerobics Research in Dallas is correct. He believes, as the Harvard alumni studies indicate, that sudden bursts of energy output provide an added benefit in heart attact prevention over the benefit derived from an equivalent amount of energy expended at a more leisurely pace. Thus, a general recommendation or exercise prescription might include a minimum of three or four stints of activity weekly in which the individual gets his heart rate up to three-quarters of maximum and maintains that level for 20, or preferably, 30 min. It is my firm belief that such a program will provide the kind of heart attack protection that the studies of the London transport workers, the British civil servants, the San Francisco longshoremen and the Harvard alumni suggest.

Dr. Vanner: So your alumni, if they have been sedentary over 10–15 years could then theoretically over a year or so get their risk factor down to the maximal protective level by at least exceeding Cooper's recommendation?

Dr. Paffenbarger: Extrapolating from the epidemiologic evidence indicating an inverse association between physically active lifestyle and heart attack incidence, one might logically conclude that taking up an active way of life would lower heart risk. I believe this to be the case. But we must be guarded in how we recommend that patients and the public begin an exercise program. Certainly no individual should convert from a sedentary to an active life pattern by beginning with an attempt to better his 440 track time of many years ago. A safe beginning would recommend a walking program of increasing distance and decreasing time until the individual could walk comfortably 3½ or 4 miles in an hour, that is without pain, dyspnea or excessive fatigue. Then and only then should a more active program be undertaken. Progression thereafter from walking, to striding, to walk-jogging, to slow jogging of increasing distances might be recommended as the individual's tolerance permits. Cardiologists and exercise physiologists usually prefer to perform an exercise tolerance (treadmill) test before recommending a physical activity program, but it should be noted that such tests often give either false positive or false negative results. Moreover, treadmill testing is not always feasible, particularly on a mass basis.

Dr. Gould: Perhaps I can supplement this streptokinase data as to whether it works. In 50 consecutive patients, we do all MIs. In those patients who have occlusion due to clot, who have a low ejection fraction and who open, the mean ejection fraction of 19–32 goes to normal. Every patient gets better. In those patients who fail to open and have low flow lesions with tight stenosis and no clots none of the ejection fractions gets better. Clearly the streptokinase patients do get dramatically better, and we showed some nice pictures showing why, but it does work on ventricular function.

Dr. Spann: Dr. Wolf, you have done approximately 17–18 of these people here in Philadelphia; would you like to add your comments to those of a Texas experience?

Dr. Wolf: Our experience is not as optimistic. What is the time period from the onset of pain until the vessel is opened?

Dr. Gould: We take all kinds up to 18 hours and we have seen an 18-hour ejection fraction dramatically improve.

Dr. Wolf: Do you measure your ejection fractions before and after streptokinase during that catheterization? And do you have control of what happens to a normal infarct that is not improved?

Dr. Gould: We measure ejection fractions three times: Before streptokinase, immediately after and 10 days later at discharge. It can take about a week for it to maximize. In a number of patients, even at 6 weeks, it still continues to improve, although the figures that I just mentioned are within 10 days.

Dr. Wolf: One final question. How are you measuring ejection fraction using what modality?

Dr. Gould: The first two angiograms and then simultaneously three measurements or more with radionuclide angiography.

Section VI

Symposium Summary

Alfred A. Bove and William P. Santamore

Current Concepts About Coronary Artery Disease: Symposium Summary

Alfred A. Bove and William P. Santamore

The goal of the 1981 Richards Symposium was to review the recent aspects of coronary disease related to the pathophysiology of the large coronary vessels. The symposium was arranged to cover a spectrum of interests in the subject, beginning with smooth muscle physiology and its application to large coronary arteries, and ending with an analysis of the epidemiology of coronary disease.

Smooth muscle physiology has made a number of recent advances. A thorough knowledge of the biochemical mechanisms of contraction, the actin-myosin interaction and the role of calcium in contraction is needed to understand the response of the large coronary vessels to hormonal, autonomic and drug influences. The question of how myosin phosphorylation contributes to the contractile process is still unanswered. Some primitive muscle requires phosphorylation for contraction but there is as yet no clear link between contraction and phosphorylation in mammalian smooth muscle. However, the role of calcium in smooth muscle contraction is becoming somewhat clearer. There appears to be a calcium-dependent resting tone, which is energy efficient; energy needs fall over time even though the resting tone is maintained.

Crossbridge cycling is known to be slower in smooth muscle. Thus, the contraction, as well as the relaxation phases, are slower. Butler (Chapter 1) finds actin-myosin crossbridge cycling in smooth muscle to be 150 times slower than in skeletal muscle. To relate these findings to coronary artery physiology, Butler points out three phases of smooth muscle contraction. The first is an attached phase of actin-myosin where cross-bridges do not cycle but resting tone is maintained. The second is the cycling crossbridge phase, where force is generated by repeated actin-myosin linking. During a prolonged tetanus, a third phase emerges where crossbridges are attached but not cycling and energy requirements fall in spite of the continued maintenance of force. The characteristics of a prolonged tetanic contraction are interesting because a mechanism for sustained contraction or spasm of a coronary artery could involve this relatively oxygen- and energy-independent tetanic contraction in the smooth muscle of the arterial wall.

To extend the concepts derived from studies of contractile properties of vascular smooth muscle cells, it is necessary to examine the active and passive mechanical characteristics of segments of blood vessels in vitro and in vivo. The studies presented by Cox (Chapter 2) describe the characteristics of intact arterial segments and provide the link between the smooth muscle cell and the functioning artery in vivo. Active vascular responses to autonomic stimuli and other smooth muscle stimulating agents are variable and depend on the type of artery (large versus small coronary arteries, for example), the degree of sympathetic activation and the amount of smooth muscle in the arterial wall. Arteries from spontaneously hypertensive rats have thicker smooth muscle layers and generate greater force when stimulated in vitro. Tonic activation is known to be present in coronary arteries, and the state of autonomic tone determines the diameter and stiffness of these arteries. Passive characteristics are also important in understanding the mechanical properties of blood vessels. The passive stiffness properties depend on elastin and collagen and vary as a function of the degree of stretch imposed on the artery. The minimally distended artery demonstrates the lower stiffness characteristics of elastin, while the distended artery is stiffer because of recruitment of collagen fibers.

Changes in active and passive stiffness may be important in coronary arteries because of changes with age, amount of smooth muscle, degree of atherosclerosis and vessel diameter. Variations in active and passive characteristics contribute to the pressure-flow relationship, which is important, especially in the partially stenosed large coronary arteries.

Regulation of coronary vascular bed is addressed in Chapter 3 by Dr. Berne. Several different levels of regulation must be considered. Mechanical forces in the myocardium that are produced during systole cause cyclic changes in flow, while autonomic control seems to be less important. Berne points out that there is alpha-adrenergic (vasoconstrictor) tone in the coronary vascular bed and that sympathetic stimulation can cause large coronary artery vasoconstriction. Control at the microvascular level is dependent on O_2 demand, while CO_2 and pH play minimal roles in regulation of coronary flow. An important mediator in microvascular flow regulation appears to be adenosine. This agent is released by ischemic cells and is a potent coronary arteriolar smooth muscle relaxant. Modulation of flow based on work demands of the myocardium remains a fundamental concept in coronary flow. When myocardial blood flow is compromised, the subendocardial region becomes ischemic earliest. The effect of proximal coronary stenosis on local function of myocardial cells continues to be an important area for research. Microscopic infarcts may occur in the subendocardial region when flow is compromised even though obvious clinical infarction is not evident.

The first three chapters encompassing basic coronary physiology provide a significant review of the current understanding of smooth muscle, large and small coronary control and myocardial flow regulation.

The next section of the symposium covers the pharmacology of the coronary circulation. Chapter 4 by Winbury delineates the two components of the coronary vascular bed—the large and small coronary vessels. It is the difference between these two types of vessels and their responsiveness to physiologic and pharmacologic stimuli that is the basis for the findings presented in later chapters on the dynamics of the coronary circulation in the presence of a stenosed artery. Winbury points out that drugs must be classed as affecting either the proximal large coronary arteries or the distal small arteries and arterioles. Nitroglycerin, for example, acts mainly on large coronary vessels and has minimal effect on the coronary microcirculation. Thus, nitroglycerin clearly causes an increase in caliber of the large, proximal arteries, which may be the primary means by which nitroglycerin relieves angina. On the other hand, drugs that dilate the distal vascular bed such as adenosine or dipyridamole do not dilate proximal arteries and may produce paradoxical effects in the presence of a proximal stenosis. Other constrictors such as ergonovine and angiotensin constrict both large and small coronary arteries. The calcium channel blockers act mainly on the large coronary arteries and provide an alternate or adjunctive drug to nitroglycerin. Beta-adrenergic stimuli also dilate large coronary arteries, while alpha-adrenergic agents constrict the large arteries. Winbury also points out the important observation that increased low density lipoproteins and several cholesterol precursors increase the sensitivity of large coronary atherosclerosis and clinical coronary artery disease.

The interaction of blood and blood vessels is further explored in Chapter 5. The studies by Aiken presented in this chapter suggest that narrowed coronary arteries may be subjected to intermittent occlusion by platelet clumps forming in the coronary arteries. Constrictor prostaglandins released by platelets (thromboxanes) may contribute to the occlusion process once the platelets are activated by the mechanical trauma and surface stimulation taking place in the stenotic area. The use of thromboxane A_2 inhibitor in Aiken's studies reduced the cyclic occlusion in the dog coronary artery. This finding suggests that specific inhibitors of thromboxane may be useful in treating the stenosed, unstable coronary artery that is undergoing intermittent platelet plugging or vasoconstriction. These studies also raise several questions concerning the dynamics of a coronary stenosis. Is platelet plugging a near terminal event that leads to total occlusion, distal thrombosis and myocardial infarction? Or do platelets activated in a stenosis release vasoconstrictors which, in the presence of a compliant stenosis, shut off the vessel and cause thrombosis and infarction? Later chapters point out that stenoses can be unstable even when no platelets are present and when the artery is not viable and thus unable to constrict. Platelet plugging, active constriction and passive narrowing of the stenosis must all be considered in the dynamics of coronary artery lesions.

We could not conduct this coronary artery disease symposium without including a discussion of the calcium entry blocking agents. These drugs have been the subject of much research and at the present time (1981) are becoming available for clinical use in the United States. Chapter 6 reviews the pharmacology of these agents. These drugs block calcium entry into vascular smooth muscle cells and inhibit constriction of the vessel. Because their action differs from nitroglycerin, they are useful adjuncts to nitroglycerin therapy and have proven to be effective in therapy of coronary disease. Their effectiveness in coronary disease is thought to be due to their ability to inhibit large vessel vasoconstriction. Perhach makes clear that there is a spectrum of action of these agents that is now being tested. These drugs have many other actions, which vary from drug to drug. The variety provides a choice that can be tailored to individual therapeutic needs. The application of these drugs to coronary disease are discussed in the section on clinical aspects of coronary disease and in Chapter 7, which deals with the physiology and pharmacology of human coronary arteries.

Chapter 7 by Ginsburg provides data on the response of human coronary arteries to various vasoconstrictor mediators and to vasodilating and constricting drugs. These data were obtained from coronary arteries removed from the hearts of patients undergoing heart transplantation. The data are derived from classic pharmacologic studies in vascular rings from these arteries. Besides the observation that all the human coronary arteries had some degree of atherosclerosis, Ginsburg reports spontaneous rhythmic contraction of these arteries with a cycle time of 1–2 min. These rhythmic contractions have been seen in coronary arteries of other species, but their presence in man has only recently been mentioned. The basal tone of the arteries seems to depend on calcium but not on catecholamine or histamine concentration. This study also demonstrates that human coronary arteries contain H1-type histamine receptors.

Vessels with significant atherosclerosis demonstrated an increased sensitivity to histamine; a finding which is similar to the data presented by Winbury in Chapter 4. Ginsburg also demonstrated a variability in local vasoconstrictor response to histamine and suggested that this variation may be an explanation for local coronary spasm.

The above studies on physiology and pharmacology of the coronary vascular bed are a prelude to the studies directed toward the clinical and experimental problem of the etiology of atherosclerosis, large coronary spasm and the hemodynamics of coronary stenosis.

Texon presented a discussion of the hydraulic characteristics of coronary and other large arteries, pointing out the characteristics that make certain regions prone to atherosclerosis. Curves in arteries usually have atherosclerotic lesions on the inner curvature. This finding is consistent enough to warrant mechanical explanation. Chapter 8 contains Texon's review of the hydraulics of curved vessels and the application of these principles to the atherosclerotic process. The following chapter by Ross (Chapter 9) discusses the reaction to injury concept of atherosclerosis. These hydraulic effects may be a contributing factor to the initial injury postulated by Ross to preceed the actual development of an atherosclerotic plaque. Texon suggests that the low pressure zones produced on the inner curvature of arterial bends or at branch points lift the endothelial damage. The degree of injury in this case would then depend on the flow velocity. The higher the local velocity, the lower the pressure. Thus, more endothelial damage would occur if velocity were chronically increased. These data lead to the question of how endothelial injury might result in atherosclerosis. Chapter 9 by Ross reviews the various theories of atherosclerosis. Of the three theories presented, the "reaction-to-injury" hypothesis seems most tenable. Ross shows that increased cholesterol causes endothelial damage. Once endothelial injury occurs and endothelial cells are separated, blood platelets adhere to exposed collagen in the medial layer. The platelets release a smooth muscle growth factor, which causes proliferation of smooth muscle in the area of damaged endothelium and institutes the pathologic process that results in an atherosclerotic plaque. Macrophages are attracted to the area by platelet-released chemotaxins and become part of the atherosclerotic process by taking up lipid to form foam cells. Ross suggests that the proliferation and migration of smooth muscle cells from the media to the endothelial region of the artery wall is the process that initiates the atherosclerotic process. An agent that blocked the platelet-derived growth factor (PDGF) would then be highly desirable for prevention of atherosclerosis. The chemical characteristics of PDGF have been worked out, and studies of this compound should provide further understanding of the atherosclerotic process and suggest new types of therapy.

The dynamics of coronary stenoses were the next topic of the symposium. Chapter 10 from our laboratory presents a review of the active and passive characteristics of stenoses. Chapters 10–12, which deal with this subject, all contain statements and inferences that a coronary stenosis is not always a fixed, rigid narrowing but rather can be a compliant, flexible region that changes dimension under a number of stimuli. There is now ample evidence that stenotic resistance varies with the degree of vasoconstriction in compliant stenoses. This change is important in understanding the clinical data on coronary spasm presented later, where change in caliber of the stenosis appears to be the most significant component of the ischemic process. Besides active vasoconstriction, stenotic resistance is dependent on the perfusion pressure to keep the artery distended. Lowering proximal pressure causes a reduction in vessel and stenosis diameter and increases the stenotic resistance. Perfusion pressure distal to the stenosis may fall precipitously in this case. In several animal studies, we have found an instability in the stenosis when the cross-sectional area is less than 85% of the original artery area. When distal resistance falls, pressure in the distal arterial segment falls, the artery narrows, causing the stenosis to become narrower. This is a positive feedback system and can result in total closure of the artery and cessation of flow. Based on these studies, the effect of distal resistance appears to be significant in maintaining hemodynamic stability in stenoses. Gould has also examined these concepts and has been able to calculate the pressure drop across the stenosis by careful consideration of the fluid dynamics of narrowed regions and with careful angiographic measurements with which to perform the calculations. Chapters 11 and 12 are both addressed to this hydraulic problem, and both demonstrate a useful relationship between flow, pressure and vessel geometry. The method and results therefrom are based on well-established fluid mechanics principles. Gould's data also support the concept of compliant stenoses and demonstrate some of the characteristics of such stenoses in his intact dog model. Chapter 12 by Brown et al. provides interesting data on the application of fluid mechanics principles to human coronary arteries. They found a variety of responses in stenoses. About one-third of human lesions are compliant, while two-thirds are fixed. In all lesions, a 60% reduction in diameter causes exertional angina, and a 75–80% diameter reduction causes subendocardial infarction. The 60% lesion, however, is capable of becoming an 80% lesion under vasoconstrictor stimuli, and they feel that ordinary vasomotor tone is sufficient to explain most unstable angina. Dr. Brown suggests that behavioral patterns may be important in the development of angina, especially with the knowledge that coronary stenoses can become critical under catecholamine stimulation, and that isometric handgrip has been found to cause narrowing of the large coronary vessels. Dr. Brown also shows in Chapter 12 that vessels distal to a tight stenosis become narrower when distal resistance falls. With dipyridamole, distal resistance decreased, distal arterial and stenotic diameter decreased and stenotic resistance increased markedly. In the presence of stenosis, there are apparently some patients who demonstrate little or no increase in flow with decreased distal resistance, while other patients actually show a fall in flow with decreased distal resistance.

The concluding portion of the symposium was addressed to the clinical problems associated with coronary artery stenosis. The studies presented in Chapters 13, 14, and 15 are as important to understanding coronary physiology in coronary disease as those done in vitro or in animals. The human model still remains unique and different from the animal models used to study the physiology of coronary disease. Dr. Maseri's A. N. Richards Memorial address deserves mention here because in it he reviewed the history of coronary disease and presented the current pathophysiologic mechanisms and understanding of the disease process. The fixed lesion concept, held since the 1930s, has been dispelled in the past 20 years by several studies that clearly demonstrated that local spasm of coronary arteries could cause angina, myocardial infarction and sudden death. Since these early observations, it has become evident that vasomotion of coronary arteries is an extremely important component of clinical coronary disease. Vasoconstriction of already present lesions is commonplace and accounts for changing anginal patterns, unstable angina, sudden death and indeed may result in ischemia with no clinical symptoms. Ischemic ECG changes were demonstrated in the absence of symptoms and occurred clinically. That these changes truly represent ischemia was proven by observed oxygen saturation changes in the coronary sinus, which occur in synchrony with the ECG changes and synchronous changes in left ventricular end diastolic pressure. The process is one of decreased blood supply with unchanged demand and not a limit on blood supply in the presence of increased demand. In this light, therapy of coronary disease must be strongly oriented toward controlling large coronary vasomotion. Maseri's successful experience with this type of therapy verifies the validity of this concept. To date, however, the mediators of coronary vasoconstriction are unknown. Alpha-adenergic antagonists and platelet inhibition with aspirin do not relieve angina, while calcium entry blocking agents and nitroglycerin drugs, which are nonspecific coronary dilators, are highly effective. The clinical experience presented by Pepine (Chapter 14) also supports Maseri's concepts of coronary disease. Of note is the need to demonstrate reactive coronary segments with a constrictor such as ergonovine to detect the presence of spasm in patients. Misleading data may result when minor narrowing of the coronary arteries is considered unimportant, while ergonovine would show a conversion of these minor lesions to significant narrowing under increased vasomotor tone. Drs. Pepine and Maseri both pointed out that hyperactivity of the coronary arteries is periodic. That is, there are periods of days or weeks where patients demonstrate coronary instability, followed by prolonged trouble-free periods, requiring no drug therapy. The value of combined calcium entry blockers and nitroglycerin in treatment is also stressed in Chapter 14. Either drug alone seems to have lesser effect, and potentiation of the action of these drugs by one another seems to be the case.

Chapter 15 reviews the current status of platelet-stenosis interaction in coronary disease. Dr. Walinsky has found thromboxane B2, the stable product of the platelet-derived vasoconstrictor prostaglandin thromboxane A2(TXA_2) to be elevated in venous blood of patients with angina pectoris. The earlier suggestion that TXA_2 caused angina and infarction can be questioned from studies that demonstrate unchanged anginal patterns after inhibition of platelet release of TXA_2. In any case, elevated TXB_2 is found in unstable angina and myocardial infarction, but the connection of these findings with the cause of angina and infarction is unclear. It is well known that platelet activation occurs whenever an acute inflammatory reaction is underway, and one would expect inflammation after an acute infarction.

Further clinical aspects of coronary disease were presented by Dr. Spann, who reviewed the recent findings of coronary thrombosis in myocardial infarction and the use of thrombolytic therapy in the early phase of myocardial infarction. This new therapy shows promise in preventing permanent death of myocardial tissue when the therapy is applied early in cases of acute infarction. A review of the various trials of platelet inhibitors is also presented in Chapter 16. There is little data to recommend these treatments to date, although some improvement in long term prognosis may occur with either sulfinpyrazone (anturane) or with combined aspirin and dipyridamole. In addition, beta-adrenergic blocking drugs may also provide a better long term prognosis. None of these drugs, however, appears to produce large scale effects in the studies done to date.

The culmination of the symposium was the presentation by Paffenbarger (Chapter 17), which documented the behavioral aspects of coronary disease. This is an important area to consider because the newer concepts of coronary disease presented in this symposium cast a different light on the epidemiologic studies of coronary disease than previously considered. Instead of examining the effects of smoking, hypertension and exercise on blood lipid levels and composition, it may be more important to examine the effects of these factors on coronary vessel reactivity. Paffenbarger has clearly shown that exercise reduces coronary disease risk; while obesity, psychologic stress, diabetes mellitus, hypertension and smoking all increase the risk of coronary disease. The relationship between these risk factors and large coronary physiology has not been carefully examined and requires extensive study. Exercise is known to alter large coronary artery diameter, change blood-lipid profile, affect platelet aggregation and fibrinolytic activity. With the data presented in the symposium, one could postulate a variety of mechanisms whereby exercise could interact with systems that affect coronary reactivity.

It is clear from the data presented here that the nature of coronary disease involves coronary artery vasomotion. It is possible that most of coronary disease involves this process. But it is more likely that a spectrum exists ranging from hard, fixed stenoses, which respond according to well-established principles of fluid mechanics, to highly compliant, highly reactive stenoses, which change diameter frequently as a daily occurrence producing minor or major ischemia as the degree of constriction varies. In the latter case, coronary artery dilator drug therapy shows promise in altering the entire course and prognosis of coronary disease; while with fixed stenosis, intraluminal angioplasty and coronary bypass surgery provide the major modes of therapy.

The 1981 A. N. Richards Symposium also served to point out the fact that coronary disease has become a new and highly mobile area of research after several decades of stable thought, which may have disregarded the true nature of the disease process.

Index

ABRM (*see* Anterior byssus retractor muscle)
Acetylcholine, 122, 124
  in coronary arteries, 73
  in human coronary artery, 106, 109–110
Actin, 17
  in active arterial mechanics, 31
  in hypertension, 54
  in smooth muscle, 4, 6, 8–10
Adenosine, 53, 58–59
  in coronary arteries, 67, 72
  in coronary blood flow regulation, 46–48, 56–58, 284
Adenosine 3′, 5′-cyclic monophosphate
  platelets and, 81
Adenosine deaminase, 58
  effect on vascular resistance, 57
  in coronary blood flow regulation, 48
Adenosine 5′-diphosphate, platelet aggregation and, 80–81
Adenosine monophosphate, 53, 58
  in coronary blood flow regulation, 48
Adenosine nitrates, in coronary arteries, 70
ADP (*see* Adenosine 5′-diphosphate)
Aminophylline, in coronary arteries, 69
AMP, cyclic (*see* Adenosine 3′, 5′-cyclic monophosphate)
AMP (*see* Adenosine monophosphate)
Anatomy, coronary, 223–224
Angina, pacing-induced, and thromboxane A_2, 250–251
Angina pectoris, thromboxane A_2 and, 248–249
Angiotensin, 122
Anterior byssus retractor muscle of *Mytilus edulis*, 53
Arterial mechanics, 19–36, 53–54, 284
  active, 26–35, 284
    elastometric approach, 27–28
    muscle approach, 28–35
    sympathetic stimulation, 35–36
  calcium in, 55
  collagen in, 55
  elastin in, 55
  isotonic contraction in, 55–56
  nonlinear properties, 20–26
  passive, 20–26, 284
  pressure-diameter in, 56
Arteries
  coronary
    large, mechanical aspects of, 19–36
    proximal and distal, 63–75
  human coronary, pharmacologic effects on, 103–114
Arteriography, coronary, and stenosis, 185–191, 205–206
Atherogenesis, 140
Atherosclerosis, 54–55, 74–75, 113–114, 123, 287
  coronary artery spasm and, 221–229
  coronary, hemodynamic basis, 127–137
  dipyridamole in, 152
  fluid mechanics, 129–133
  implications, 135–137
  localization, 133–134
  pathogenesis of, 139–145, 149
    hypercholesterolemia, 140
    lipid infiltration hypothesis, 140–141
    monoclonal hypothesis, 142–143
    response-to-injury hypothesis, 141–142, 152
  platelet-derived growth factor in, 144, 150–151, 153
  prostacyclin in, 151
  response-to-injury hypothesis, 287
  role of endothelium, 143
  role of monocyte/macrophage, 145
  role of platelets, 144–145, 150
  role of smooth muscle, 144
Autoregulation, in coronary arteries, 67
Basal tone, human coronary artery, 104–106
Bepridil, as calcium blocker, 94–98, 100–101
Beta blockers, coronary artery spasm and, 243

291

Blood, interaction with blood vessel wall, 79–91
Blood flow, coronary, regulation, 39–49
Blood vessel wall, interaction with blood, 79–91
Bronchospasm, 123, 245
　calcium blockers and, 100
Caffeine, coronary heart disease and, 278–279
Calcium
　in arterial mechanics, 55
　in coronary blood flow regulation, 49
　in human coronary artery, 106–108
　regulation, in smooth muscle, 8
Calcium blockers, 123, 125, 286
　bepridil, 94–98, 100–101
　bronchospasm and, 100
　cardiac output and, 99
　coronary artery spasm and, 239–242, 276
　coronary blood flow and, 97
　diltiazem, 94–98, 100, 112
　hypertension and, 100
　in ischemic heart disease, 93–101
　myocardial oxygen consumption and, 98–99
　nifedipine, 94–97, 100, 112, 150
　perhexiline, 94–96
　platelet aggregation and, 100
　verapamil, 94–96, 100, 112, 150
Calmodulin, in smooth muscle, 8
Carbon dioxide, in coronary blood flow regulation, 45
Cardiac output, calcium blockers and, 99
Catecholamines, in coronary arteries, 70
CBF (see Coronary blood flow)
CHD (see Coronary heart disease)
Cholesterol, in coronary arteries, 74–75
Chromonar, in coronary arteries, 69
Cigarette smoking
　coronary heart disease and
　　in college men, 270
　　in longshoremen, 266
Cold pressure test, for coronary artery spasm, 238
Collagen, in arterial mechanics, 21–26, 55
College men, coronary heart disease in, 268–271
Coronary anatomy, 223–224
Coronary arteries drug responses, 63–75
　acetylocholine, 73
　action potential, 72
　adenosine, 67, 72
　adenosine nitrates, 70
　autoregulation, 67
　catecholamines, 70
　cholesterol, 74–75
　dipyridamole, 66
　hypoxia, 67–68
　ischemia, 70–71
　isoproterenol, 69, 73
　methoxamine, 73
　nifedipine, 69, 73
　nitrates, 64, 69–71
　nitroglycerin, 72–73
　potassium, 73–74
　reactive hyperemia, 67
　sympathetic stimulation, 70
effect of methoxamine on, 35
effect of nitroglycerin on, 35
human, 121, 124
　acetylcholine in, 106, 109–110
　basal tone, 104–106
　calcium in, 106–108
　diltiazem in, 106
　ergonovine in, 106, 111
　histamine in, 106, 110
　ibuprofen in, 104
　indomethiacin in, 104
　nitroglycerin in, 106, 113
　norepinephrine in, 106, 108–109
　pharmacologic effects on, 103–114
　pH in, 106
　potassium in, 106
　prostacyclin in, 104–105
　prostaglandins in, 110–111
　rhythmic activity in, 105–106
large, mechanical aspects of, 19–36
proximal and distal, 63–75
species differences, 108
stenosis, 64–66
sympathetic stimulation, 35–36
Coronary arteriography, stenosis and, 185–191, 205–206
Coronary artery disease, thromboxane A_2 in, 247–251
Coronary artery spasm, 122–123, 221–229, 275–276, 288–289
　atherosclerosis and, 221–229
　beta blockers and, 243
　calcium blockers and, 239–242, 276
　clinical clues, 224
　cold pressure test, 238
　criteria for, 234–235
　definition, 227
　diagnosis and treatment, 233–245
　diltiazem treatment, 241
　ergonovine and, 275
　ergonovine testing, 236–238
　hazards, 237
　nifedipine and, 276
　nifedipine treatment, 241–242
　nitrates and, 239, 275
　nitroglycerin and, 239, 276
　passive changes, 225–226
　perhexiline treatment, 240–241
　platelets and, 243–244
　propranolol and, 243

prostacyclin and, 228, 243–244, 275
prostaglandins and, 243–244
thromboxane A_2 and, 244
vasoconstriction, 225–227
verapamil treatment, 242
vessel wall and, 227–228
Coronary artery stenosis, 157–171, 173–198, 199–212, 215–219, 287, 288
  active characteristics, 158–159, 166–171, 202–203, 207–210, 287
    animal model, 158–159
  animal model, 215
  arteriography, 185–191, 205–206
  diagnosis, 210–211
  dipyridamole in, 208–211
  fluid mechanics, 174, 200–201
  geometric changes, 168–170
  hemodynamics of, 173–198
    animal model, 175–180
  isometric handgrip in, 207–208
  isoproterenol in, 164
  mathematical model, 160–162
  methoxamine in, 164
  nitroglycerin in, 209–210, 216
  passive characteristics, 160–171, 202, 208, 215–216, 287–288
    animal model, 163–164
  pressure-flow relation, 185, 188, 193–198
  patient studies, 204–205, 207–208, 218–219, 288
  pressure-velocity relation, 195–198
  therapy, 211
  vasoconstriction, 158–159, 166–168, 171
Coronary artery vasoconstriction, 158–159, 166–168, 171
Coronary atherosclerosis, hemodynamic basis, 127–137
Coronary blood flow
  calcium blockers and, 97
  mechanical factors, 40–41
  metabolic factors, 44–49
  neural factors, 42–44
  regulation, 39–49
    adenosine, 46–48, 56–58, 284
    carbon dioxide, 45
    extravascular compression, 40–41
    oxygen, 44–47
    parasympathetic stimulation, 44
    pH, 45
    potassium, 45
    sympathetic stimulation, 42–43, 56
    vascular waterfall phenomenon, 41
Coronary heart disease, 278–279, 290
  caffeine and, 278–279
  college men, 268–271
  cigarette smoking, 270

exercise, 269–70
hypertension, 270
diet and, 272
exercise and, 278–279
lifestyle patterns and, 263–273, 290
longshoremen, 264–267
  cigarette smoking, 266
  exercise, 264–266
  hypertension, 267
obesity and, 271
stress and, 272
Coronary steal, 277
Coronary vasomotion, 225
Crossbridge cycle
  in isometric contraction, 13–14
  in smooth muscle, 7–8, 10, 16–17, 283
Cyclic AMP (*see* Adenosine 3', 5'-cyclic monophosphate)
Cyclooxygenase inhibitors, 120–121
  platelets and, 81–82, 84–86
Diet, coronary heart disease and, 272
Diltiazem
  as calcium blocker, 94–98, 100, 112
  in human coronary artery, 106
  treatment, of coronary artery spasm, 241
Dipyridamole, 285
  in atherosclerosis, 152
  in coronary arteries, 66, 69
  in coronary artery stenosis, 208–211
DP (*see* Dipyridamole)
Elastic modulus
  in active arterial mechanics, 27–28
  in passive arterial mechanics, 20–25
Elastin
  in arterial mechanics, 55
  in passive arterial mechanics, 21–26
Elastometric approach, in active arterial mechanics, 27–28
Endothelium, role of, in atherosclerosis, 143
Energetics, in smooth muscle, 10–16
Epinephrine, in coronary arteries, 70
Ergonovine, 117, 122
  coronary artery spasm and, 227, 275
  in human coronary artery, 106, 111
  testing
    for coronary artery spasm, 236–238
    for coronary artery spasm, hazards, 237
Exercise
  coronary heart disease and, 278–279
  in college men, 269–270
  in longshoremen, 264–266
Extravascular compression, in coronary blood flow regulation, 40–41
HDL (*see* High density lipoproteins)
Heparin, 257–260
High density lipoproteins, 140

Histamine, 122, 286
  in human coronary artery, 106, 110
Hypercholesterolemia, atherosclerosis and, 140
Hyperlipoproteinemias, 140
Hypertension
  actin in, 54
  calcium blockers and, 100
  coronary heart disease and
    in college men, 270
    in longshoremen, 267
  myosin in, 54
Hypoxia, in coronary arteries, 67–68
Ibuprofen
  in human coronary artery, 104
  platelets and, 86
Indomethiacin
  in human coronary artery, 104
  platelets and, 84, 86, 88
Inosine, 58
Interstitial fluid, in coronary blood flow regulation, 46
Ischemia, in coronary arteries, 70–71
Ischemic heart disease, calcium blockers in, 93–101
ISF (see Interstitial fluid)
Isometric contraction
  energetics of, in smooth muscle, 11–14
  in active arterial mechanics, 29–33
Isometric force development, in active arterial mechanics, 29–31
Isometric handgrip, in coronary artery stenosis, 207–208
Isometric relaxation, energetics of, in smooth muscle, 14–15
Isoproterenol
  in coronary arteries, 69–70, 73
  in coronary artery stenosis, 164
Isotonic contraction, in arterial mechanics, 55–56
Isotonic shortening, in active arterial mechanics, 31–33
Latch state, of crossbridges, in smooth muscle, 10
LDL (see Low density lipoproteins)
Leiotonin, calcium regulation and, in smooth muscle, 8
Lidoflazine, in coronary arteries, 69
Lifestyle, patterns, coronary heart disease and, 263–273
Lipid infiltration hypothesis, 140–141
Longshoremen, coronary heart disease in, 264–267
Low density lipoproteins, 140
Macrophage, role of, in atherosclerosis, 145
Methoxamine
  effect on coronary artery, 35
  in coronary arteries, 73
  in coronary artery stenosis, 164
Monoclonal hypothesis, 142–143
Monocyte, role of, in atherosclerosis, 145
Myocardial infarction
  thrombolysis therapy, 255–261
  thromboxane A_2 and, 250, 252
Myocardial oxygen consumption, calcium blockers and, 98–99
Myosin, 17
  in active arterial mechanics, 31
  in hypertension, 54
  in smooth muscle, 3–6, 8–10
Myosin ATPase, in smooth muscle, 8
Muscle
  smooth
    physiology of, 3–17
    role of, in atherosclerosis, 144
Muscle approach
  in active arterial mechanics, 28–35
  isometric force development, 29–31
  isotonic shortening, 31–33
  series elasticity, 33–35
Nerves
  parasympathetic, in coronary blood flow regulation, 44
  sympathetic, in coronary blood flow regulation, 42–43
Nifedipine
  as calcium blocker, 94–97, 100, 112, 150
  coronary artery spasm and, 276
  in coronary arteries, 69, 73
  in thrombolysis therapy, 256
  treatment, of coronary artery spasm, 241–242
Nitrates, 245
  coronary artery spasm and, 239, 275
  in coronary arteries, 64, 69–71
  thromboxane A_2 and, 278
Nitroglycerin, 285
  coronary artery spasm and, 239, 276
  effect on coronary artery, 35
  in coronary arteries, 72–73
  in coronary artery stenosis, 209–210, 216
  in human coronary artery, 106, 113
  thrombolysis therapy and, 257–258
Nitroprusside, in coronary arteries, 69
Norepinephrine, 122
  in coronary arteries, 70
  in human coronary artery, 106, 108–109
Obesity, coronary heart disease and, 271
Osmolarity, in coronary blood flow regulation, 49
Oxygen, in coronary blood flow regulation, 44–47
Papaverine
  in coronary arteries, 69
  in coronary artery stenosis, 177, 185

Parasympathetic stimulation, in coronary blood flow regulation, 44
PCr (see Phosphocreatine)
PDGF (see Platelet-derived growth factor)
Perhexiline
 as calcium blocker, 94–96
 treatment, of coronary artery spasm, 240–241
 in coronary arteries, 69
PG (see Prostaglandin)
PGI_2 (see Prostacyclin)
pH
 in coronary blood flow regulation, 45
 in human coronary artery, 106
Phosphocreatine, in coronary blood flow regulation, 48
Phosphorylation, 6, 8, 17
 in isometric contraction, 12–13
Platelet aggregation, calcium blockers and, 100
Platelet-derived growth factor, 286
 in atherosclerosis, 145, 150–151, 153
Platelets, 79–91, 118–121, 285–286
 animal model, 82–84, 118–120
 coronary artery spasm and, 243–244
 cyclooxygenase inhibitors and, 81–82, 84–86, 120–121
 ibuprofen and, 86
 indomethacin and, 84, 86, 88
 prostacyclin and, 79–82, 85–91, 119–120
 role of, in atherosclerosis, 144–145, 150
 thromboxane A_2 and, 81–91, 120, 277
Potassium
 in coronary arteries, 73–74
 in coronary blood flow regulation, 45
 in human coronary artery, 106
Prenylamine, in coronary arteries, 69
Pressure-diameter, in arterial mechanics, 26–27, 56
Pressure-flow relation, in coronary artery stenosis, 185, 188, 193–198
Pressure-velocity relation, in coronary artery stenosis, 195–198
Propranolol, coronary artery spasm and, 243
Prostacyclin, 119–120, 117–118
 coronary artery spasm and, 228, 243–244, 275
 in atherosclerosis, 151
 in human coronary artery, 104–105
 platelets and, 79–82, 85–91
 thromboxane A_2 and, 247–249
Prostaglandins, 104–105, 121–122
 coronary artery spasm and, 243–244
 in coronary blood flow regulation, 49
 in human coronary artery, 110–111
Reactive hyperemia, 57–58
 in coronary arteries, 67

Relaxation, energetics of, in smooth muscle, 14–15
Response-to-injury hypothesis, 141–142, 152, 287
S-Adenosylhomocysteine, in coronary blood flow regulation, 48
SAH (see S-Adenosylhomocysteine)
Series elasticity, in active arterial mechanics, 33–35
Serotonin, 122
Shortening, energetics of, in smooth muscle, 15–16
Smooth muscle, 283–284
 actin-myosin interaction in, 8–10
 calcium regulation, 8
 crossbridge cycling, 283
 energetics in, 10–16
 physiology of, 3–17
 role of, in atherosclerosis, 144
 ultrastructure, 3–8
Species difference in coronary arteries, 108
 passive arterial mechanics and, 26
Stenosis, coronary artery, 64–66, 157–171, 173–198, 287–288
Streptokinase, 279–280
 in thrombolysis therapy, 255–261
Stress
 coronary heart disease and, 272
 relaxation, in smooth muscle, 9–10
Sympathetic stimulation
 in active arterial mechanics, 35–36
 in coronary arteries, 70
 in coronary blood flow regulation, 42–43, 56
Synthesis inhibitor, thromboxane A_2, in platelets, 83–91
Thrombolysis therapy, 290
 for myocardial infarction, 255–261
 nitroglycerin and, 257–258
 streptokinase, 255–261
Thromboxane A_2, 120, 124–125, 247–251, 277–278, 285, 289
 angina pectoris and, 248–249
 as synthesis inhibitor, in platelets, 83–91
 coronary artery spasm and, 244
 in coronary artery disease, 247–251
 myocardial infarction and, 250, 252
 nitrates and, 278
 pacing-induced angina and, 250–251
 platelets and, 81–82, 277
 prostacyclin and, 247–249
TXA_2 (see Thromboxane A_2)
Vascular waterfall phenomenon, in coronary blood flow regulation, 41
Vasoconstriction
 in coronary artery spasm, 225–227
 of coronary artery, 158–159, 166–168, 171

Vasomotion, coronary, 225
Verapamil
 as calcium blocker, 94–96, 100, 112, 150
 in coronary arteries, 69
 treatment, of coronary artery spasm, 242

Very low density lipoproteins, 140
Vessel wall, coronary artery spasm and, 227–228
VLDL (*see* Very low density lipoproteins)
Warfarin, 257–259

DATE DUE

OCT 11 84			
APR 1 3 1991			
OCT 1994			
OCT 2 9 1994			
NOV 0 1 1995			
FEB 2 1 1996			
Mar 14			
OCT 1 8 1996			
Nov 8 1996			
OCT 2 6 1997			
FEB 2 2 1998			
APR 1 3 1998			
DEC 1 3 1998			

616.123   C81   112574

CORONARY   ARTERY   DISEASE

College Misericordia Library
Dallas, Pennsylvania 18612